Plant Secondary Metabolites

NIPA® GENX ELECTRONIC RESOURCES & SOLUTIONS P. LTD.
New Delhi-110 034

Plant Secondary Metabolites

by

Y. M. SHUKLA *(Associate Professor),* **JITENDRA J. DHRUVE**
(Assistant Research Scientist), Main Vegetable Research Station
N.J. PATEL *(Assistant Professor),* Department of Bichemistry
B.A. College of Agriculture, **RAMESH BHATNAGAR** *(Head)*
Department of Biochemistry, B.A. College of Agriculture
J. G. TALATI *(Professor),* Department of Biochemistry
B.A. College of Agriculture, **K. B. KATHIRIA** *(Head)*
Main Vegetable Research Station

Anand Agricultural University, Anand-388 110 (Gujarat) India

nipa®

NIPA® GENX ELECTRONIC RESOURCES & SOLUTIONS P. LTD.
New Delhi-110 034

NIPA® GENX ELECTRONIC RESOURCES & SOLUTIONS P. LTD.

101,103, Vikas Surya Plaza, CU Block
L.S.C. Market, Pitam Pura, New Delhi-110 034
Ph : +91 11 27341616, 27341717, 27341718
E-mail: newindiapublishingagency@gmail.com
web: www.nipabooks.com

For customer assistance, please contact
Phone: + 91-11-27 34 17 17
Fax: + 91-11- 27 34 16 16
E-Mail: feedbacks@nipabooks.com

ISBN: 978-81-19254-61-3

Composed and Designed by NIPA®.

Prof. M.C. Varshney
Vice Chancellor
Anand Agricultural University
Anand-388 110
Gujarat

Foreword

Plant secondary products have always been of interest in the context of pharmacology, but within the last fifteen years there has been a substantial growth in interest in secondary products from plant physiologists and molecular biologists interested in plant defense and in signaling processes. There is also increasing attention paid to these compounds as dietary constituents and particularly as actual or potential antioxidants. Secondary products are therefore at last widely recognized as a legitimate topic of mainstream interest, rather than as an arcane speciality. Plant cell produce far more chemical compound that is necessary for their basic functions, i.e. biochemical pathway for survival and propagation. Basic or primary metabolism refers to all biochemical process for the normal anabolic and catabolic pathway which results in assimilation, respiration, transport, and differentiation. By and large, basic, or 'primary" metabolism is shared by all cells, while "secondary metabolism" generate divers and seemingly less essential or non-essential byproduct called "secondary product". The secondary products are what give plants the colors, flavors, and smells. These produces are sources of fine chemicals, such as drugs, insecticides, dyes, flavors, and fragrances, and the phytomedicines found in medicinal plants. Rapid development in the field of the biochemistry has given great importance in the secondary metabolites and its importance in the plant sciences. Plant secondary metabolites play very important role in the plant metabolisms, medicines and biotechnology.

The present text deals with most of the secondary metabolites such as alkaloids, terpenoids, glycosides, etc. The method of their extraction and qualification have also been discussed. The biochemical approaches for enhancement of these constituents have also been highlighted. The book would be useful for Phytochemists, Agriculturists, Medicos, Home sciences, Veterinary science, Ayurvedic and Naturopathy students as well as teachers teaching in these branches of sciences.

April, 2009

M.C. Varshney

Dr. A.R. Pathak
Director of Research and Dean P.G. Studies
Anand Agricultural University
Anand-388 110
Gujarat

Message

Secondary plant products have for thousands of years played an essential role in medicine. Traditionally, they have been directly used as food and herbs. Plant secondary metabolites represent tremendous resources for scientific and clinical research and new drug devolvement. These secondary metabolites are the major sources of pharmaceuticals, food additives, fragrances and pesticides. Secondary products are the compounds which, whilst not essential to the survival of the individual cell, nevertheless fulfill an important - even essential - role in the life and survival of the organism as a whole. Secondary metabolites are apparently multifunctional in nature. The most disconcerting feature of secondary compounds is their frequent presence in plants as complex mixtures of structures which increases the difficulty of establishing a unique function.

Overall, their pharmacological value not only remains undiminished until today, but is increasing due to constant discoveries of their potential roles in health care and as lead chemical for the new drug development. In the present text an attempt has been made to provide glimpses of most of the secondary metabolites present in medicinal and spice crops. The assay protocols of their extraction and qualification has been also discussed. The Biochemical approaches for enhancement of these constituents have been also highlighted. This book would be useful for faculties, students and researchers in the disciplines of Agriculture, Medicinal and Aromatics plants and associated other disciplines. One of the purposes of this book is to provide an essentially biochemical context to these developments, directing the reader to specialized information which can be found rarely elsewhere.

April, 2009

A.R. Pathak

Preface

Organic chemists of the nineteenth century were among the first to recognize and study the diversity of plant secondary metabolites and to analyze them both in terms of structure and function. Nowhere in the plant kingdom do ecology, evolution, and human affairs come together as intricately as phenomena involving secondary metabolites. The importance of these compounds is apparent in some of the earliest annals of human history. Past 60 years have seen the development, testing and refinement of secondary substances. With the functional roles of these compounds broadly acknowledged, several challenges presented themselves to scientists interested in their ecological and evolutionary dynamics. Most obviously, the details of the processes underlying the interactions between each of these compounds and their target pest or pathogen became one of the most vibrant topics in research. Secondary metabolites are compounds biosynthetically derived from primary metabolites but more limited in occurrence in the plant kingdom and may be restricted to a particular taxonomic group. Secondary metabolites are apparently multifunctional in nature. The most disconcerting feature of secondary compounds is their frequent presence in plants as complex mixtures of structures which increases the difficulty of establishing a unique function. In the present account of secondary metabolite functions, substances with growth regulatory properties and those involved in pollination and seed dispersal, as antifungal agents and anti-herbivore agents have been discussed. Beside this, biotechnological aspects for enhancement of secondary metabolites and assay procedures for some important commercially vibrant secondary metabolites have also been covered. We hope that the book would be useful for researchers and teachers associated with vivid biological fields. It is also hoped that the present text will improve and immense value for research workers, planners and above all farmers and individual who are eager to know biochemistry of plant products.

Anand
May, 2009

Authors

Contents

Chapter 1

Introduction

Plants are used for many purposes apart from food such as industrial products like perfumes, pharmaceuticals, agrochemicals, food additives, cosmetics and also for rectifying the side effects of allopathic medicines, etc. Interest was taken in the chemical constituents of plants in the very early days of modern science. Plants were used for very many purposes besides providing food, such as for treating medical ailments and for dyeing in textiles.

To the agricultural chemists, any biological organism is ultimately constituted from the elements like C, H, O, N, P, Ca, Mg, S etc. Two or more elements combine to form complex organic compounds such as carbohydrates, fats, proteins, enzymes, alkaloids, glycosides, organic acids and many more complex compounds. These biomolecules can be classified into two main major metabolites. (1) Primary metabolites and (2) Secondary metabolites.

Primary Metabolites

They are defined as the metabolites universally present in all living systems which play important role in energy linked life processes and metabolism. They are essential to the cell for life which, include amino acids of proteins, simple sugars of carbohydrates, the purines and pyrimidines of nucleic acids, Fatty acids of lipids etc.

Secondary Metabolites

They are defined as the substances produced in little amount from the primary metabolites, play a non-essential role which are specialized chemicals, having enormous chemical diversity and doing a specific job of either protection, reserve food energy or germicidal effect etc. They vary in distribution in microorganism, plants, insects etc. The secondary metabolites include antibiotics, alkaloids, gums, mucilage, oleoresins, terpenes, phenols, phytoalexins, glycosides, and so on.

- About 120,000 have been identified
- Often accumulated and stored in high concentrations - 1% to 3% of dry weight
- Hydrophilic compounds stored in vacuoles
- Hydrophobic compounds stored in resin ducts, laticifers, trichomes, oil cells, or in cuticle
- Sites of synthesis and sites of storage often different - transported in the plant.

Secondary metabolites can be distinguished from the primary metabolites by the following criteria:

Primary Metabolites	Secondary Metabolites
Wide spread distribution in all living organisms	Restricted distribution found mostly in plants and microorganisms
Characteristics of all living cells such as bacteria, fungi, plants, insects, frog, etc.	Characteristics of individual genera, species or strains (Nicotine from tobacco, Erucic acid from mustard, Cynogenic glycosides from sorghum)
Major biochemical pathway for energy generation and synthesis Essential for life processes	Subsidiary specialized pathways from the primary metabolites Non-essential for basic life processes
Generally endogenous in nature	Many are secreted outside the cell (gums, mucilage, antibiotics)
Produced in energy generation and biosynthesis of important bio-molecules	Specific functions e.g. Protection, antibiosis, reserve food energy
Produced from carbohydrates, proteins and lipids	Produced from handful of primary metabolites such as α–amino acids, acetyl Co-A , mevalonic acid etc.

Primary metabolites and their functions have been studied in detail	Their synthesis, functions and importance yet to be understood thoroughly.
Fairly large amounts are produced in the cell	They are produced in small amounts.
Examples: Intermediates of TCA cycle, Glycolysis, Fatty acid synthesis/oxidation, purine/pyrimidine biosynthesis	Examples: antibiotics, mucilage, gum, oleoresins, alkaloids etc.
Often accumulated and stored in high concentrations as seed reserve materials in specialized tissues	Often accumulated and stored in high concentrations – 1% to 3% of dry weight
1. Hydrophilic compounds stored in specialized tissues 2. Hydrophobic compounds stored in oil bodies	1. Hydrophilic compounds stored in vacuoles 2. Hydrophobic compounds stored in resin ducts, laticifers, trichomes, oil bodies, or in cuticle
3. Sites of synthesis and sites of storage often different - transported in the plant	3. Sites of synthesis and sites of storage often different - transported in the plant

In general, primary metabolites obtained from higher plants for commercial use are high-volume, low-value bulk chemicals. They are primarily used as industrial raw materials, foods or food additives; examples: vegetable oils, fatty acids (used for making soaps and detergents) and carbohydrates (sucrose, starch, pectin and cellulose).

Although secondary plant products are very common, this does not mean that every plant can produce every product. Some compounds are restricted to single species, others to related groups. But they are nearly always found only in certain specific plant organs, often in just one type of cell (and there again only in a certain compartment). Also, they are often generated only during a specific developmental period of the plant.

Secondary metabolites produce by plant cells. Many of these are highly toxic and are often stored in specific vesicles or in the vacuole. Several studies indicate that this kind of storage functions on one hand as a detoxification of the plant itself and generates on the other hand a reservoir of, e.g., nitrogen-rich molecules. Some secondary plant products can be reversibly degraded and are fed into the basic metabolism while others cannot.

Secondary metabolites are compounds biosynthetically derived from primary metabolites but more limited in occurrence in the plant kingdom and may be restricted to a particular taxonomic group (genus, species or family). As mentioned above, secondary metabolites are mostly accumulated by plant cells in smaller quantities than primary metabolites. These secondary metabolites are synthesized in specialized cells at particular developmental stages, making their extraction and purification difficult (compared to the primary product produced by the whole plant or organ).

Since the medicinal plants are those rich in secondary plant products their compounds are termed as 'medicinal' or 'officinal'. These secondary metabolites or products exert in general a profound physiological effect on the mammalian system and thus are known as the active principle of that plant. The physiological effect of these active principles is used for curing ailments and therefore these are drugs of plant origin or natural drugs. The use of crude medicines of plant origin (unpurified preparations of active principles, plant extract or sometimes powdered plant material) is used in the Indian system of medicine or 'Ayurveda'. A large number of medicines of plant origin are still used in Western medicine (Table 1.1 & 1.2). Though some of the medicines are obtained by synthesis for commercial uses, others are still obtained from natural sources.

Table 1.1 : Applications of some secondary metabolites.

Active compound	Plant source	Proposed therapeutic use
Alkaloids		
Atropine, hyoscamine, scopolamine	*Solanaceous spp.*	Anticholinergic
Vinblastine, Vincristine	*Catharanthus rosesus L*	Antineoplastic
Nicotine	*Nicotiana spp.*	Smoking cesssation
Codeine, morphine	*Papaver somniferum L.*	Analgesic, Antitussive
Quinine	*Cinchona spp.*	Antimalarial
Quinidine	*Cinchona spp.*	Cardiac depressant
Terpenes and steroids		
Artimisin	*Artimisia annua L.*	Antimalarial
Diosgenin, hecogenin, stigmasterol	*Dioscoria spp.*	Oral contraceptives, hormonal drugs
Taxol and other taxoids	*Taxus brevifolia Nutt.*	Antineopalstic

Active compound	Plant source	Proposed therapeutic use
Glycosides		
Digoxin, digitoxin	*Digitallis spp.*	Cardiotonic
Sennosides A and B	*Cassia angustifolia Vahl.*	Laxative
Others		
Ipecac	*Cephaelis ipecacuanha (Brot.) A. Rich*	Emetic
Podophyllotoxin	*Podophyllum peltatum L.*	Antineoplastic

Table1.2. : Some secondary metabolites as plant medicines.

Acetyldigoxin	Digitoxin	Papain	Reserpine
Aescin	Digoxin	Papaverine	Scillarenes
Ajmalicine	Emetine	Physotigmine	Scopolamine
Allontoin	Ephedrine	Picrotoxine	Sennosides
α-Lobeline	Hyoscyamine	Pilocarpine	Sperteine
Atropine	Khellin	Protoveratrinies	Strychnine
Bromelain	Lanatosides	Pseudoephedrine	Tetrahydrocannabinol
Caffeine	L-Dopa	Quabain	Theobromine
Codeine	Leurocristine	Quinidine Quinine	Theophylline
Colchicine	Morphine	Rascinnamine	Tubocuramine
Danthron	Narcotine		Vincaleukoblastine
Deserpidine			Xanthotoxine

With the discovery of the physiological effects of a particular plant, efforts are made to know (i.e. chemical properties) the exact chemical nature of these medicines (i.e. active principles) and subsequently to obtain these compounds by chemical synthesis. To determine the chemical nature of such a compound, isolation of the substance in pure form using various separation techniques, chemical properties and spectral characteristics are prerequisite to establish its correct structure. Purified secondary products are used in exact proportions in allopathic medicines. Thus, medicinal plants are used in crude or purified form in the preparation of drugs in different systems.

Besides secondary plant products, there are several examples of primary metabolites exerting strong physiological effects. In this category proteins are principal compounds having as diverse functions as blood agglutinants from *Fabaceae*, hormones (e.g. insulin), various snake venom poisons, ricin from *Ricinus communis* and abrine and precatorine from *Abrus precatorius*. Other examples of primary metabolites exerting a strong physiological effect include antibiotics, vaccines and several polysaccharides acting as hormones or elicitors.

Besides medicines, mankind is almost completely dependent on plants for requirements such as food, shelter and clothing. However, most of the natural secondary products are compounds biosynthetically derived from primary metabolites such as amino acids, carbohydrates and fatty acids. These secondary metabolites are the major sources of pharmaceuticals, food additives, fragrances and pesticides. Secondary products are the compounds which, whilst not essential to the survival of the individual cell, nevertheless fulfill an important - even essential - role in the life and survival of the organism as a whole.

Classification of Secondary Metabolites

It has been observed that, the secondary metabolites can not be classified using a single criteria but should be classified on the basis of several criteria depending upon the metabolites.

1. They can be classified depending on whether or not they have an essential role in plant metabolism. But this classification has certain disadvantages. Secondary metabolites suggest them to be less important, but many secondary metabolites are important in protecting the plants. They also sometimes act as reserve food material. e.g. Erucic acid which is a fatty acid acting as reserve food for primary metabolism.

2. They can be classified according to its carbon skeletal type and the functional groups present and accordingly naming can be done. But the problem with a chemical nomenclature for plant products is that they are cumbersome for practical use.

3. They can be classified on the basis of plant source e.g. piperine is obtained from *piper* plant.

4. They can be classified using either generic or species name as basis such as Strychnine from Strychnos, or Parthenolide from Parthenium. But this system also has problems. Neem produce an alkaloid called azadirachtin (Earlier it was thought that only

one alkaloid is produced, but recent studies has shown six other closely related molecules).

5. The most satisfying system for classifying plant constituent is according to their biogenesis and biosynthetic origins. There are several classes of secondary metabolites having varied functions (inhibitory, stimulating, involved in pollination, seed dispersal, antifungal, herbivory, reserve food energy etc.). They have been broadly classified into terpenoids, alkaloids, derivatives of phenolic compounds and carbohydrate containing secondary products such as glycosides, gums and mucilages.

Major Functions of Secondary Metabolites

Secondary metabolites are apparently multifunctional in nature. Salicylic acid, for example, is regarded as a signal molecule often produced when a plant is stressed, e.g. by pathogen attack. It is a metabolic signal for heat production during pollination in the *Arum* lily. Salicylic acid accumulates in various bound forms in leaves of *Salix* spp. and has been shown to protect these trees from herbivory.

The most disconcerting feature of secondary compounds is their frequent presence in plants as complex mixtures of structures which increases the difficulty of establishing a unique function. For example, well over eighty alkaloids have been described from the Madagascar periwinkle, *Vinca rosea*, over fifty flavonoids may be characterized from a plant of the *Compositae* while over 150 volatiles have been identified in the floral fragrance of an orchid. Furthermore, there is also evidence of selective advantage in plants which accumulate mixtures of several related substances over the presence of just one of those substances. It has been shown that a mixture of six furanocoumarins in the leaves of the wild parsnip, *Pastinaca sativa* is more effective against insect herbivory than one of those compounds, xanthotoxin, at the same concentration as the mixture of six furanocoumarins.

In the present account of secondary metabolite functions, substances with growth regulatory properties and those involved in pollination and seed dispersal, as antifungal agents and anti-herbivore agents have been discussed. There are several classes of secondary metabolites having varied functions (inhibitory, stimulating, involved in pollination, seed dispersal, antifungal, herbivory, reserve food energy etc.).

Role of Plant secondary metabolites in defense

Plant Secondary Metabolites

- Defense
  - → Herbivores
  - → Microbes
  - → Competing Plant
- Attraction
  - → Pollinating Insects
  - → Seed Dispersing Animals
  - → Root Nodule Bacteria
- UV Protection

Specialists

Herbivores

- → Avoidance of toxic plants, except host plants
- → Cutting laticifers and resin ducts filled with allelochemicals
- → Non-resorption or fast intestinal food passage
- → Resorption followed by detoxification and elimination (faeces, urine)
  - Hydroxylation
  - Conjugation
  - Elimination
- → Resorption and Accumulation
  - Specific compartments/cells/tissues for sequestration
  - Evolution of insensitivity

  Ultilisation of dietary secondary products
  - Defence against predators (e.g. cardiac glycosides, indule glycosides, cyanogenic glycosides, pyrrolizidine alkaloids, quinolizidine alkaloids, aconitine)
  - Signal molecule pheromones (e.g. pyrrolizidine alkaloids)
  - Morphogen (e.g. pyrrolizidine alkaloid)

Microorganisms

- → Inactivation of allelochemicals
- → Evolution of insensitivity

Fig. 1.1 : Adaptations of specialist herbivores and pathogens.

Antiherbivore Agents

Majority of secondary metabolites in plants is to provide a defense against animal herbivoroy. Such herbivory is a major threat to plant survival and as a consequence of plant-animal co evolution, plants have developed various defense strategies including the ability to accumulate chemicals that are hostile to animal feeding. It is the flexible response of herbivores to detoxify these chemicals or otherwise circumvent their effects that allows the limited grazing that can be witnessed today in the natural world.

Plant chemicals may be apparently targeted to affect one particular type of herbivore (e.g. cardiac glycosides against mammals), although they may also be toxic to all forms of life, including the plant itself (e.g. cyanogenic glycosides). To avoid auto toxicity, plant chemicals are therefore usually located on the surface of plant tissues or sequestered in bound form within the plant in the cell vacuole. Some examples of plant chemicals that have been established as hostile to mammalian herbivory are given in Table 1.3 to 1.5.

Table 1.3 : Secondary metabolites as plant-pollinator interactions.

Compound	Plant	Role
Delphinidin 3,5-diglucoside	*Delphinium nelsonii*	Blue flower colour attracts bumble bee and humming bird
Delphinidin and cyaniding 3,5-diglucoside	*Phlox drummondii*	Violet flower colour attracts butterfly pollinator
Pelargonidin 3,5-diglucoside	*Ipomopsis aggregata*	Scarlet flower colour attracts humming bird pollinator
Patuletin and carotenoids	*Rudbeckia hirta*	Visible yellow and UV patterning increases efficiency of bee pollination
Indole and r-cresol	*Arum maculatum*	In scent attracts fly away from cow dung
Geraniol, geranoil and others	*Ophrys lutea*	Attracts male bee for "pseudocopulation"
Carvone oxide	*Catasetum* spp.	Attracts Euglossine male bees, which use it as a pheromone
Dimethyl disulphide and 2,4-dithiapentane	*Crescentia cujete*	Attractive to bat pollinators
Methyl anthranilate and isoeugenol	*Cimifuga simplex*	Synergies to attract butterfly pollinators
Ethyl acetate	*Zygogynum* spp.	Attracts moth pollination

Table1.4 : Some plant chemicals hostile to mammalian herbivory.

Compound and source	Animals affected
Fluoracetic acid in *Dichapetalum cymosum*	Most mammals (respiratory poison) Cattle
Miserotoxin in *Astragalus atropubescens*	Cows and man Most mammals (heart poison)
Oenanthetoxin in *Oenanthe crocata*	Snowshoe hares Western hare
Ouabain in *Acokanthera oubaio*	Livestock (liver poison) Livestock
Papyriferic acid in *Betula resinifera* Salicin in *Salix* spp. Senecionine in *Senecio jacobaea* Sinigrin in *Brassica* spp.	Some *spp.* of mammals

Terpenoids, alkaloids and phenolics have all been implicated as antiherbivore agents and there is almost no class or subclass of secondary metabolite that does not have an effect on herbivore feeding. Within a given class, some molecules may be more effective than others; among monoterpenoids, oxygenated derivatives are usually more toxic than the hydrocarbons. Nevertheless, almost every secondary compound which accumulates in plant tissue is potentially hostile to herbivory.

Table1.5 : Some plant chemicals hostile to insect and molluscan herbivory.

Compound and source	Animals affected
Demissine in *Solanum demissum*	Colorado beetle
L-DOPA in *Mucuna* spp.	Bruchid beetles
Lactupicrin in *Cichorium intybus*	Locusts
Linamarin in *Lotus corniculatus*	Slugs
b-Ocimene in *Astronium graveolens*	Leaf-cutting ants
Rotenone in *Derris elliptica*	Insects
Tannins in *Quercus robur*	Aphids and moths
Xanthotoxin in *Pastinaca sativa*	Army worms

Plants have evolved their own complex defense mechanisms against both herbivores and pathogens.

During the initial stage of insect attack, the wound caused by insect bite generates a signal within the plant body heralding the danger. The defense signaling against insect attack involves the production of two kinds of signaling molecules in the plant, *viz.*, systemin and jasmonates. The signaling system involving these two kinds of molecules leads to the production of proteinase inhibitors in the plant cell. These proteinase inhibitors inhibit the digestive enzymes (proteinases) which digest the proteins in the insect gut. As a result, the insects which feed on the leaves of these plants develop the problem of improper digestion of their food, resulting in stunted growth followed by reduced reproduction. It has been recorded that a potato leaf accumulates proteinase inhibitors up to 2% of its soluble protein content within 48 hours of initial leaf damage by wounding. Interestingly, the Colorado beetle, which normally feeds on these leaves, is able to detect the presence of proteinase inhibitors and avoids further feeding and moves on to another plant. In their chemical nature, the proteinase inhibitors are themselves proteins. Crop plants like potato and tomato produce two general classes of proteinase inhibitor molecules referred to as proteinase inhibitor I and II of molecular mass 39,000 Da and 21,000 Da, respectively. In addition, proteinase inhibitors are well-known constituents of many plant seeds where they play a similar protective role in deterring insect feeding. However, the production of these inhibitors in seeds is constitutive (not induced by any internal or external factors) and also not controlled by the jasmonate signaling system.

Reaction to Injury

It has been shown that the initial wounding caused by insect bites finally leads to the production of proteinase inhibitors in the plant cell. The jasmonate signaling system mediates this process. The wounding causes production of prosystemin which is a protein consisting of 200 amino acid residues. This large molecule is then processed (trimmed), leading to the formation of systemin, an 18 amino acid-long oligo peptide. The systemin molecule is systemic in nature, which means that it is readily transported from one part of the plant to the other through the conducting tissue (phloem). The systemin molecule induces the synthesis of jasmonates in the cell by initiating a cascade of metabolic events. This initiation begins with the recognition and binding of the systemin to a receptor molecule in the plasma membrane. For example, in tomato, the receptor is a systemin-binding membrane protein (SBP50) of molecular mass 50,000 Da. The systemin-receptor complex appears to induce the activity of the enzyme phospholipase which hydrolyzes the membrane lipids and liberates their fatty acid components into the cytoplasm. These fatty acids then become the substrates for the synthesis of jasmonates. A series of enzymes acts on these substrate molecules, resulting in the synthesis of jasmonic acid structurally, jasmonic acid (JA) consists of a cyclopentanone ring with acetyl and n-pentenyl group substitutions in positions 3 and 7 of the ring jasmonic acid is also methylated to produce the highly volatile methyl jasmonate (MeJA).

Resistance Against Insects

Injury caused by insects → systemin production

Insect bites → volicitin → Jasmonate biosynthesis

pin gene induction Production of proteinase inhibitors Resistance to insects. Jasmonates are able to induce (turn 'on') a large number of genes in plants. The products of the jasmonate induced gene expression are commonly termed as jasmonate-induced proteins' (JIP). Proteinase inhibitors are one of the kinds of JIPs. The proteinase inhibitor I and II genes (*pin*1 and *pin*2) are coordinately expressed, and their expression is stimulated by wounding which may be due to a simple mechanical shearing of leaves, or herbivore-induced injury. In either case,there occurs the release of systemin which is followed by jasmonate synthesis finally leading to the induction of *pin* gene expression. In addition to the systemin-mediated stimulation, the jasmonate-induced *pin* gene expression is also stimulated by insect oral secretions. The chemical compound, volicitin [N-(17- hydroxylinolenoyl)-L-glutamine which is a component of insect oral secretion has also been found to be an inducer of jasmonate biosynthesis. Therefore, insect attack may stimulate the biosynthesis of jasmonates in two different ways, one through the wound induced systemin production, and the other through the insect oral secretion. In both the cases it leads to the expression of *pin* genes resulting in the production of proteinase inhibitors. Methyl jasmonate is highly volatile, and is transmitted through air.

The signal is perceived at the level of the plasma membrane by the membrane-associated receptors. The signals from the herbivore injury in the form of systemin, and the insect oral secretion which contains volicitin are perceived. Similarly, elicitors formed by pathogen invasion (oligogalacturonides and chitosan) are also able to induce jasmonate biosynthesis. The jasmonates thus produced in the cytoplasm stimulate the expression of specific genes in the nucleus. Jasmonates induce the genes which express the synthesis of proteinase inhibitors, phytoalexins, or the volatile terpenoids that attract the carnivorous insects. In addition, other jasmonate induced proteins (JIPs) involved in other functions may also be induced. Jasmonates are also transported from cell to cell across the membranes, and from organ to organ through phloem.

Communication Between Plants

The methyl ester of jasmonic acid, methyl jasmonate is highly volatile, and it is readily transmitted through air. In fact, this compound was first isolated from the essential oil of jasmine (*Jasminum grandiflorum*) as the fragrant component, and its name is derived from the plant from which it was first isolated. Methyl jasmonate is transmitted through air and induces the production of proteinase inhibitors in uninduced plants growing at a distance. Therefore, it appears that the insect attack on plants may send out a signal through air to other plants growing in the neighboring area, and induce insect resistance in them. By doing this, plants can give out warning signal to their neighbouring community. Using this principle, there have been attempts to develop methods to control insects by growing plants which emit methyl jasmonate.

The plant, *Artemisia tridentata* (a member of Asteraceae) produces methyl jasmonate, and growing rows of this plant in tomato fields was considered to be effective in inducing proteinase inhibitors in tomato plants. However, it should also be remembered that insects are able to produce a variety of proteinases,and as the result they can produce proteinases that are insensitive to proteinase inhibitors I and II to which they are exposed. This leads to development of resistance to these proteinase inhibitors. However, a careful study of different proteinase inhibitors induced in a wide variety of plants, and judicious use of these inhibitors may lead to the design of suitable pest management methods.

Response to Plant Pathogens

Invasion of the plant body by microbial pathogens like fungi or bacteria also leads to damage and disintegration of the host plant cells in the infected regions. The disintegration of the plant cell wall results in the liberation of broken wall components such as oligogalacturonides (obtained from the cell wall pectin degradation) and oligosaccharides (products of cellulose degradation). It appears that the insect attack on plants may send out a signal through air to other plants growing in the neighboring area, and induce insect resistance in them.

Infection of plants by pathogens → production of elicitors → synthesis of jasmonates → jasmonate-induced gene expression → increase in the levels of the enzymes of phenylpropanoid metabolism → production of phytoalexins → inhibition of pathogens.

In addition, some fungal wall components such as chitosans are also liberated. It has been discovered that these wall components are also able to initiate the biosynthesis of jasmonates. These wall components are collectively known as elicitors, and they appear to exert their influence in a manner similar to that of systemin, leading to the release of fatty acids from membrane lipids which results in the biosynthesis of jasmonates in the cytoplasm. In the infected plants, the jasmonates then stimulate the production of phytoalexins. Phytoalexins are the antimicrobial, low molecular weight chemical compounds produced by the host plants against the invading pathogens and they inhibit the growth of the pathogens in the plant body, thereby offering protection to the infected plant. It has been discovered that the jasmonates are able to induce the expression of genes which produce the enzymes involved in phenylpropanoid metabolism. The phenylpropanoid metabolic pathway in turn leads to the synthesis of certain coumarin compounds which act as phytoalexins in some plants.

Apart from the direct way of defending themselves against insects by producing proteinase inhibitors, plants are also able to defend themselves by indirect methods. Plants can respond to damage caused by herbivorous insects by producing volatile chemical compounds that attract carnivorous insects which prey upon the herbivores. Carnivorous insects depend heavily upon information-conveying chemicals originating from the herbivore, from the plant, or from an interaction between herbivore and plant to guide them to their prey. Plants can respond to damage caused by herbivorous insects by producing volatile chemical compounds that attract carnivorous insects which prey upon the herbivores. The most intriguing fact is that a single chemical compound is able to control a large number of diverse metabolic events in plants. Besides their action in plant defense against both insects and pathogens in entirely different ways, jasmonates are also able to induce quite a few growth characteristics in plants. In fact, jasmonates are able to regulate diverse developmental events in plants such as senescence, tuberization, bulb formation, tendril coiling, induction of vegetative storage proteins, etc. On the other hand, the same signaling and defense mechanisms discussed above are also influenced by other plant growth regulators as well as abiotic stresses. Many of the chemicals described here are deterrents to invasion by pathogens. Some of the chemicals are produced and accumulated constitutively (that is at low levels constantly throughout the life of the plant), while others are produced as part of the inducible defense system. Secretion of an elicitor (a protein involved in pathogen invasion, or a sugar derived from cell wall breakdown) by a pathogen and its recognition by a plant resistance (R) gene triggers a series of responses in plants that repress the growth of the pathogen. The activated R gene triggers Ca^{2+} influx and (separately or in concert with Ca^{2+} this point is not clear yet) then triggers a plasma membrane response leading to cell wall reinforcement and cellular response leading to defense gene activation. The defensive (pathogenesis related or PR) genes include proteins that degrade the cell walls of bacteria and fungi as well as proteins that are involved in synthesizing secondary chemicals. In the plasma membrane the system that generates reactive oxygen species (ROS, superoxide and H_2O_2) together with peroxidase enzymes leads to lignin formation to reinforce the walls of cells near the site of infection. The ROS may also exert a direct anti-microbial effect on the invading pathogen. The gene induction system also leads to the production of salicylic acid (SA), a by-product of the phenyl propanoid pathway. SA is transported through the phloem to healthy, uninfected cells where it triggers the induction of defensive responses by a process known as systemic acquired resistance (SAR).

Plant Growth Substances

One clear function of secondary metabolites in plants is in the control of growth and development. Over the years, a variety of structures have been recognized as growth substances or plant hormones. Five main groups are widely recognized based on ethylene, indole-3-acetic acid, gibberellic acid, zeatin and abscisic acid. More recently, two further classes have been added: the brassinosteroids based on brassinolide and the polyamines based on spermine.

In addition to the recognized classes of growth substance, there are many other secondary constituents that have individually been shown to produce an effect on plant growth or development. This is commonly in only one or two plants and the effect is often one of growth inhibition or of interacting with one of the established plant hormones. Some examples of those putative hormones are listed in Table 1.6. One illustration is gallic acid (3,4,5-trihydroxybenzoic acid) which has been described as a flowering inhibitor from its occurrence in leaves of *Kalanchoe blossfeldiana*. Another case is dihydroconiferyl alcohol, which synergises with gibberellic acid in inducing hypocotyl elongation in the lettuce plant.

Table 1.6 : Plant hormones and other growth substances.

Structural class	Chemical variation; effect on growth*
Established hormones	
Ethylene	Single structure; ripening hormone
Indole-3-acetic acid	Some 30 conjugates known; growth hormone
Gibberellins	102 structures; stem elongation hormone
Cytokinins	18 structures; cell division hormone
Abscisic acid	2 structures; stomatal opening hormone
Brassinosteroids	14 structures; cell elongation factor
Polyamines	4 structures; interacts with ribosomal RNA
Putative hormones (growth inhibitors)	
Phenolic acids	e.g. gallic acid
Phenylpropanoids	e.g. chlorogenic acid, dihydroconiferyl alcohol
Coumarins	e.g. coumarin, umbelliferone
Lactones	e.g. parasorbic acid
Stilbenoids	e.g. batatasin I
Sesquiterpene lactones	e.g. xanthinin
Diterpene lactones	e.g. podolactone E
Fatty acids	e.g. palmitic, oleic acids

* All established hormones have several effects on plant growth and interact with each other to control the various aspects of plant growth and development.

Secondary compounds may also have an indirect effect on plant growth, by mediating in the regulation of hormones synthesis or turnover. Phenolic compounds have been implicated in IAA turnover in some plants through an effect on the enzyme of degradation, IAA oxidase. This enzyme is stimulated *in vitro* by monophenols and inhibited by catechol-derived biphenols. How important this effect is *in vivo* is still controversial.

Floral Pigments and Odours

A bewildering array of volatile chemicals have been encountered in the scents of angiosperm flowers. As many as 150 scent constituents may be produced by an orchid flower, such as *Ophrys lutea*. Orchids are a particularly rich source of different odour compounds and many species of this family have now been analyzed. Among the more unusual chemical constituents encountered in plants other than orchids are the presence of p-cresol, 2-heptanone, indole and germacrene B in the floral odour of the cuckoo pint *Arum maculatum*. Mono and sesquiterpenoids are among the most common of flower volatiles but they may well be accompanied by aliphatic (e.g. pentadecane) and aromatic (e.g. eugenol) components. *Cimifuga simplex*, which is butterfly-pollinated has 15 terpenoids, accompanied by methyl anthranilate and isoeugenol. In some forms of this plant, there two latter volatiles are replaced by benzenoids, e.g. methyl benzoate.

Antifungal Agents

Some examples of lipophilic plant constituents present at the surface of leaf, stem or fruit are illustrated in Table 1.7, with an indication of their fungitoxicity. In many cases, more than one secondary metabolite may be involved. In the case of *Lupinus albus*, for example, a range of other fungitoxic isoflavonoids in addition to luteone have been characterized on the leaf or root surface. Again, a mixture of oxygenated fatty acids together with epoxylinoleic acid on rice leaves have been suggested as providing resistance to rice blast, *Pyricularia oryzae*. Some of these compounds are also probably effective against bacterial infection, and this has been demonstrated in the case of parthenolide and its occurrence in leaf glands of feverfew, *Tanacetum parthenium*.

Other secondary metabolites may be present in the vacuole of upper epidermal cells of the leaf and undergo enzyme hydrolysis to yield the free antifungal agent. The occurrence of different saponins in the leaf and the root of the oat plant *Avena sativa* is noteworthy. In both cases, the original saponin loses one of its sugars to give the antifungal agent, which may then undergo further metabolism by fungal enzymes to produce an inactive sapogenin. In the case of 1-tuliposide A in tulip bulbs, during infection this undergoes isomerisation to 6-tuliposide A and then hydrolysis and lactonisation to tulipalin A before it is an effective fungal toxin. It is not clear yet how widespread bound toxins are, but a recent study of plants of Rosaceae suggested that they are commonly present in this family. Two examples – the flavone chrysin 7-glucoside and the simple hydroquinone glucoside arbutin – are shown in Table 1.7.

Table 1.7 : Constitutive antifungal agents in plants.

Compound and source	Fungus affected
Surface Constituents	
Catechol in *Allium cepa*	*Colletotrichum circinans*
12,13-Epoxylinoleic acid in *Oryza sativa*	*Pyricularia oryzae*
Luteone in *Lupinus albus*	*Helminthosporium carbonum*
Nobiletin in *Citrus* spp.	*Deuterophoma tracheiphila*
Parthenolide in *Tanacetum parthenium*	*Botrytis cinerea*
5-Pentadecylresorcinol in *Mangifera indica*	*Alternaria alternata*
Sakuranetin in *Ribes nigrum*	*Botrytis cinerea*
Sclareol in *Nicotina glutinosa*	*Alternaria longipes*
Vacuolar Constituents*	
Arbutin in *Pyrus communis*	*Nectria cinnabarina*
Avenacin AI in *Avena sativa* root	*Gaeumannomyces graminis*
Avenacoside A in *Avena sativa* leaf	*Fusarium avenaceum*
Chrysin 7-glucoside in *Malus sieboldii*	*Phomopsis perniciosa*
Sinigrin in *Brassica oleracea*	*Peronospora parasitica*
Tomatine in *Lycopersicon esculentum*	*Fusarium solani*
1-Tuliposide A in *Tulipa* cultivars	*Fusarium oxysporum*

* Bound toxins which undergo enzymic hydrolysis (usually with β-glucosidase) to release the true antifungal agents.

The structures are similar to constitutive antifungal agents but the compounds are universally lipophilic in nature. In some families such as the Leguminosae, the phytoalexins are nearly always isoflavonoids and are very similar to isoflavonoids which occur constitutively within the family. In other cases, the phytoalexins are uniquely produced as a result of the infection processes. This is true of the sulphur indole-based phytoalexins of the Cruciferae and of some of the dibenzofuran phytoalexins of Rosaceae. Two other chemicals changes that occur during infection deserve brief mention. Firstly, the synthesis of some plant constituents can be increased during infection so that substances such as the coumarin scopoletin, normally present in trace amount, may increase several-fold in infected tissue. Secondly, new toxins produced by the fungal invader may be formed in the infected plant. These phytotoxins are often responsible for the damaging symptoms (e.g. wilting) which appear in the leaf as the disease takes hold of the plant. Another class of fungal metabolite - the mycotoxins - may be specifically produced in plant storage tissue (fruits, seeds) following infection and these mycotoxins may be poisonous to animals (birds, farm animals, man) when nuts or seeds (e.g. cereal grain) are eaten.

Plant Compounds with Animal Hormonal Activity

One of the most surprising discoveries in plant science, made about 30 years ago, was the fact that insect moulting hormones are present in plant tissue. Relatively massive amounts of the sterol 20-hydroxyecdysone, which had just been characterized in trace amounts in the silkworm, were found in the leaves of the common yew *Taxus baccata* and the fronds of the fern *Polypodium vulgare*. Plant surveys were initiated and these steroidal hormones were found to occur regularly in ferns and gymnosperms. Subsequently, they were also found in angiosperms and a recent review indicates that these are present in 27 families of ferns, 10 families of gymnosperms and 74 families of angiosperm.

In addition to the presence of the actual moulting hormones of insects, such as ecdysone and 20-hydroxyecdysone, a range of ecdysones unique to plants were uncovered. About 100 of these phytoecdysones have been characterized. A fascinating property of many phytoecdysones is their enormous hormonal activity and some are 20 times as active as zooecdysones. As a result, they can have very damaging effects on insect development. There is thus good evidence that at least for sensitive insect species, they exert various harmful effects in insects feeding on plants containing these constituents. There is thus a reasonable argument that they are produced specifically to protect plants from insect herbivory, although much further work is needed to confirm this hypothesis.

During metamorphosis, insects also have a requirement for a second terpenoid-based hormone, juvenile hormone. Four closely related structures based on farnesol have been characterized from insects. Again, it is remarkable that one of these four compounds, juvenile hormone III, has been found in a plant in large amounts, in the sedge *Cyperus iria*. In addition, several related structures have been encountered in plants which disrupt metamorphosis at this critical juvenile stage. These plant substances may cause precocious metamorphosis and hence have fatal effects on insects feeding on plants containing them. Their ecological purpose, again, would seem to be one of protecting plants against insect herbivory.

Yet another hormonal link between plants and animals lies in the record of oestrogen-like molecules in plants. In fact, the mammalian hormones oestriol and oestrone have been described in trace amounts from several plant sources, including the seeds of the apple and the pomegranate. More effective quantities of oestrogen-mimic structures have also been encountered, notably the isoflavone formononetin in legume forage plants. This compound is responsible for continual reduction in lambing percentages in Australian sheep, because of its presence in significant amount in the Australian clover plant *Trifolium subterraneum*. Other sources of plant oestrogen include the shrub, *Pueraria mirifica*, which contains the oestrone-mimic miroestrol and which is a potent abortifacient in humans.

Plant Chemicals in Symbiotic Associations

Higher plant symbioses include the familiar legume-*Rhizobium* interaction, where a bacterium initiates nitrogen fixation in the roots of clover and other legumes. The chemistry of nitrogen-fixing plants is not noticeably different, however, from that of the same plants lacking *Rhizobium* infection. Theoretically, higher plants might exist in symbiosis with fungi, without necessarily showing disease symptoms. Such a hypothetical symbiosis was proposed for the composite shrub *Baccharis megapotamica*, when it was found to contain several complex trichothecins, macrocyclic molecules only otherwise known to be synthesized by soil fungi belonging to the genera *Fusarium* and *Mycotheceum*. This idea became firmly established in the early literature but more careful study of the plant in the glasshouse showed that it was not infected with any micro-organisms and moreover the trichothecins were specifically produced not in the root, leaf or stem of the plant but in the seed.

The most distinctive symbioses between one higher plant and another are those in which a *Striga* or an *Orobanche* species becomes a root parasite on a suitable host plant (often a crop plant) and takes all its nourishment from that host. In such cases, there is some interesting chemistry in the signal molecules released from the host root to trigger attraction and attachment of the parasite but there is not usually any exchange in secondary chemicals, the parasite producing its own distinctive chemical constituents. However, such exchange may occur in the case of semiparasites, which attach to a host, but are also capable of photosynthesis. The uptake of host alkaloids is now well established for different species of the semiparasitic *Pedicularis*. Piperidine alkaloids may be "borrowed" from a spruce host, pyrrolizidine alkaloids from a Senecio host and quinolizidine alkaloids from a lupin host.

Aa brief introduction to the secondary metabolites of the plant kingdom in spite of the enormous structural diversity that has been revealed to date, there is still much to be rediscovered. The biosynthesis of the major classes is briefly indicated and some information is given of their functions within the plant. More detailed informations on individual plant chemicals have been discussed in subsequent chapters.

Chapter 2

History of Secondary Metabolites

Nowhere in the plant kingdom do ecology, evolution, and human affairs come together as intricately as phenomena involving secondary metabolites. The importance of these compounds is apparent in some of the earliest annals of human history. For example, *Papaver somniferum,* the original source of morphine and codeine, was known to the *Sumerians* in 4000 B.C. as *hul gil* (joy-plant). These two alkaloids, so important in human affairs for many years, probably evolved within the genus *Papaver* originally as protective compounds against herbivores. As a testament to the importance of secondary metabolites, *P. somniferum* was one the first plants to be cultivated for a reason other than its caloric or nutritive value. Sadly, its importance has only increased over the time. Organic chemists of the nineteenth century were among the first to recognize and study the diversity of plant secondary metabolites and to analyze them both in terms of structure and function. The German organic chemists developed techniques to acetylate morphine and produce what they claimed at the time to be a non addictive version of the drug. However, acetylation product of morphine trade name Heroin, was vastly more addictive. The economies of several developing nations in Asia still depend on the acetylation of this plant secondary metabolite, and tens of thousands of lives each year are destroyed by its commercial importance. In another striking example of profitable secondary metabolites, acetylation techniques to salicylic acid, derived originally from the bark of willows, *Salix*, to create aspirin. The modern appreciation of these secondary metabolites from ecological and evolutionary perspectives had its spread outside of the plant-insect ecology community. The overwhelming array of chemicals found in plants was more than simply by-products of primary metabolism that served as waste products for these organisms that lacked excretory systems.

Ecologists and evolutionary biologists soon took up the cudgels, and the past 60 years have seen the development, testing, refinement, and, in some cases, rejection of models that describe the ecology and evolution of these "secondary" substances. With the functional roles of these compounds broadly acknowledged, several challenges presented themselves to scientists interested in their ecological and evolutionary dynamics. Most obviously, the details of the processes underlying the interactions between each of these compounds and their target pest or pathogen became one of the most vibrant topics in ecological and physiological research.

Evolutionary and ecological studies of plant secondary metabolites have been closely linked because of the early recognition that many of these compounds played distinct ecological roles while also showing phylogenetic affinities, such that details of the distribution of chemical structures among taxa could not be explained without considering evolutionary relationships. However, it soon became apparent that phylogenetic relationships among plants were not sufficient to predict functional roles of secondary compounds. For example, chemically similar secondary metabolites such as terpenes can serve a range of functions, including herbivore deterrence, fungal toxicity, and pollinator attraction; they can also function as solvents for higher molecular mass compounds that would otherwise solidify and clog transport systems in plants. Ecological and evolutionary models have focused on the origin and maintenance of plant chemical diversity and on the regulation of chemical concentrations within plants. There has been less effort to date on formal models of the evolution of secondary metabolite function and of how function may change over time, though some researchers have examined these questions on the scale of particular plant clades.

Plant alkaloids such as strychnine, brucine and quinine were first isolated in crystalline form during 1817-1820. The triterpene betulin from birch bark was first described in the scientific literature in 1788.

Anthocyanin pigments were first investigated by Robert Boyle in 1664, while the co-occurring flavones present in many plants used for dyeing were extensively studied by British chemists in the mid-nineteenth century. Brief outline of historical development has been presented in Table 2.1.

Table 2.1 : Historical development of secondary metabolites.

Adam Lonicer (1528-1586)	:	Gave the nature and importance of essential oils
J.R. Glauber (1604-1670)	:	I[st] industrial chemist to work on essential oils
M. Charas (1618-1698), N.Lemery, Demachy, J.F (1728-1803) Boerhave (1668-1738)	:	Pioneers in the research on volatile oils.
Gildemeister, E and Hoffman, F (1643)	:	Gave the term "Volatile Oils".
Robert Boyle (1664)	:	First investigated anthocyanins pigments
Sertüner F.W. (1805)	:	Isolation of morphine from opium.
Pelletier and Caventoü (1817-1820)	:	Studied plant alkaloids (Strychnine, brucine, quinine) were first isolated and crystallized
Meissner C.F.W. (1819)	:	Proposed the term alkaloid for alkali like substances
1900-1950	:	True development of study of plant chemicals in several universities started in several countries on the production of antibiotics by different groups of microorganisms such as penicillin, streptomycin, Nyastatin, aureofungin, bacitracin etc.
Post World War (After 1945)	:	Development of chromatographic techniques gave a great momentum to the research on plant chemicals. New structures were described even though they were present in minute quantity and in non - crystalline form.
Karrer (1957)	:	Published a comprehensive dictionary of 2750 compounds excluding alkaloids produced by various plants. The list including alkaloids was around 5000.
1990 onward	:	Total number of plant product identification has crossed 18,000 mark.

With the advent of radio tracer techniques, isotope labeling studies, mutation research and many other new advanced techniques has made it possible to study the secondary metabolites and their synthesis pathways. During the last 20 to 30 years, the analysis of secondary plant products has progressed a lot. The use of modern analytical techniques like chromatography, electrophoresis, isotope techniques and enzymology succeeded in the elucidation of exact structural formulas and the most important biosynthetic pathways.

Chapter 3

General Biosynthetic Pathways

Plant cells contain far more compounds than are produced by the basic metabolism. Terpenes, waxes, alkaloids and pigments are just some key words that illustrate what is meant. The term basic metabolism comprises all pathways necessary for the survival of the cells, while secondary plant products are such that occur usually only in special, differentiated cells and are not necessary for the cells themselves but may be useful for the plant as a whole. Examples are flower pigments and scents or stabilizing elements. Both metabolisms are overlapping since it is often not understood why a certain compound is produced. Furthermore, no typical cell exists so that some compounds may be necessary for the survival of some cells but not for that of others.

Arguments in support of important functions for plant secondary products are underlined by the organizational complexity and specificity which characterizes many aspects of their biosynthesis. Furthermore - with the very important exception of substances produced in response to stress or pathogen attack - much of secondary metabolism is reproducible from one individual of a species to another and, to a remarkable degree, produces the same principal compounds in broadly the same relative proportions. For example, an *Atropa* plant extracted for alkaloids can confidently be predicted to contain predominantly atropine, rather than its immediate precursor, tropine, or a more distantly-related alkaloid, nicotine - just as the passenger boarding a train for Mumbai at Anand can be reassured that his train will not terminate prematurely at a "precursor station" (Surat), or even adopt an "alternative pathway" (to Poona). On the other hand, the evolutionary circumstances leading to the development of atropine formation in *Atropa*, rather than to the formation of other alkaloids with comparable activity (for example, nicotine) remain substantially unknown. A similar question has been discussed regarding two families of plant pigments with apparently similar functions, the anthocyanins and the betalains. With regard to defense (and similarly but perhaps less obviously protection against ionizing radiation), a general hypothesis argues that plants evolved a broad defensive strategy based upon a diversity of antimicrobial and anti feedant substances from which, as a result of chance mutation, more potent substances conferring additional selective advantage from time to time arose. It is conceivable that in some cases enzymes evolved or became adapted to catalyse reactions of benefit which could already occur to some extent (though in a non-stereospecific manner) non-enzymically. Mutation will then have led to the development of modified enzymes able to catalyse reactions with new or different substrates, or to catalyse alternative reactions with existing substrates.

Characterization of metabolic pathways is a multi-disciplinary activity. It requires the identification of metabolic intermediates and the demonstration of a plausible reaction sequence, followed by the isolation and characterization of the individual enzymes responsible and the determination of their tissue and subcellular localization. It requires control to be studied at the metabolic level, to investigate the relationships between biosynthesis and further metabolism or degradation and to identify reactions and metabolite movements which may contribute to rate-limitation. Thirdly, it involves the study of transcriptional and post-transcriptional control - in particular, of the coordinated expression of genes in response to environmental or ontogenic factors (which may be more- or less-defined), and of the signal-transduction pathways which lie behind the transcriptional responses observed. We know today of a range of metabolic compounds that have developed in parallel in non-related species and are produced by different biosynthetic pathways, such as Caffine (Fig. 3.1), acetate-mevalonate, shikimate, homogentisate and hydroxybenzoate pathway.

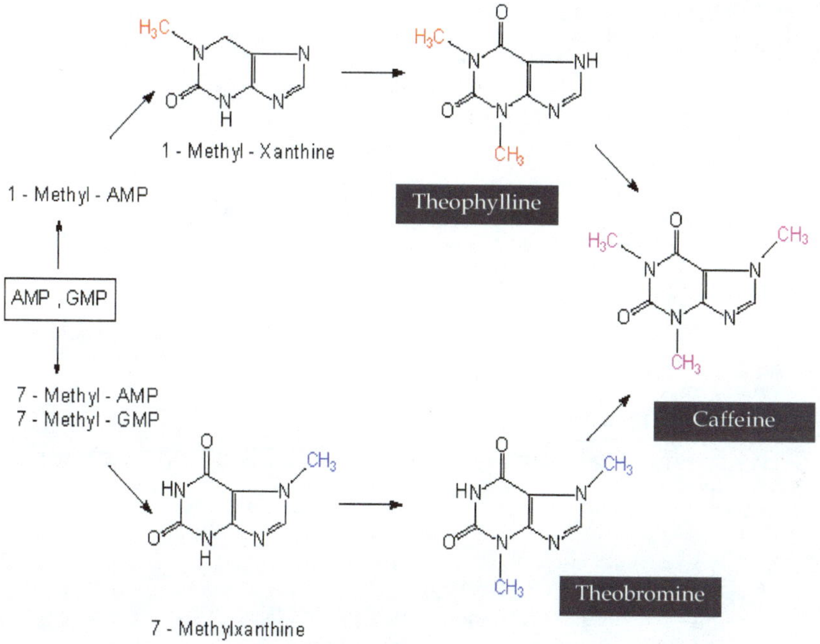

Fig. 3.1 : Pathway for the synthesis of caffeine

The acetate-malonate pathway

Synthesis of plumbagin (*Plumbago*, Plumbaginaceae)

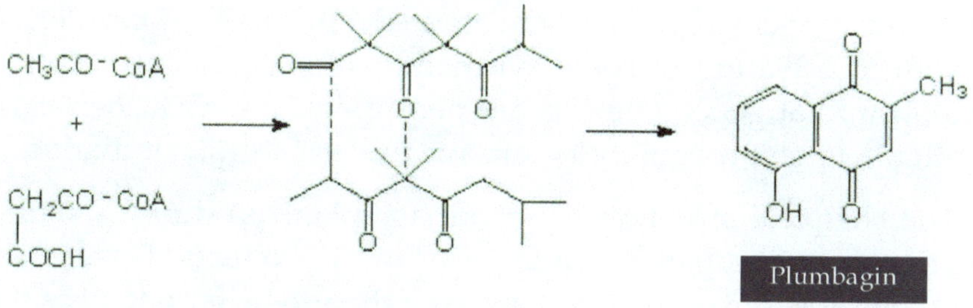

The shikimate pathway

Synthesis of juglon (*Juglans*, Juglandaceae)

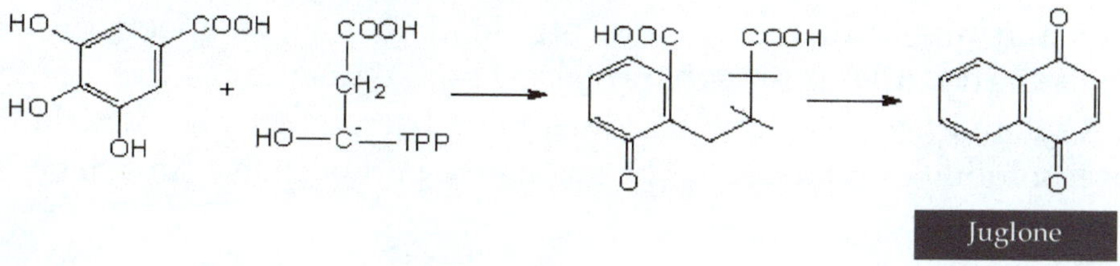

The homogentisate pathway

Synthesis of chimaphylline (*Chimaphila*, Pyrolaceae)

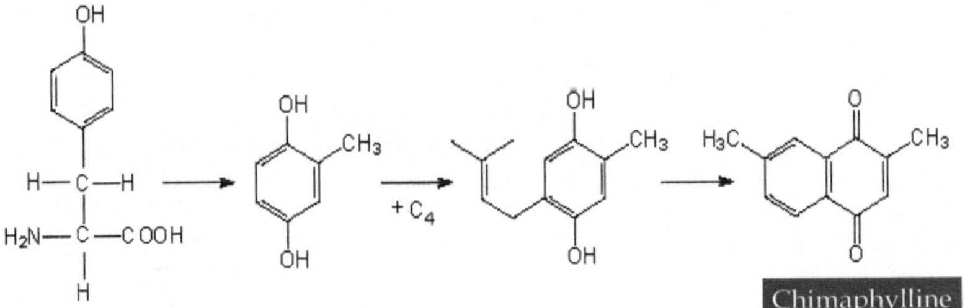

Chimaphylline

The hydroxybenzoate pathway

Synthesis of alkannin (*Plagiobothrys*, Boraginaceae)

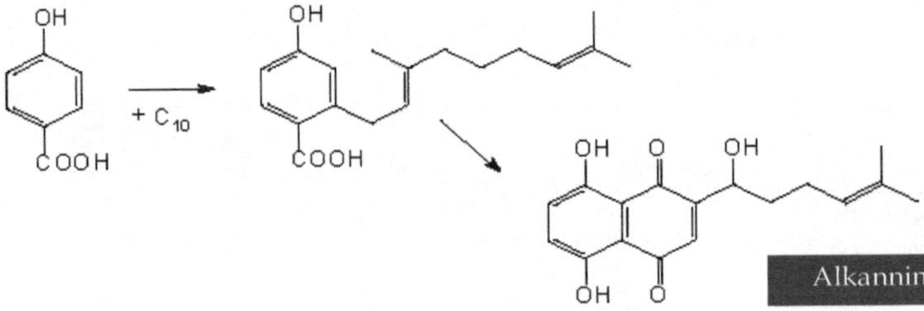

Alkannin

A number of mutants are unable to synthesize certain products due to a blocked metabolism. A classic example is the white-flowering varieties of species with otherwise coloured, often red flowers. Perhaps, it is indeed a feature of some synthetic pathways of the secondary metabolism that genetic defects are permissible and that their carrier has often a large probability to survive under natural conditions.

The chemical structure of secondary plant products is without exception more complex than that of primary products. This becomes comprehensible remembering that many though by far not all of them are derived from amino acids or nucleotides. Most of the compounds found in plants belong to rather few families of substances. Only small chemical modifications like methylations, hydroxylations, intercalations with metal ions, etc. lead to a wide spectrum of functionally different substances. These substances are often glycosylated (certain sugar residues have been added) so that their water solubility is increased. The sugar-free part of such a substance is called an aglucon.

Among the largely unanswered questions are those after the compartment a certain substance is produced in, is that whether all steps of the biosynthetic pathway take place in this compartment or only the first and the last, whether synthesis and storage occur in different compartments, how organ-specific occurrence can be explained and how biosynthesis is controlled. Are the biosynthetic pathways ramified, do they lead to several, related products, exists a feedback inhibition? Why do the pathways of related species differ? How are the synthesis and the activity of the necessary enzymes controlled? Are they monomerous proteins or multienzyme complexes, do they occur in a free state or are they bound to a membrane? How are they transported within the cell and are they possibly excreted?

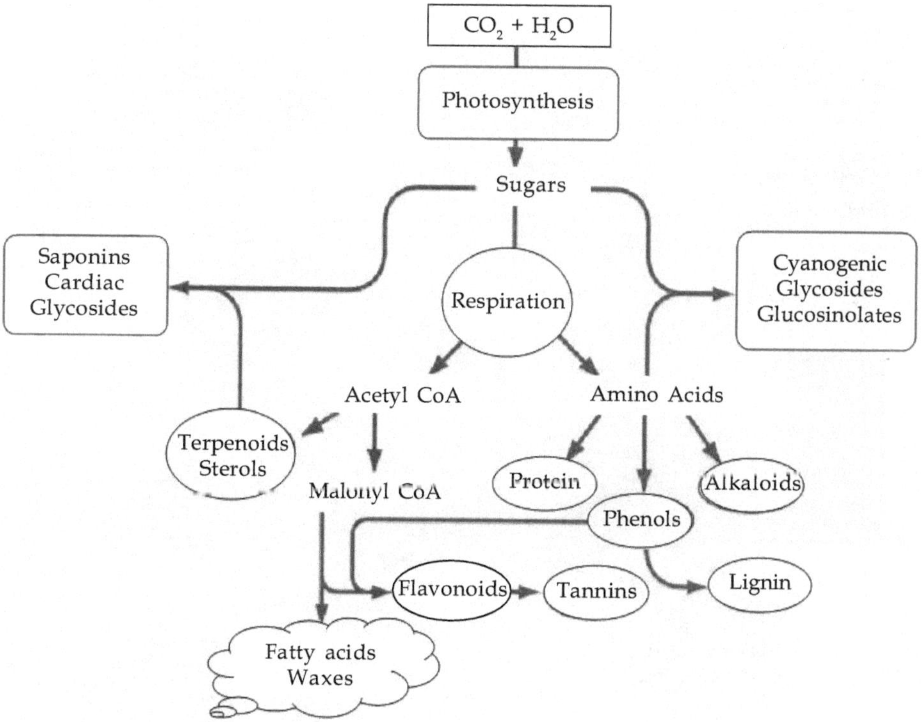

Fig. 3.2 : Biosynthetic relationship among primary and secondary metabolites.

Central metabolic pathways for some secondary meta-bolite produ-ctions have been studied and presented here under (Fig. 3.2 to 3.8).

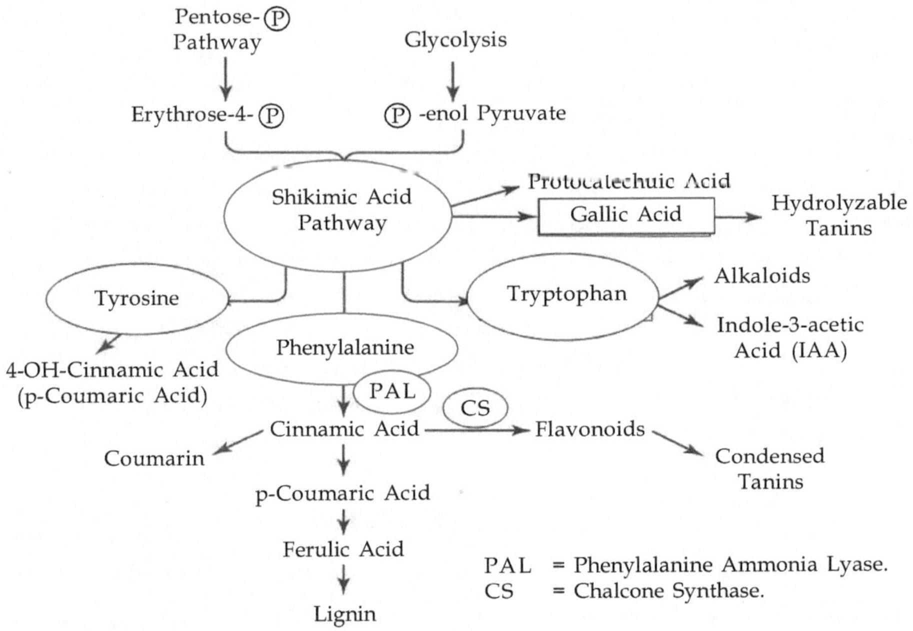

Fig. 3.3 : Shikimic acid pathway in the synthesis of various primary and secondary metabolites.

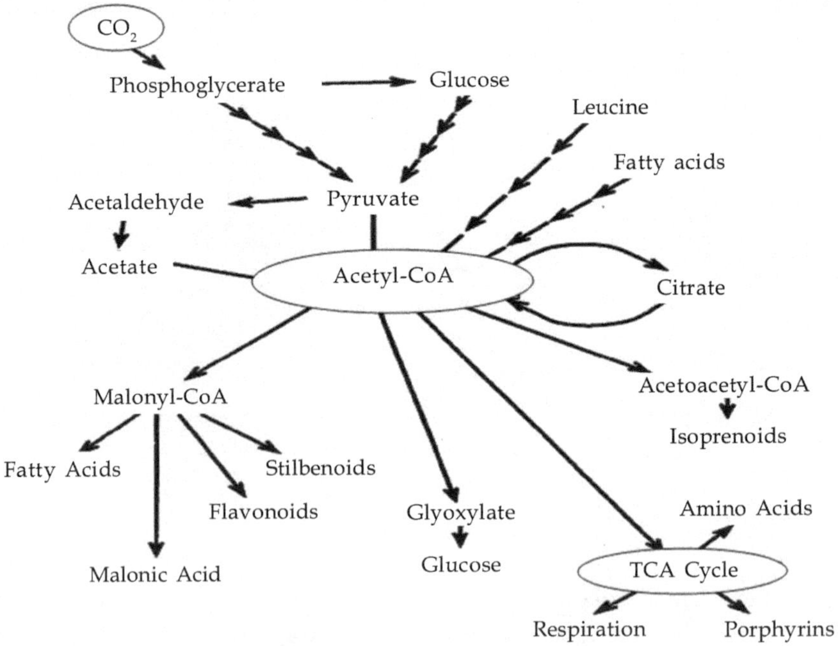

Fig. 3.4 : The metabolism of Acetyl CoA; various process

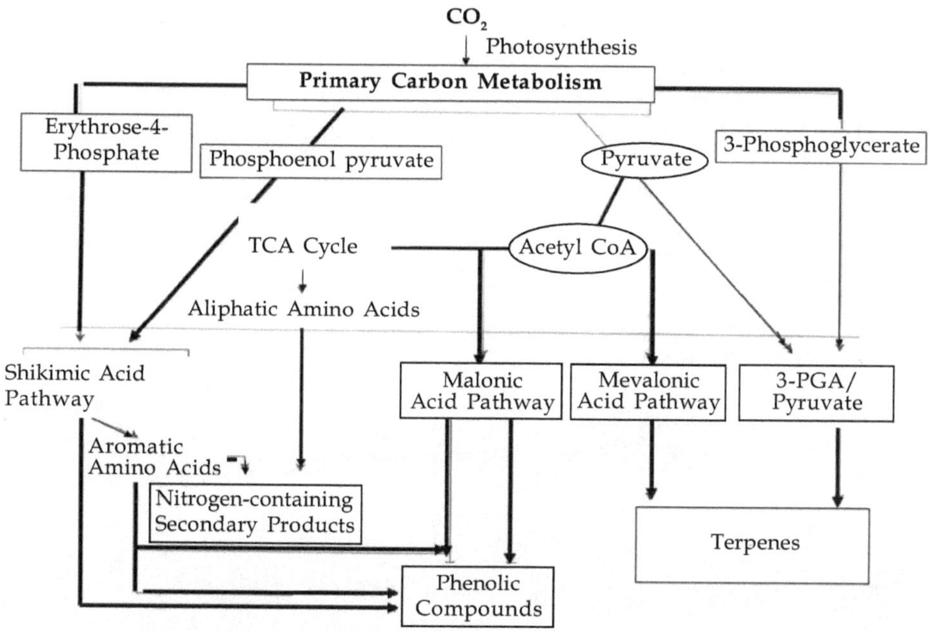

Fig. 3.5 : Phenolic compounds and terpenes from primary carbon metabolites

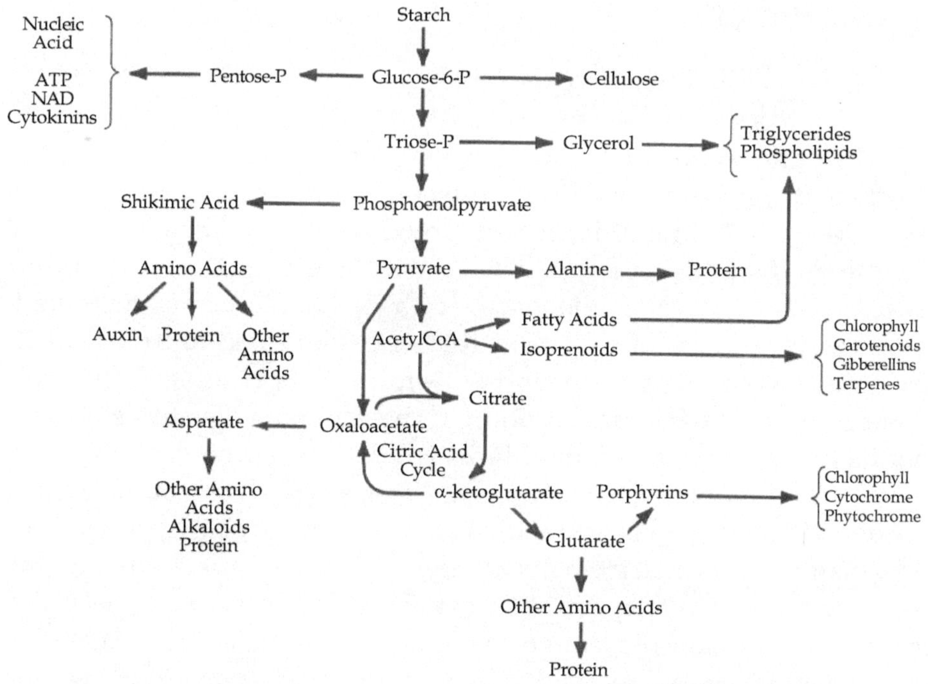

Fig. 3.6 : Glycolysis pathway and its role in synthesis of protein.

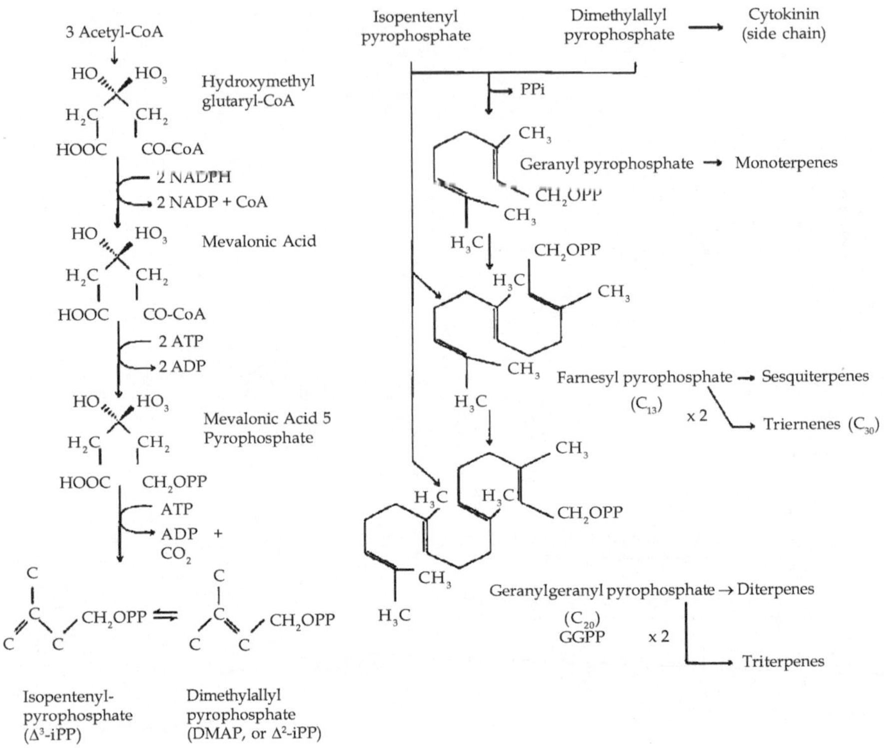

Fig. 3.7 : Biosynthesis of Terpenoids from the mevalonic acid pathway

Tropane alkaloids and nicotine are derived from diamine putrescine produced from ornithine by ornithine decarboxylase (ODC), arginine, or both. Putrescine is *N*-methylated by PMT then oxidatively deaminated by diamine oxidase to the 1-methyl-D1- pyrrolinium cation. This cation is condensed with a derivative of nicotinic acid, forming nicotine in tobacco, or is further metabolized to tropinone in tropane alkaloid-producing plants. Hygrine is formed nonenzymatically by condensation of the cation and acetoacetic acid, but its involvement in alkaloid biosynthesis has not been established. Tropinone is reduced by tropinone reductase I (TR-I) to tropine, which condenses with phenylacetic acid or its derivative, giving hyoscyamine. Scopolamine is formed from hyoscyamine via 6b-hydroxyhyoscyamine by the bifunctional enzyme hyoscyamine 6b-hydroxylase (H6H). The nicotinic acid moiety of nicotine is supplied from the pyridine nucleotide cycle, in which quinolinic acid phosphoribosyltransferase (QPT) serves as the entry-point enzyme.

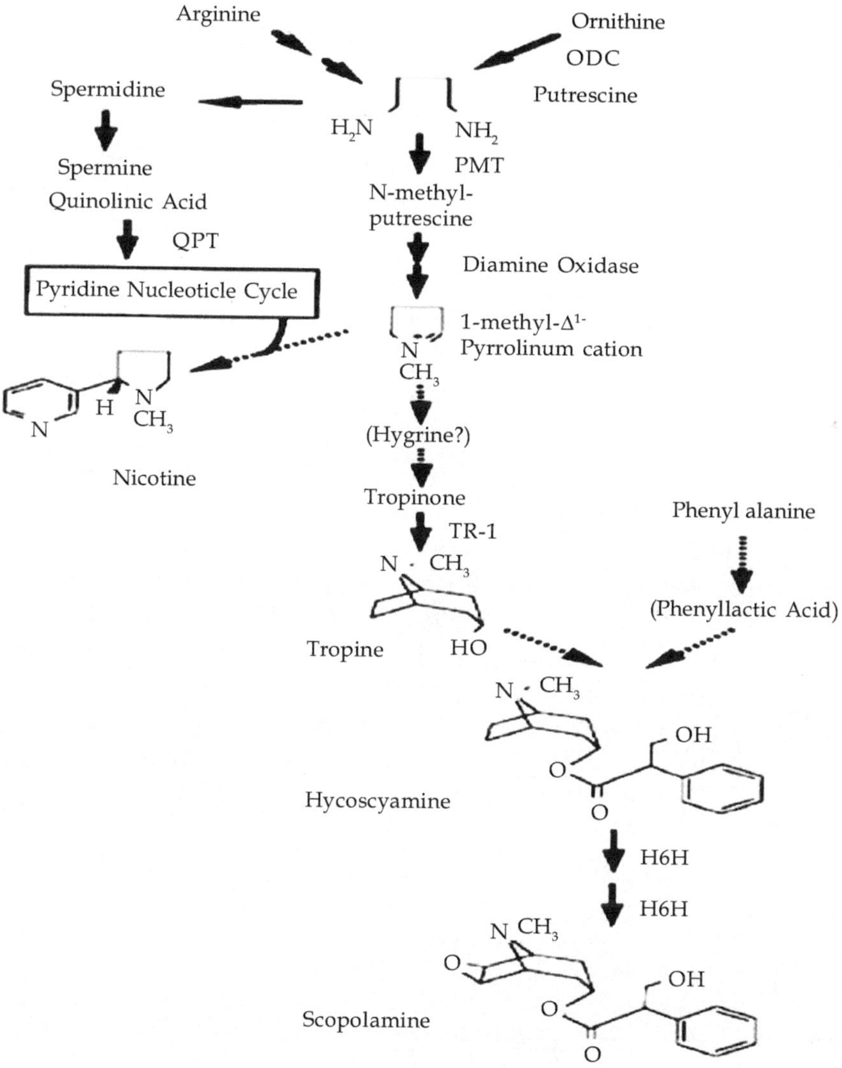

Fig. 3.8 : Pathways for Tropane and nicotine alkaloids biosynthesis

Biosynthesis of Phenolics

Phenolic compounds are aromatic structures bearing one or more hydroxyl groups. Most are polyphenols, having several hydroxyl group substituents, one or more of which may be substituted by methyl or glycosyl groups. Phenolics share a common biosynthetic origin from phenylalanine (Fig. 3.9), one of the three protein amino acids formed from sedoheptulose via the shikimate pathway.

These flavonoids are the best known group of polyphenols, sharing the same carbon skeleton of flavone or 2-phenylbenzopyrone and comprise some 4000 structures. The total number of phenolics including all the non-flavonoids is well over 8000. The vast majority of these are of plant origin, although a few simple phenols (e.g. m-cresol) are found in the pheromonal secretions of elephants and some flavonoids (e.g. quercetin) are stored in butterfly wings after dietary ingestion.

The different classes of Polyphenol range in molecular weight from simple compounds such as phenol itself and salicylic acid (2-hydroxybenzoic acid) through complex anthocyanin pigments with molecular weights of 2000 or more to the polymeric condensed tannins where the molecular weight may reach 30,000.

The flavonoid pathway is part of the larger phenylpropanoid pathway, which produces a range of other secondary metabolites, such as phenolic acids, lignins, lignans, and stilbenes. The key flavonoid precursors are phenylalanine, obtained via the shikimate and arogenate pathways, and malonyl-CoA, derived from citrate produced by the TCA cycle. Most flavonoid biosynthetic enzymes characterized to date are thought to operate in enzyme complexes located in the cytosol. Flavonoid end products are transported to various subcellular or extracellular locations, with those flavonoids involved in pigmentation generally being transported into the vacuole.

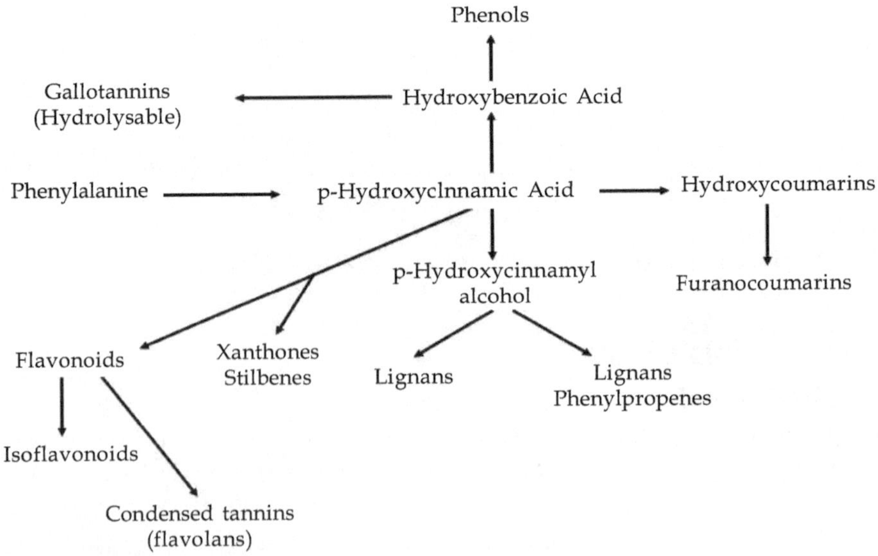

Fig.3.9 : Different phenolic classes and their relationship

There are many branches to the flavonoid biosynthetic pathways, with the best characterized being those leading to the colored anthocyanins and proanthocyanidins (PAs) and the generally colorless flavones, flavonols, and isoflavonoids. Genes or cDNAs have now been identified for all the core steps leading to anthocyanin, flavone, and flavonol formation, as well as many steps of the isoflavonoid branch, allowing extensive analysis of the encoded enzymes. In addition, several DNA sequences are available for the modification enzymes that produce the variety of structures known within each class of compound.

Significant recent advances in our understanding of flavonoid biosynthesis include characterization of the formation of anthocyanidin 3-O-glucoside from leucoanthocyanidin, clarification of PA monomer formation, progress toward elucidating aurone and 3-deoxyflavonoid formation, the molecular characterization of several genes encoding enzymes that modify the flavonoid core structures, analysis of enzyme function, the determination of enzyme structures by x-ray crystallography and homology modeling, and the identification of several different groups of transcription factors regulating anthocyanin and PA biosynthesis. Data are also starting to emerge on the subcellular organization of the biosynthetic enzymes within the cytosol (and the role this may play in metabolic channeling), and transport mechanisms for the flavonoids within the cell. However, there are still major areas where data are lacking. Tertiary structures are available for only a few of the biosynthetic enzymes, little is known about the turnover or degradation of flavonoids, and details of post-transcriptional regulatory mechanisms are limited. Furthermore, the range of genes encoding secondary modification enzymes that have been characterized is still limited compared to the great array of known flavonoid structures. Nor have cDNAs or genes been published for some of the enzymes carrying out hydroxylation of the core flavonoid structure, such as at the C-8 and C-2′ positions.

The key enzymes involved in the formation of the hydroxycinnamic acids (HCAs) from phenylalanine and malonyl-CoA are now discussed in detail, while later sections address the branches of the flavonoid pathway leading to anthocyanins, aurones, flavones, flavonols, PAs, and isoflavonoids. This is followed by brief reviews of the regulation of flavonoid biosynthesis.

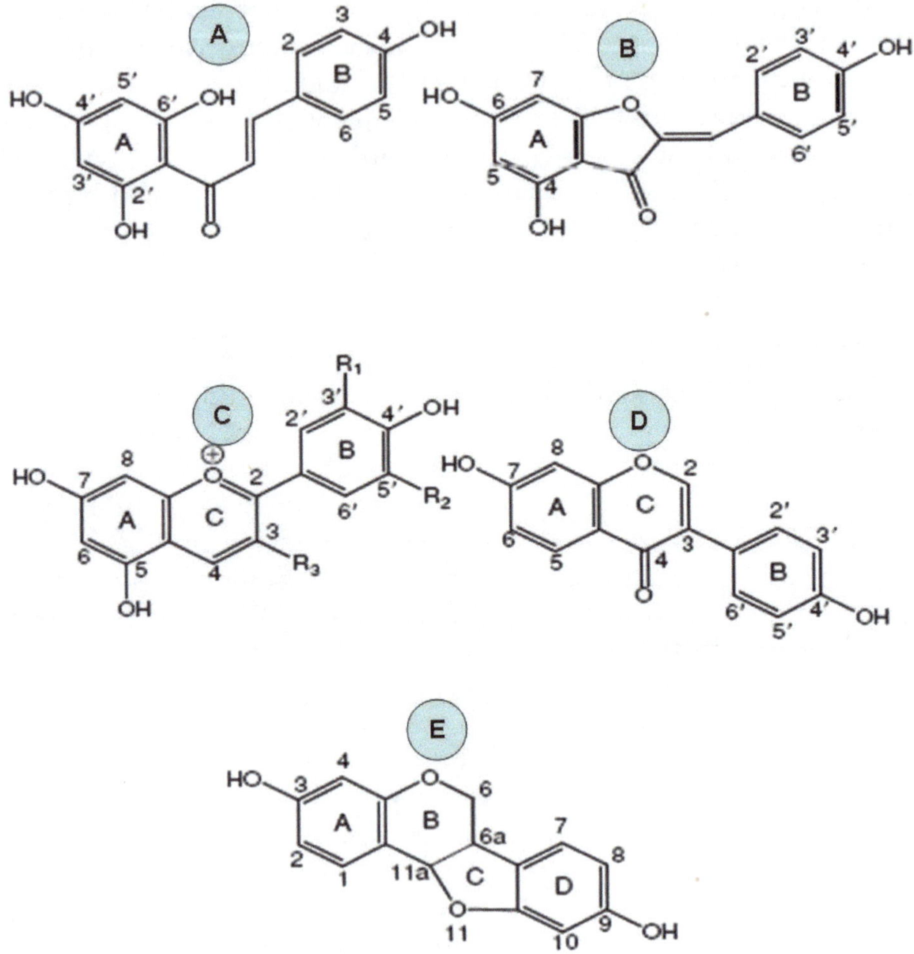

Base structures of a chalcone (A), an aurone (B), the main anthocyanidins (C), an isoflavonoid (D), and a pterocarpan (E). The lettering of the carbon rings is shown, as well as the numbering of the key carbons. Here note that the numbering is different for each type of compound. For the majority of flavonoid types the numbering is as for the anthocyanidins, and for the cinnamic acids it is as for the chalcones. R1, R2, and R3 substitutions determine the various common anthocyanidins. The common 3-hydroxyanthocyanidins (R3=OH) are pelargonidin (R1 and R2=H), cyanidin (R1=OH and R2=H), delphinidin (R1 and R2=OH), peonidin (R1=OCH3 and R2=H), petunidin (R1=OCH3 and R2=OH), and malvidin (R1 and R2=OCH3). The rare 3-deoxyanthocyanidins (R3=H) are apigeninidin (R1 and R2=H), luteolinidin (R1=OH and R2=H), and tricetinidin (R1 and R2=OH).

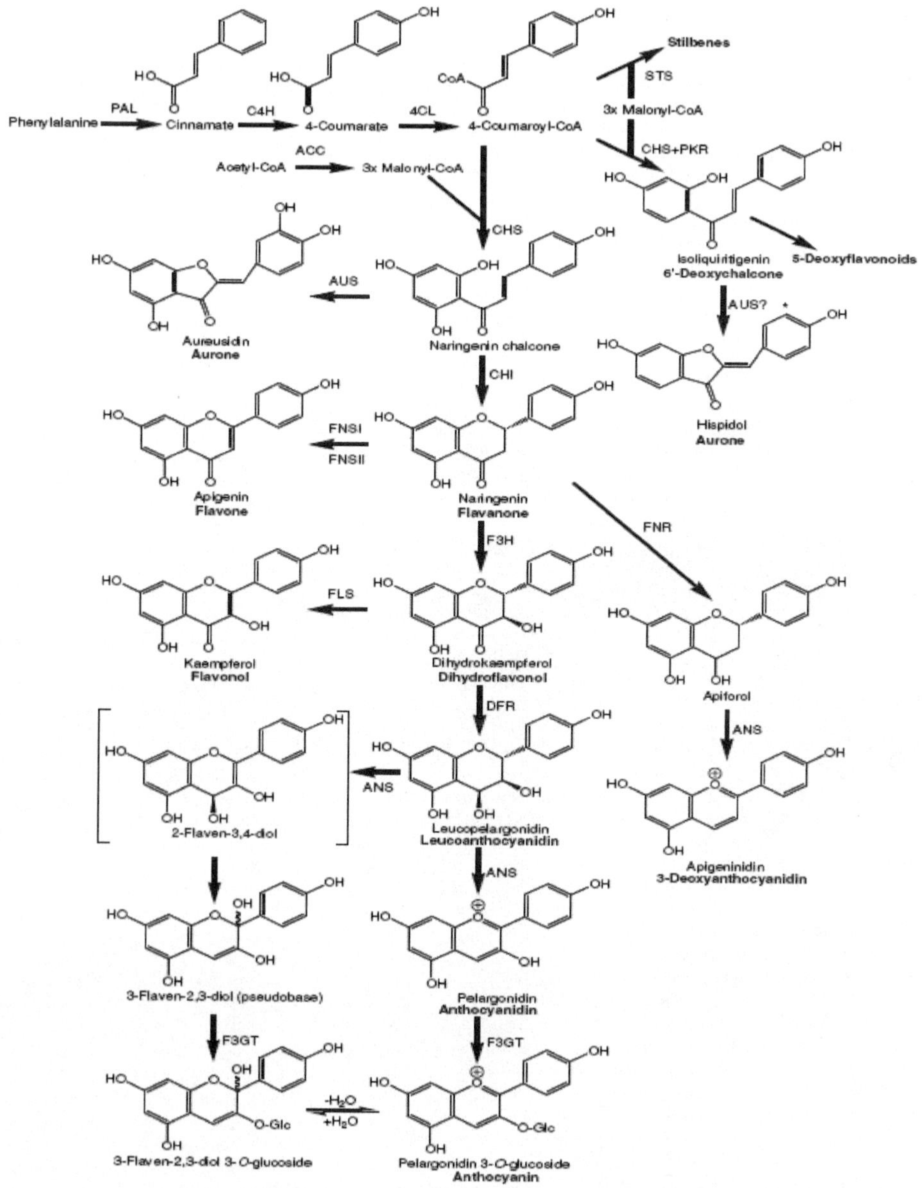

PAL – Phenylalanine ammonia lyase C4H- Cinnamate 4 hydroxylase 4CL- 4 coumarate: CoA Ligase STS- Stilbene synthase CHS- Chalcone synthase CHI- Chalcone isomerase FNS- Flavon synthase FLS- Flavonol synthase F3H- Flavanone 3β-hydroxylase DFR- Dihydroflavonol 4 reductase ANS- Anthocyanidin synthase FNR- Flavanone reductase FLS- Flavonol synthase F3′5′H- Flavonoid 3′,5′-Hydroxylase F3GT- Flavonol glucose transferase.

Fig.3.10 : General phenylpropanoid and flavonoid biosynthetic

Chapter 4

Essential Oils Terpenes / Terpenoids

The functional diversity of chemicals within plants is best demonstrated by terpenoids. More than 30,000 terpenoids have been identified, each one composed of 5-carbon (prenyl diphosphate) building blocks added together to make 10-carbon, 15-carbon, and even 2000–500,000-carbon chains, as is the case for rubber. Terpenes are functionally diverse, and many are integral to primary metabolism, e.g., hormones such as gibberellins and abscisic acid, electron carriers such as plastoquinone and ubiquinone, terpene-derived compounds that form structural parts of membranes such as phytosterols, and photosynthetic pigments such as carotenoids.

Plant terpenes are also available as essential oil or ethereal oil. Essential oil is defined as the volatile oil obtained by the steam distillation of plants. There is a distinction between fixed or fatty oils and volatile oils. Their volatility (boiling point) and plant origin are characteristic properties of these oils.

Bitter almond and Mustard oil	→	Obtained enzymatically followed by steam distillation
Lemon oils and orange oils	→	Obtained by pressing the fruits.
Ocimum or eucalyptus oil	→	Extraction by organic solvents.

All are included in essential oils.

The oldest of volatile oil 'EAU DE COLOGNE' prepared in 1725 by Johann Maria Farina in Cologne is still extracted in same fashion and is being used in the cosmetics. It was found that the oil contains chiefly liquid and more or less volatile compounds of many classes of organic substances. Thus, we find, acyclic and isocyclic hydrocarbons and their oxygenated derivatives. Some contain sulphur or nitrogen. Essential oil can be broadly classified in to four groups depending upon the reactive groups, which are as under.

1. Esters : This group include methyl esters of salicylic acid; Oil of winter green.
2. Aldehydes : This group include cinnamic aldehyde of cinnamon.
3. Ethers : This group contain oil of clove (eugenol)
4. Terpenes : Camphor, menthol , oil of lemon etc. are included in this group.

There are basic differences between fixed or fatty oils and volatile or essential oils.

How essential oil differs from fixed oil ?

S.No.	Essential/volatile oil	Fixed/fatty oil
1	Boiling points are less than 60 °C	Boiling points are higher than 100 °C
2	Can be steam distilled without prior to volatilisation.	Decompose any change in its biological property
3	Produce temporary greasy spot on paper	Produce permanent greasy spot on paper.
4	Example:Eugenol, cinnamic aldehyde etc	Example: Linoleic acid, Arachidonic acid etc.
5	Uses: Fragrance, perfume medicine etc	Uses: Edible oil in food preparation

There are four classes of essential oils

1. Terpenes related to isoprene or isopentene.
2. Straight chain compounds not containing any side chain
3. Benzene derivatives
4. Miscellaneous group having varied structures not included in first three groups.

Terpenes

They are either hydro carbons ($C_{10}H_{16}$) or oxygen containing compound ($C_{10}H_{16}O$) or ($C_{10}H_{18}O$). The name terpene was given by KEKULE. Major terpenoid source and different classes of terpenoids are given in Table 4.1 and 4.2

There are compounds which have less number of carbon and hydrogen. The common isoprene i.e. (C_5H_8). Members of the C_{10} group are often referred as mono-terpenes. Compounds having a more distant connection with the terpenes, but still containing features which link them with terpene structures are sometimes called terpenoids or isoterpenoids.

O.Wallach who is considered as 'MESIAH OF TERPENES' differentiated around 500 essential oils on the basis of their crystallisation properties.

Hemi-terpenes		C – C – C – C | C	C_5
Terpenes		C – C – C – C C – C – C – C | | C C	C_{10}
Sesqui-terpene	3 x	C – C – C – C | C	C_{15}
Di-terpene	4 x	C – C – C – C | C	C_{20}
Tri-terpene	6 x	C – C – C – C | C	C_{30}
Tetra-terpene	8 x	C – C – C – C | C	C_{40}
Ppoly-terpene	n x	C – C – C – C | C	C_n

Geraniol ($C_{10}H_{18}O$)	Chief constituent of rose and geranium oil
Linalool ($C_{10}H_{18}O$)	Component of lavender oil
α - Terpeniol	Oil of hyacinth
Thymol	Thyme camphor
Menthol	Peppermint

There are several isomers of geraniol also. Lycopene, a red pigment of tomato also falls under the group of terpene. It is a tetra-terpene having a molecular formula of C_{40} H_{56} having 32 carbon atoms in the ring with 8 methyl side chain having 14 double bonds. The β- carotene and Vitamin E also falls under this group of terpenes with several isoprene ring structure. Their presence have been reported in scent of eucalyptus, the flavour of cinnamon, colour of yellow flower.

While terpenes with more than five isoprene units are quite universal, many of the simpler terpenes are restricted to certain plant groups. Sesquestiterpenes, for example, are common in mosses but occur in higher plants, too. They can be found with *Magnoliales*, but not with *Ranunculales*. This example shows, why the presence of certain secondary plant products has proven to be a useful taxonomical feature. The same is also true for monoterpenes (iridoid compounds, iridians). Among the diterpenes are the gibberellins, a group of phytohormones.

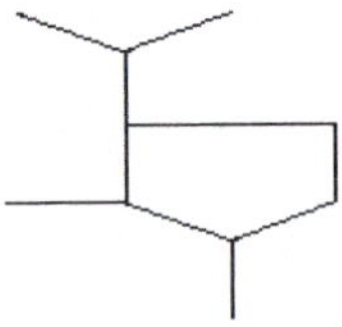

Iridane skeleton
basic unit
of the monoterpenes

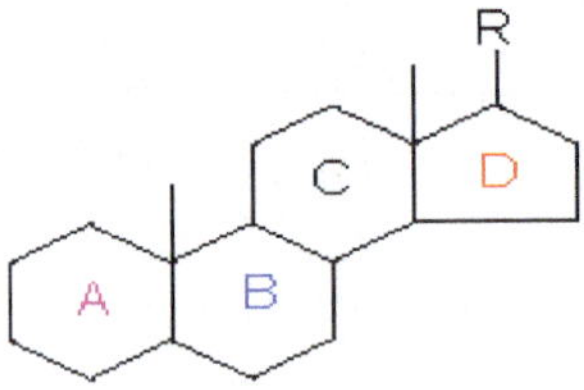

Sterane skeleton
basic unit
of a steroide

Steroids are triterpenes or triterpenoids. Triterpenes are a group of molecules that contain 30 C- atoms and are generated by the polymerization of six isoprene units although a number of derivatives, some with more but most with less C-atoms are also counted among this group. Steroid molecules consist of four rings marked A, B, C and D that have a number of additional residues R. It is of some importance whether two of these are in a cis- (i.e. at the same side of the cyclic system) or in a trans-position (at opposite sites). Steroids have been shown to occur both in gymnosperms and in angiosperms.

Carotenoids are very common both in the plant and the animal kingdom though they are always of plant origin. All of them are tetraterpenes, i.e. they contain 40 C-atoms in eight isoprene residues.

The pictures below show that they all have a centre of symmetry. They are formally derived by the subsequent hydration, dehydration, ring formation, shifting of double bonds and / or methyl groups, chain elongation or shortening and the incorporation of oxygen into a non-cyclic $C_{40}H_{56}$ compound. Carotenoids can be further classified into carotenes (pure carbohydrates without additional groups) and the xanthophylls (carotenoids containing oxygen).

beta-carotene

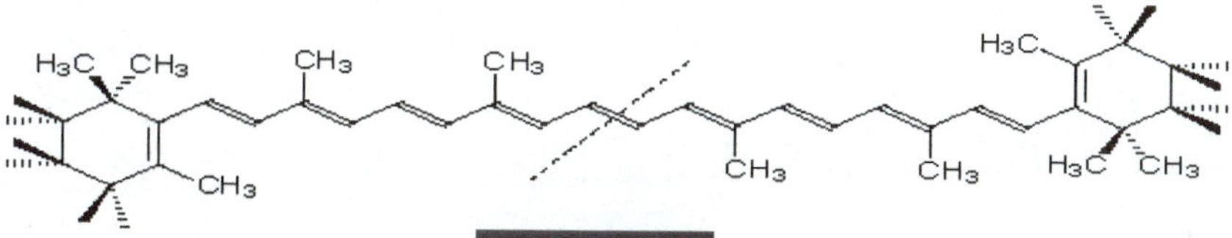

β-carotene

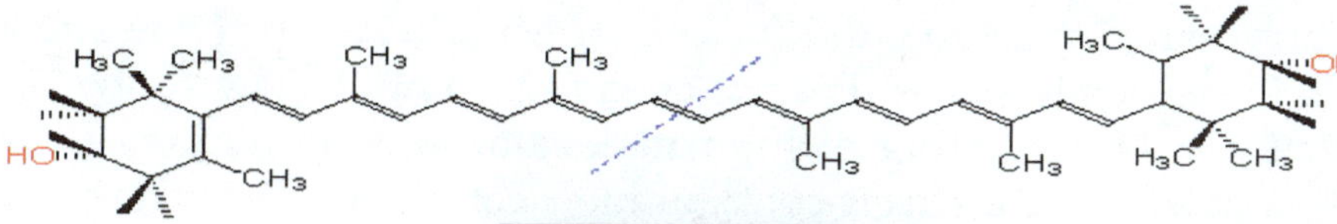

Lutein (xanthophyll)

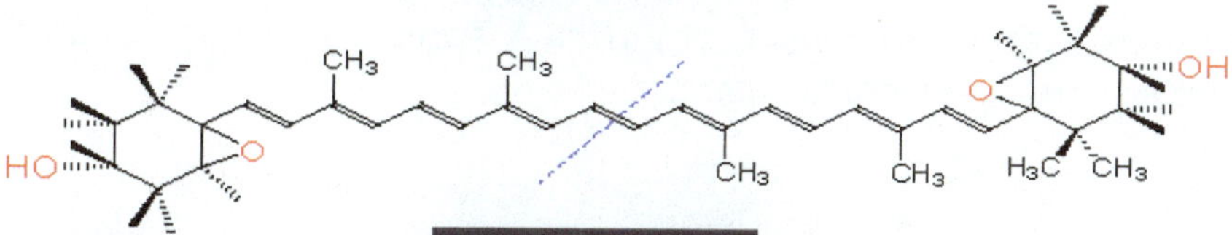

Violaxanthin

Members of both groups are components of the pigment systems (the light traps) of chloroplasts and are involved in the primary light absorption and the photon canalization of photosynthesis. Moreover, they also function as light receptors in a number of further light-induced plant processes. Some representative absorption spectra are shown below. The yellow colour of many flowers is caused by carotenoid-containing chromoplasts that are usually devoid of chlorophyll. Carotenoids are also common in fruits. The red colour of ripe tomatoes and of pepper is caused by the presence of lycopene. It is a linear molecule with 13 double bonds, 11 of which are conjugated. Many carotenes (and xanthophylls) are cyclic at their termini and loose as a consequence the terminal double bond(s).

If such a ring is formed at just one terminus, then the result is *gamma*-carotene, if they occur at both, either *alpha*- or *beta* - carotene is formed depending on the type of ring generated. *Beta*-carotene is best-known as the pigment of the carrot (*Daucus carota*). It occurs mostly as a crystal. One of its most important derivatives is vitamin A (a precursor of visual purple).

Xanthophylls like the common xanthophyll of green leaves or lutein are derived from carotenes. Violaxanthin, for example, is a derivative of *alpha*-carotene. The yellow pigment of corn, zeaxanthin is a *beta*-carotene derivative. Fucoxanthin, the brownish pigment of brown algae and diatoms, is another xanthophyll. Among the catabolic products of xanthophyll is the pigment of saffron, the crocetin.

Rubber-Like Polymers / Polyisoprenes

The first record mentioning the use of rubber goes back to the 11th century. Since this time, the Indians of Middle America use rubber balls in their ball games. From a chemical point of view rubber is a carbohydrate consisting of high molecular weight chains of 1,4 - polyisoprene residues in cis-configuration (catachnic). The main source is *Hevea brasiliensis*. Gutta-percha consists of 1,4 - polyisoprene residues in trans-configuration. Its molecular weight is far below that of rubber. The main source is *Palaquium gutta*. A similar substance, balata, is obtained from *Mimosops balata*.

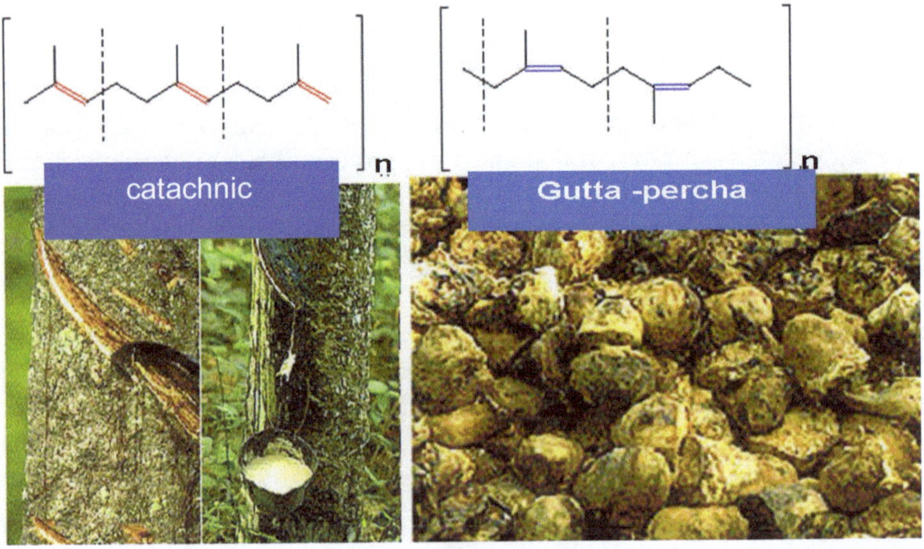

Chicle (obtained from *Achras sapota*), finally, is a polymer containing both cis- and trans-bonds (in the ratio 1:2). It is the basic substance of bubble gum.

Altogether, more than 1800 plant polyisoprenes have been identified. Their cellular concentrations are usually small, and their molecular weights are relatively low.

Polyisoprenes occur in certain plant cells as small latex particles. They can be seen in the electron microscope as clearly defined, cytoplasmatic inclusions specific for the respective species.

Characteristics of Terpenes

- Derivatives of terpene have common biosynthetic origin from isoprene (C_5H_8).
- Lipophilic in nature.
- Found in leaf glandular trichomes, bud exudates, bark resins.
- Mainly flavonoids, carotenoids, chlorophylls.
- May mimic insect growth hormones.
- Include cardiac glycosides which affect the heart.
- Toxic to most fungi and insects.

There are several difficulties in studying the terpenes.

1. Terpenes are unstable and tend to re-arrange intra-molecular groups. This property is an obstacle in their studies.
2. They are liquids so that thorough fractionation is necessary to separate the constituents, which boil within a restricted range.
3. The boiling point difference between several essential oils is varying narrow leading to improper purification of active principles.

Table 4.1 : Major terpenoids with their source.

Terpenoids	No. Found	Source	Plant Part
Monoterpenoids	2500	Conifer	Bark
Sesquiterpenoids	5000	Cotton	Leaf
Ditepenoids	2500	Taxus	Leaf
Triterpenoids	5000	Neem Tree	Leaf
Tetraterpenoids	500	Carrot	Bark

Table 4.2 : Different classes of Terpenoids and their characteristics.

Terpenoid class	Characteristics
Monoterpenoids	Volatile, essential oil constituents
Iridoids	Bitter tasting lactones, usually in glycosidic
Sesquiterpenoids	form Higher boiling essential oil constituents
Sesquiterpene lactones	Characteristic of the family compositae
Diterpenoids	Resin acids and gibberellins
Triterpenoid saponins	Haemolytic glycosides
Steroid saponins	Haemolytic glycosides
Cardenolides and	Heart poisons and toxins
Bufadienolides	Membrane constituents
Phytosterols	Bitter principles, especially of the
Cucurbitacins	Cucurbitaceae
Nortriterpenoids	Limonoids and quassinoids
Other triterpenoids	Lupanes, hapanes, ursanes, etc.
Carotenoids	Yellow to red pigments

The number of fully characterized terpenoids is now probably in excess of 20,000.

Biosynthesis of Terpenes

Several thousand different types of molecules from very different plant groups have been isolated and characterized. Despite their varied structures, all of them are synthesized by only a few pathways.

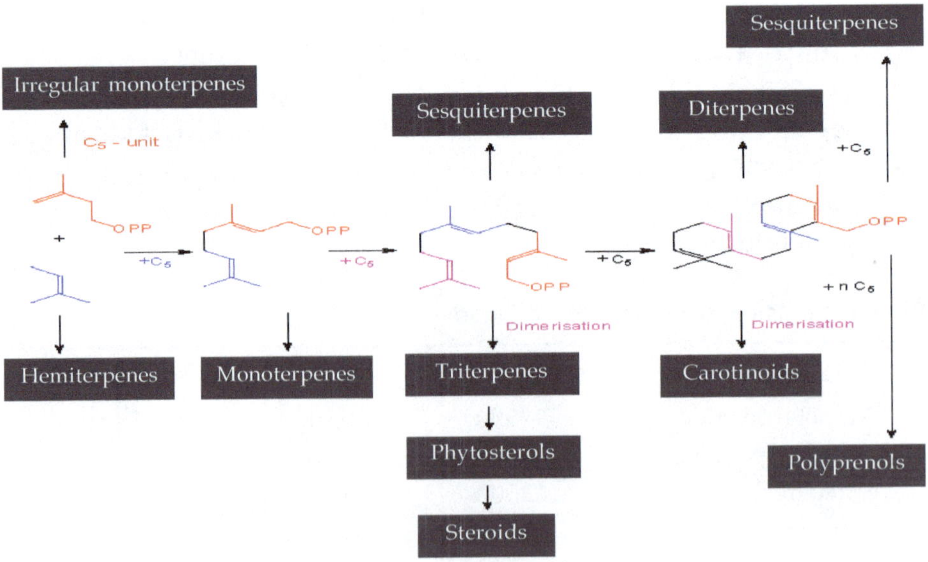

Fig. 4.1 : Biosynthesis of Terpenes

The starting product of all the different groups of compounds shown in the illustration above is mevalonic acid that is transformed into a phosphorylated isoprene upon phosphorylation. This isoprene polymerizes subsequently. In the course of polymerization, the number and position of the double bonds are fixed. All green plants are able to generate linear isoprenoids in this way.

In plants there are two subcellular locations for the synthesis of terpenes, the cytosol and the plastids. There are two biochemical pathways responsible for the synthesis of terpenoids (Fig. 4.1 to 4.6) In both prenyltransferases act in the condensation of an isoprene unit, IDP (isopentenyl diphosphate), with an IDP isomer, DMADP (dimethallyl diphosphate), in a head-to-tail addition. The result, prenyl diphosphates of varying lengths, is then modified through dimerization and cyclization by TPSs (terpene synthases) to produce a diverse array of terpenoids with an almost equally diverse array of functions. The first pathway described, one that is common to bacteria, fungi, mammals, and plants, is the mevalonic acid pathway. Recent pathway, the deoxy xylulose phosphate/methylerythritol (DOXP/MEP), is identical to that discovered in bacteria a few years earlier and probably is a legacy of prokaryotic endosymbiotic ancestors. Thus, in higher plants there are two pathways for generating terpenes. The classic mevalonic acid pathway produces the precursors of sesquiterpenes (C15) and multiples thereof, for example, the triterpenes (C30), via the cytosol; and the plastidic DOXP/MEP produces units of C10, such as the precursors of monoterpenes (C10) and diterpenes (C20), etc. Recent evidence suggests that there may well be sharing of intermediates across these pathways, a sort of biosynthetic cross talk. A common ancestor has been implicated for both prokaryotic and eukaryotic enyltransferases. Evidence for the common heritage of the plant terpene synthases comes from the similar reaction mechanism, as well as from sequence similarity, including exon and intron size and conserved sequence motifs. Phylogenetic analysis of 33 TPSs from angiosperms and gymnosperms established that the origin of TPSs occurred before the splitting off of the angiosperms. Synthases from angiosperms and gymnosperms functioning in primary metabolism are more closely related than angiosperm synthases. However, the specific functions of monoterpene, sesquiterpene, and diterpene synthases involved with secondary metabolism evolved after the divergance of the gymnosperms and the angiosperms. Another path to diversification involves enzymes that synthesize multiple products depending on protein environment. In some cases only a single product is formed, while in other cases numerous products are generated by the same synthase. For example, in grand fir, *Abies grandis*, the substrate farnesyl diphosphate (FPP) leads to an extraordinary diversity of end products when acted on by constitutive synthases such as γ-humulene synthase (three major and 52 minor sesquiterpenes) or δ-selinene synthase (three major and 34 minor sesquiterpenes). In contrast, inducible synthase enzymes such as δ-cadinene synthase and (*E*)- α-bisabolene synthase each produce a single end-product These two single-product enzymes are induced in response to herbivore damage, suggesting perhaps a general pattern of constitutive terpene synthases leading to multiple end-products, while those that are induced in response to damage have fewer end-products. Induction by wounding or by fungal elicitors may also lead to an upregulation of TPSs and prenyltransferases.

Biosynthetic Pathway for Terpenoids

The terpenoids are conveniently listed in order of increasing molecular weight. Within the monoterpenoids and sesquiterpenoids, it is usual to separate those structures with lactone substitution as iridoids (monoterpene lactones) and sesquiterpene lactones. The latter classes are particularly numerous, with well over 3000 structures. Among the diterpenoids are the gibberellins, a group of natural plant growth regulators. These have been systematically numbered from 1 to 102 in order of discovery. The best known is gibberellic acid or GA_3. The largest single class of terpenoid are the triterpenoids, with many saponins being known. Within the triterpenoids are several subclasses, described as nor triterpenoids to indicate that some degradation has occurred during the latter stages of biosynthesis, with progressive loss of four to eleven carbon atoms. Thus, there are the C_{26} limonoids, the C_{24} bufadienolides, the C_{23} cardenolides (or cardiac glycosides), and the C_{20} and C_{19} quassinoids.

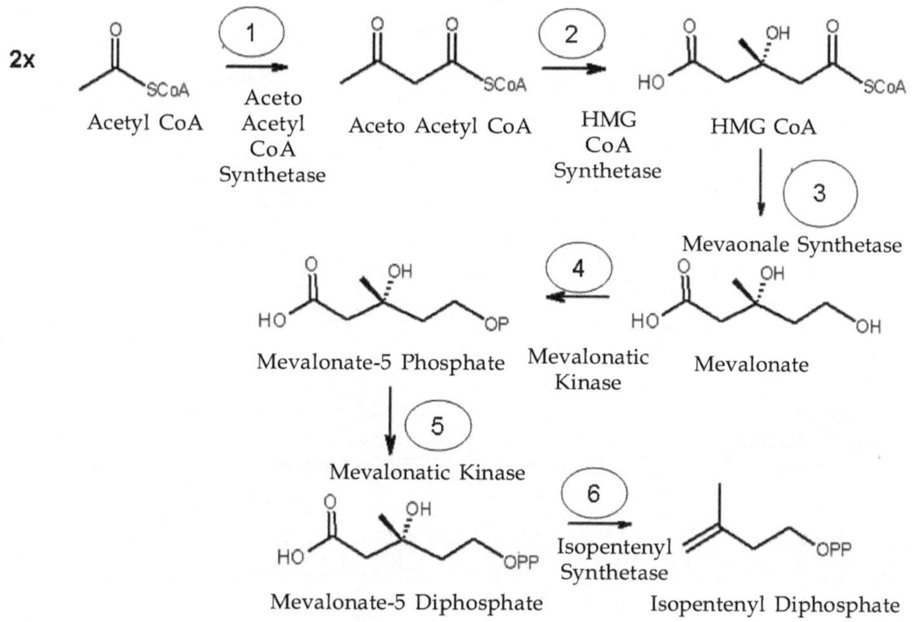

Fig. 4.2 : Biosynthetic pathways for terpenoids.

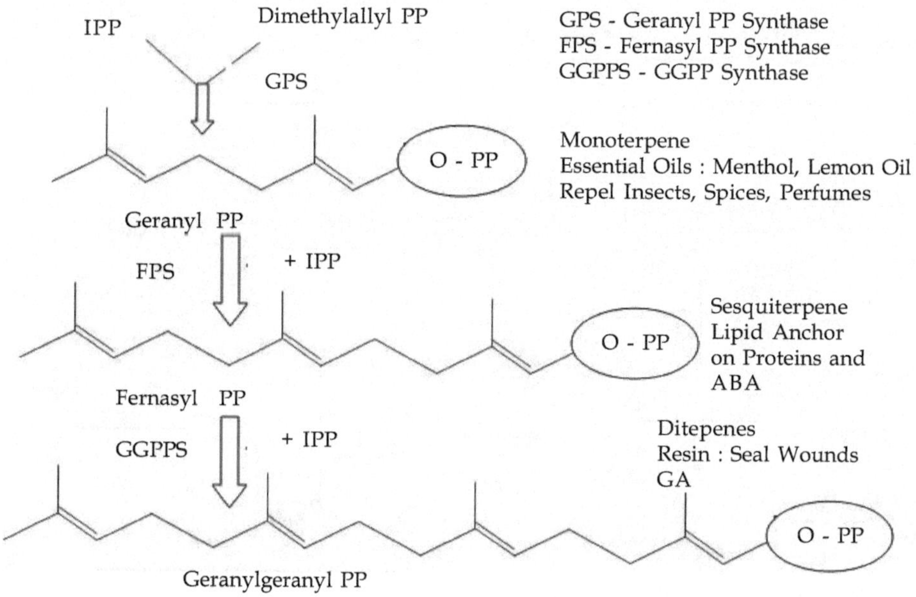

Fig 4.3 : Biosynthesis of plant growth regulator precursors.

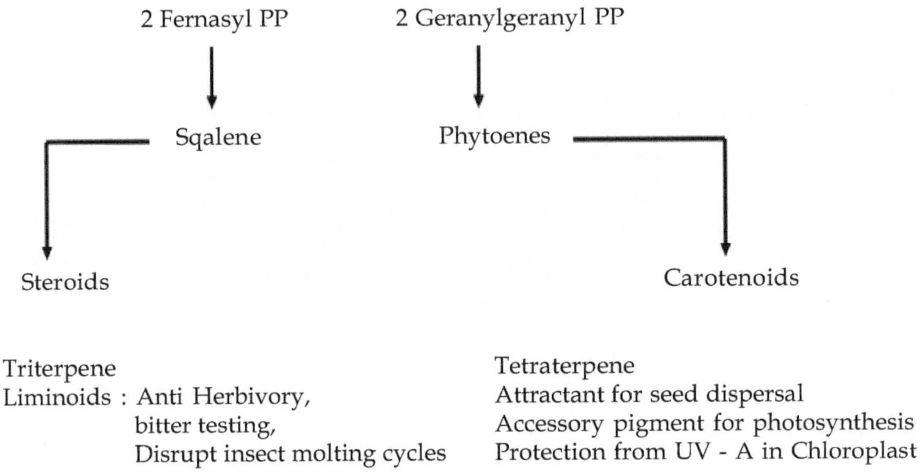

Fig 4.4 : Biosynthesis of plant volatiles in response to herbivory.

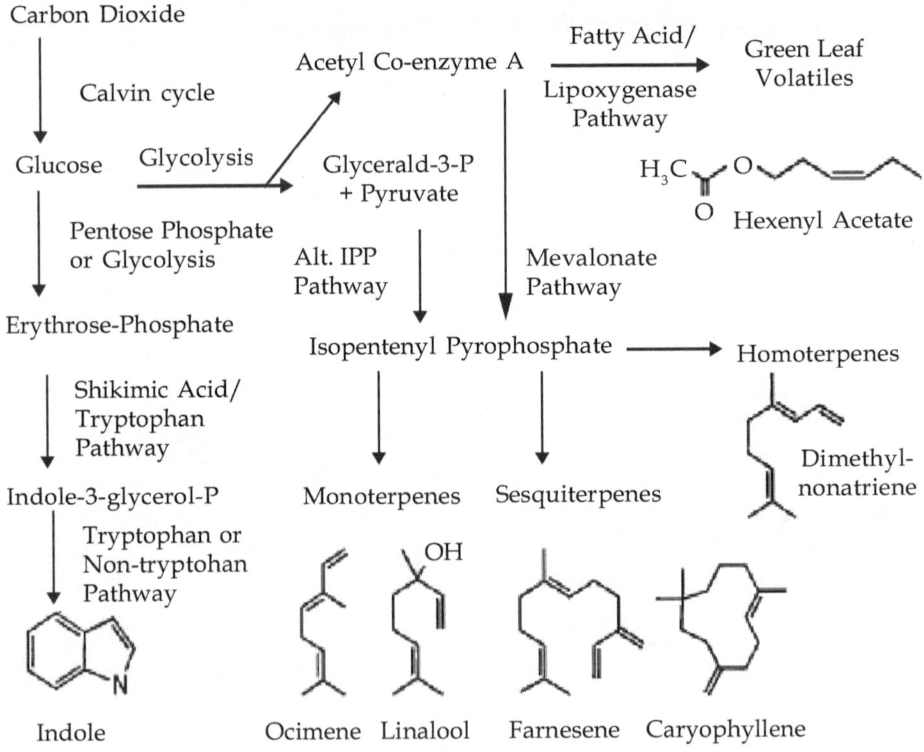

Fig 4.5 : Biosynthetic pathway of different terpenes.

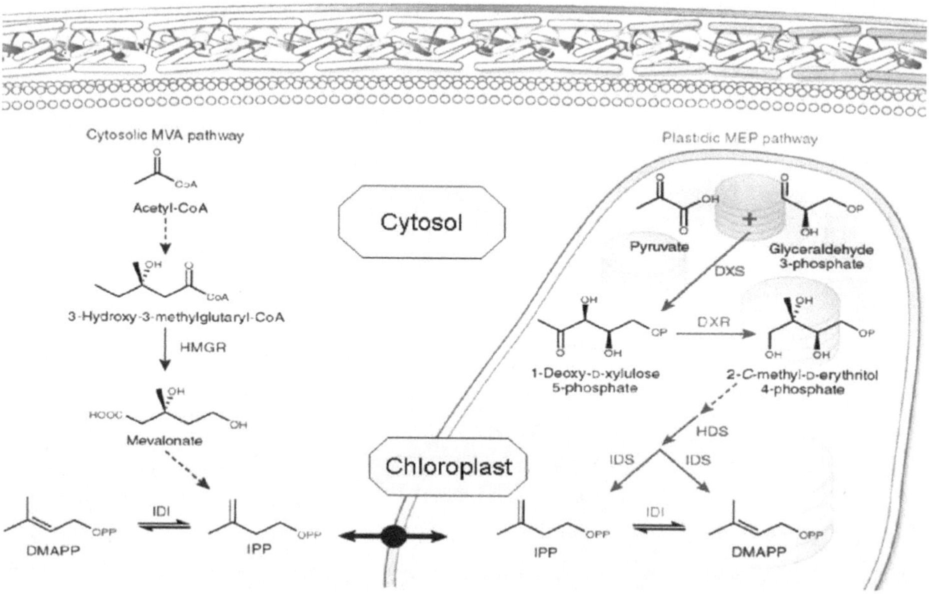

Fig 4.6 : Biosynthetic MVA and MEP pathway of different Terpenes in cytosol and chloroplast

Functions of Essential Oils Terpenoids in Plants

Functions of attractants for natural enemies of herbivores

- Activate genes responsible for the production of phytoalexins and proteinase inhibitors.
- Act as antioxidants.
- Formation of tropospheric ozone.
- Attractants for pollinators.
- Play role as growth hormone.
- Some of the oil-bearing plants are attractive to certain animals/ insects, whereas, some are repellent. This property is useful in more effective cross-pollination through insects' frequent visits.
- Some of the essential oil producing plants imparts protection against insect/animal predation. The presence of essential oils in the plant makes the plant unpalatable e.g. there is little insect/ animal damage to *Ocimum* plants because of the presence of eugenol.

- In some cases, these oils act as reserve food material.
- It also helps in sealing a wound of the plant.
- It acts as varnish (oily layer) to prevent excessive evaporation of water. They cause reversible lowering of permeability of water and water-soluble substances, thereby decreasing the transpiration in plants.
- Act as bactericidal/fungicidal agent in some cases.

Production of volatile terpenoid chemicals such as (E)-α-ocimene, 4, 8-dimethyl-1,3(E), 7-nonatriene and linalool as well as methyl salicylate produced by the plants have been found to attract the predatory mite *Phytoseilus persimilis*. The production of the volatile terpenoid chemicals by the infested plants sends out a signal through the air to the enemy of the herbivore insect (predatory mite) which senses the incoming chemical signals and directs its flight to the spot from where the chemicals are originating. Thus the plant has evolved an ingenious way of recruiting its enemy's enemy for its own protection. Similar relationships have been observed in some other herbivores and their carnivorous predators. Several different plant species, including corn (*Zea mays*) infested by caterpillars of the beet army worm *Spodoptera exigua*, take revenge on this pest by attracting the parasitoid *Cotesia marginiventris*. Cabbage plants infested by the caterpillars of the cabbage whites *Pieris brassicae* and *P. rapae* send out their 'chemical cry' to the parasitoids *Cotesia glomerata* and *C. rubecula*. In a majority of such relationships, the chemical signals transmitted through air have been found to be two of the homoterpenes, 4, 8-dimethyl- 1,3(E),7-nonatriene, and 4,8,12-trimethyl-1,3-(E), 11-tridecatetraene. In addition, (E)-α-ocimene, linalool, (E,E)-α-farnesene, and (E)- α -farnesene are also produced. It has recently been discovered that the insect oral secretion product, volicitin [N-(17-hydroxylinolenoyl)-L-glutamine] is able to induce the synthesis of volatile terpenoid chemicals in the plants. Volicitin is the product of interaction of both the plant and the herbivore insect. By using heavy isotope labelling technique it has been found that the fatty acid portion (linolenoyl moiety) of the volicitin molecule is derived from the plant, while the glutamine and 17-hydroxylation are contributed by the caterpillar. Furthermore, the induction of volatile terpenoid synthesis is linked to the jasmonate signaling system. Experiments conducted on tomato plants by spraying with jasmonic acid confirm that there occurs an increase in the production of volatiles which attract parasitoid wasps that prey upon tomato caterpillars. Therefore, jasmonic acid is able to mediate the plants' response to herbivores both directly and indirectly. The following sequence of events appears to function in the indirect defense of plants:

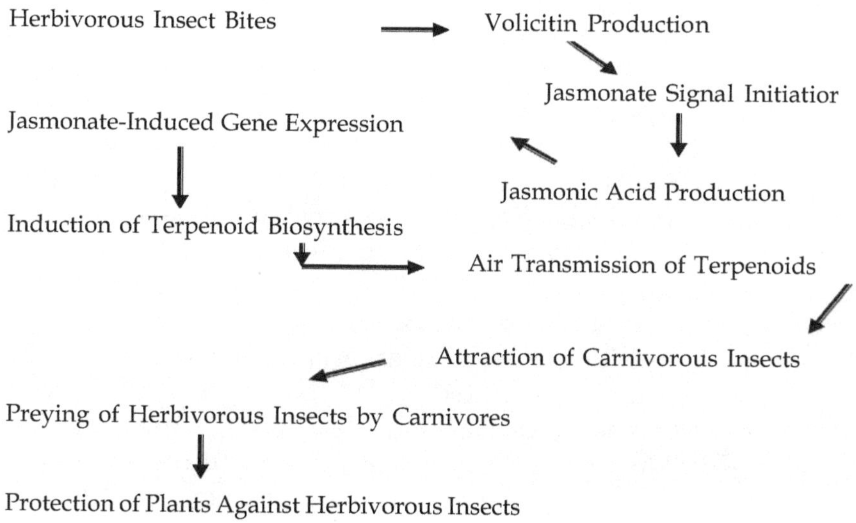

Plants have developed numerous physical (spines, thorns, tough tissues, sticky resins, and hairs) and chemical defenses that may reduce herbivory. Some of these are fixed (constitutive), whereas others are only produced (induced) when the plant is attacked. A tremendous diversity of plant biochemicals are toxic, repellent, or antinutritive for herbivores of all types. Many of these chemicals have been called **"secondary metabolites"** because roles have not been found for them in primary plant functions like growth and reproduction. Examples include alkaloids (such as caffeine and nicotine), terpenoids (terpene and pinene), glucosinolates (sinigrin), and phenolics (tannin and chlorogenic acid).

Herbivores, especially insects, have developed behavioral and biochemical mechanisms that reduce the effects of plant defenses. Plant evolution includes ongoing development of new defenses, which is thought to favor the evolution of new herbivore adaptations and promote specialisation in both plants and herbivores. This kind of reciprocal evolutionary impact is called coevolution. While all plants gain some protection from defenses, no plant escapes herbivory by at least some adapted herbivores. Plant defenses and consumer adaptation can limit consumption, and thus can determine the length and shape of **food webs**.

Terpenoid secondary metabolites occur across a wide range of plant tissue types; those serving as defensive chemicals are often secured in secretory structures. Such specialized structures minimize the risk of autotoxicity but maintain terpene concentrations at sites whose defense is crucial. In conifers, terpenoids are stored in resin ducts or lactifers under pressure, which can have a devastating impact on small herbivores. In angiosperms, glandular trichomes that contain terpenes often serve as a first line of defense against herbivores. These externally based structures enhance the effectiveness of chemical defenses because they can arrest feeding pre-emptively. In addition, pellucid glands and secretory ducts within leaves are also common. In conifers, oleoresin, a complex mixture of terpenoids that includes monoterpenes, sesquiterpenes, and diterpenes, is an important defense strategy against bark beetles and their associated fungal pathogens. There is great diversity in the manner of storage and release for this defensive blend. On one end of the continum are compounds stored in branched interconnected canals, e.g., the resin canal system of *Pinus*. Attack by an herbivore or pathogen causes very little biochemical induction of terpene synthesis in conifers with complex canal systems; the main plant response involves the transport of terpenes through the canals to the site of attack, often across several meters. At the other end of the spectrum are the simple resin cells of *Thuja* (cedar), which can be induced by attack but are normally either absent or present in very low quantities. *Abies* (true firs) have multicellular resin blisters that are less complex in *Larix*, *Picea*, and *Pseudotsuga* (larch, spruce, and Douglas fir), where the blisters are connected but also inducible. Concentrations of terpenoids are generally higher in reproductive structures and typically the highest in the foliage during and immediately following flowering. Young leaves are more important to a plant than older leaves, and the highest levels of terpenoids are found in the young organs.Variation in concentration can also vary within a tissue.

For terpenoids that are released to attract insects, specialized storage structures are far less common. These compounds are generally released as they are produced and so are maintained within plant tissues far below toxic levels. In orchids such as *Stanhopea*, *Clowesia*, and *Polycycnis*, euglossine bees are attracted to the terpene-based scent that is emitted from these structures. Specialized structures are not necessary for the establishment of spatial patterns in floral emissions. Pollen and anthers can have altogether different mixtures of volatile scents compared to the rest of the flower, and many pollen-feeding insects are adapted to discerning these scent mixtures.

Dalechampia is an excellent example of the crucial role that spatial patterns of scent emission can play in plant-insect interactions. From a phylogenetic study, determined that a triterpene resin underwent an evolutionary switch in function from a deterrent and toxin to an attractant and reward, and then back again to its deterrent role. Ancestrally, resin functioned as a defense, evenly distributed in the floral tissue. However, in a group of more derived species within the same genus, pollinated by resin-collecting bees, resin ducts are unified and positioned for optimal pollinator attraction leading to greater pollination efficiency. In the most derived species, resin ducts occur in the leaves and protect the foliage from herbivores. The chemical composition of the resins is similar in all three taxa; it is the placement of the resin responsible for defensive mechanism in plants.

Monoterpenes are chemicals that accumulate in resin ducts, secretory cavities, and epidermal glands and are considered secondary chemicals because they lack a role in basic plant processes. The specific monoterpenes present between species is highly variable, and in many cases are also different within a species due environmental conditions and herbivory pressures.

Monoterpenes have been shown to repel plant herbivores and in many cases cause herbivore death. Toxicity in some cases is due to the monoterpene vapors and not direct contact. In response, many insect plant herbivores have developed detoxifying mechanisms that allow them to feed on the plant parts containing monoterpenes. Over time this coevolutionary "arms race" has resulted in further adaptations including insect species that have adapted the use of monoterpenes as chemical cues to sense plant health. Additionally, many species of bark beetles can utilize components of the host resin to create pheromones promoting aggregation. Moreover, one copy of the gene remained conserved in structure and function. The second copy diverged to form the gene superfamily of terpene synthases involved in secondary metabolic pathways such as those that act on IPP. This is further supported by terpene synthase genomic intron/exon organization, which demonstrates that certain introns have been conserved over time. Protein-based phylogenetics and intron/exon organization also indicate that the separation between primary and secondary metabolites occurred before the separation of angiosperms and gymnosperms.

The simplest of the terpenes are the monoterpenes which consist of a ten-carbon unit. Similar to other terpenes, monoterpenes have been demonstrated to act as toxins, feeding deterrents, or oviposition deterrents to a large variety of insects. Thus it has been hypothesized that they play an important role in herbivore deterrence. A well-studied example is the pyrethroids, that are monoterpene esters, found in certain *Chrysanthemum* species leaves and flowers. The toxin causes disturbance in the nervous system and leads to paralysis. A study performed demonstrated that vapours from monoterpenes also cause mortality. They exposed the fir engraver, *Scolytus ventralis* LeConte, to various monoterpenes found in quantities similar to their host grand fir, *Abies grandis* (Douglas) Lindley. They were careful that the monoterpenes did not come in contact with the beetle. Results showed that all monoterpene vapours were toxic at both levels tested and some compounds were more toxic than others. In the laboratory, the beetle can be observed retreating from resin flow. Furthermore, monoterpenes slowed the growth of the beetle-fungal symbiont, *Trichosporium symbioticum* Wright, that is also responsible for tree death. These results indicate that monoterpenes play a major role in plant defense.

Attack behavior by tiger moth larvae, *Halisdota ingens* Hy. Edwards, also indicates a monoterpene role in plant defense. The tiger moth larvae feeds on ponderosa pine needles and consumes 1/2-2/3 of the needle, but not the base. Analysis revealed that a concentration and diversity of monoterpenes is greatest at the base of the needle, indicating that foraging may be reduced by increases in monoterpenes. However, authors caution that plant morphology may also play a role in moth feeding behavior. Tiger moth larvae also have been shown to induce secondary monoterpene production. Induction of monoterpene production by moth larvae was two- fold higher than just mechanically wounding the plant and large increases in monoterpene volatilization were observed. Recently, herbivory by the white pine weevil, *Pissodes strobi* Peck., has been shown to directly induce gene expression in Sitka spruce, *Picea* sitchensis [Bong.] Carriere. By subjecting branches to weevil attack and then harvesting and extracting RNA a two- fold increase in the monoterpene synthase gene transcripts was observed.

This evidence demonstrates a direct link between herbivory and monoterpene production. Although the mechanisms are not always the same, these studies suggest that monoterpenes can affect insect herbivores.

Variation in conifer monoterpenes not only do plants contain and produce monoterpenes for plant defense, the composition of monoterpenes has also been shown to vary in relation to insect herbivory and in response to stresses such as drought or fire. The composition of monoterpenes seems to affect the trees ability to resist insect attack. A study determined that Douglas-fir, *Pseudotsuga menziesii* var. *glauca* (Beisn.) Franco, trees differ in their resistance ability. Douglas- fir trees were found to produce different levels of terpenes and these levels conferred different levels of resistance to western spruce budworm, *Choristoneura occidentalis* Freeman. Trees that were resistant in the first year of the study were retested the second year and most remained resistant, even though the terpenes that conferred the resistance changed between years. The most important components that conferred resistance were the individual terpenoid, the acetate fraction, and the terpene evenness. This study also determined that the trees that were susceptible remained susceptible in following years and were not able to switch to resistant modes. Interestingly, preliminary data seemed to indicate that induction of secondary metabolites in Douglas- fir did not take place. Mechanical injury did not produce long-term induction of terpene production.

Studies on Scotch pine trees, *Pinus sylvestris* L., of resistant and susceptible varieties were exposed to herbivory by the Zimmerman pine moth, *Dioryctria zimmermani* (Grote), and monoterpene responses were measured. The presence of wounding did not change the proportion or ratio of monoterpenes of each variety. This is consistent with many previous studies that demonstrate that mechanical wounding does not change the monoterpene composition. However, the monoterpene composition varied significantly among varieties. Limonene was the only monoterpene that was consistently higher in both resistant varieties. Limonene acts as an oviposition stimulant for at least three members of the pine moth genera. However, for many other herbivores limonene acts as an oviposition deterrent and is toxic to many herbivore species. Therefore, the authors suggest that it may confer resistance against other herbivorous species than the pine moth. Even though many studies have shown a lack of induced secondary monoterpenes in conifers, there are some studies that do demonstrate a change of terpene composition in response to herbivory. Monoterpene content in *Pinus caribaea* Morelet needles was found to change after attack by *Atta laevigata* (Smith), leafcutter ants. Newly defoliated pines differed from undefoliated pines in both an increase and decrease of some monoterpenes. Furthermore, four months after defoliation the increases and decreases of monoterpene concentrations were greater than after the initial defoliation. This change was accompanied by the observation that no further signs of defoliation were present after the initial defoliation event. In this system it is possible that changes in terpenes are a direct defense mechanism.

Based on the evidence that differences in monoterpenes affect herbivore survival, studies began to examine if herbivores are a selective force on the evolution of monoterpene concentrations. Evidence provided suggests that western pine beetle, *Dendroctonus brevicomis* LeConte, predation has caused variation in ponderosa pine, *Pinus ponderosa* Laws., xylem resin. For example limonene, which is toxic to the pine beetle and its fungal symbionts, was found in higher concentrations in areas where pine beetle predation was continuous. Additionally, higher proportions of myrcene (needed for beetle pheromone production) and beta-pinene (the least toxic terpene) were found in populations with more destructive beetle damage. However, evidence that herbivores are not a selective force on the evolution of monoterpene concentrations. By examining cone production, resin flow rate, monoterpene composition, and herbivory with multiple regression analysis, they found that resin characteristics were not correlated with herbivory attack. Instead, the pattern between resin characteristics and fitness components suggest that other factors than herbivory are causing the association.

Other factors in addition too herbivory are also known to change plant resin composition. Water stress is one of these important factors that has been studied well. Water stress in trees reduces the resin exudation pressure and thus the rate of resin flow is lowered. Many hypothesized that this event renders the tree more susceptible to herbivores. Therefore, drought stressed trees should produce more constitutive defenses. This is also in support of the carbon-nutrient balance hypothesis that states that excess carbon not used for growth is allocated for defense. Constitutive defenses were measured after exposing Scots pine, and Norway spruce, *Picea abies* (L.) Karst., to medium and severe drought stress for two growing seasons. Concentrations of total monoterpenes and resin acids were significantly higher in the severely drought stressed trees. More specifically drought increased the concentrations of abietane-type resin acids, which are known to be strongly toxic to wood rotting fungi. Studies on loblolly pine, *Pinus taeda* L., have also demonstrated an increase monoterpenes in response to drought stress. A more recent study determined that constitutive resin flow was least during periods of rapid tree growth and most under drought conditions. However, not all plant systems fit these exact patterns. Constitutive defenses in ponderosa pine increased not only in the water stressed plants, but also in the artificially watered plants as compared to the controls (non-watered, non-stressed). Changes in constitutive defenses of water stressed loblolly pines also demonstrated an increase in some monoterpenes and a decrease in others.

In addition to constitutive defenses, inducible defenses also play a major role in herbivore resistance. Significant changes in inducible defenses under drought conditions have been shown to exist in several conifers. Inducible defenses in drought stressed Scots pine exposed to bark beetle-associated fungus were measured two weeks after the exposure to the pathogen. Inducible defenses, including the length and resin quantity, were significantly less in drought stressed trees, similar results in drought stressed ponderosa pine seedlings that produced significantly lower levels of phenols, needle nitrogen, and tannins than non-stressed seedlings. These finding support theories that stressed plants are unable to produce the level of inducible plant defense that un-stressed plants can produce. Thus, the previously discussed increase in constitutive defenses in water stressed plants serves an important role to compensate for the reduction in inducible defenses. Fire is another factor know to change plant resin composition, but has been studied far less. Measurements of resin flow on red pines, *Pinus resinosa* Ait., following a prescribed burn showed a significant increase in resin flow. Other conifers that are a subject to frequent fires also exhibit an increase in resin flow. The response of increased resin flow after a fire may be an evolved defensive response due to the increased probability of attack by some bark beetles. Alternatively, the response could be due to the wounding by the fire. Further studies of plant species, historically exposed and not exposed to fire, need to be performed to demonstrate the actual defensive mechanisms.

Many insect herbivores have evolved mechanisms to detoxify toxins they encounter. Herbivores can convert toxins into less toxic chemical compounds, sequester the toxin for its own defense or in some cases secrete the chemical compound. For instance, the weevil, *Oxyops vitiosa* (Pascoe), produces a secretion of terpenoids from its host *Melaleuca quinquenervia* (Cav.). This secretion covers the larval integument and provides defense from generalist predators. A common example of detoxification is in the Lepidopteran family. Larvae contain cytochrome P-450-dependent oxygenases in their guts and are able to convert monoterpenes to more polar metabolites that allows conjugation and excretion. In many cases cytochrome P-450 oxygenase activity is present in low levels, but is induced by ingestion of monoterpenes. Bark beetles in the family Scolytidae and the interaction with their host trees have been studied in detail due to their destructive capacity to bore into trees. Along with their symbiotic fungi, the beetles feed on the cambium of the tree and oviposit under the bark, but it is not clear if bark beetles detoxify the resin they encounter when attacking a tree. It is clear that they use monoterpenes in chemical host location and selection. Beetles in a certain area will converge upon newly exposed resin. Bark beetles use olfactory, gustatory, and visual signals to locate a suitable host. Once they locate a host, they may begin boring or decide the tree is unsuitable and take flight in search of another host. While the bark beetle is boring into the tree, it may encounter a resin duct and if the resin flow is strong enough the insect will be overcome by the resin and die. This process called "pitching-out" is one of the most important defenses a tree has against bark beetles. Once a suitable host tree is located, the bark beetle will produce an aggregation pheromone. The aggregation of many beetles over comes the trees defenses and allows successful colonization. Aggregation pheromones are usually derivatives of monoterpenes. cis-Verbenol, (+)- ipsdienol and (-)-ipsdienol were the first scolytid aggregation pheromones identified from *Ips paraconfusus* Lanier. *I. paraconfusus* converts the acyclic monoterpene myrcene to either (+) or (-) enantiomer of ipsdienol. In this species (+)- ipsdienol elicits an aggregation response. Interestingly, (-)-ipsdienol elicits the opposite response and signals that the tree has sufficient numbers of individuals and directs colonization towards adjacent trees. Monoterpene pheromones are also important as sex attractants. This indicates that beetles many have evolved the use of tree defensive compounds into a sophisticated communication system. Until recently the common belief was that free- living fungal symbionts and beetle gut bacteria converted tree monoterpenes such as alpha-pinene and myrcene to the corresponding pheromones. Studies showed the conversion of labeled monoterpenoid precursors to the corresponding pheromones .

However, a study clearly supports the recent findings of de novo synthesis of ipsdienol and ipsenol. They report the first known monoterpene synthase activity in animals found in the bark beetle *Ips pini* (Say). Furthermore, they reject that the monoterpene synthase enzyme activity is sequestered from the host tree. A biosynthetic pathway is proposed in which the insect is able to synthesize ipdienol and ipsenol via a mevalonate pathway similar to the pathway previously described in plants. Because the pathways arose through independent functional evolution in plants and animals, they expect further work to reveal that the synthases from plants will be substantially different than those found in animals. This research has exciting implications including the possibilities that other insects possess similar enzymes capable of synthesizing their own pheromones de novo.

Many other insects besides bark beetles respond to monoterpenes emitted from trees. The beetle family *Cerambycidae,* known as longhorned woodborers are attracted to dead or dying trees. Trees that have been stressed by events such as fire or logging will emit volatile monoterpenes. *Monochamus carolinensis* (Oliver) and *M. titillator* (F.) both responded terpentine solution distilled from mixed resins of slash and longleaf pines. More specifically, *M. alternatus* Hope demonstrated a strong attractiveness to alpha-pinene, beta-pinene and beta-phellandrene, which are monoterpenes components of pine trees Several other herbivores such as weevils, are also attracted to monoterpenes emitted from trees. Lastly, monoterpenes emitted from trees not only attract herbivores to the trees, but also attract insect herbivore predators. Induced plant volatiles are known to attract parasitoid wasps and predatory mites. Simple oxygenated monoterpenes produce longrange attraction of predators such as clerid beetles or *Rhizophagus* predator beetles. The attraction of predators demonstrates the complexity of plant-herbivorepredator systems. Until recently experiments examining the tree-beetle-fungus-predator/parasitoid association and the biochemistry of resin formation in conifers have largely been neglected. This neglect is probably due to the vast scope of the topic. The examples presented in this review article clearly demonstrate many interactions take place between herbivores, environmental conditions and plant resin formation. Furthermore, the plant resin formation plays a direct role in host selection and predator attraction. By understanding these interactions exciting possibilities exist for genetic manipulation of resin composition. For example, it may be possible to increase the levels of resin compounds toxic to invaders by recombinant DNA methods. Whatever the outcome, future studies will no doubt bring a better understanding to the mechanisms of resin production and regulation that confer susceptibility and resistance in conifers.

Mode of Action of Terpenoids

When wounding occurs due to secretion of volicitins from insects, a signal is generated, which subsequently activates the genes responsible for the production of volatile Terpenoids (Fig.4.8 & 4.9). These terpenoids are released from the leaf and they contain characteristic odors which attract the natural enemies of insects such as parasitic wasps. Study on emission of volatile terpenoids in response to weevil in Sitka spruce revealed that terpenoids emission is higher in infected plants than in normal plants.

Wounding also activates the wound induced protein kinase (WIPK), a gene due to presence of terpenoids, the protein produced due to gene WIPK gene play significant role in the defense mechanism against biotic stress. It was found that various terpenoids are inducers of WIPK gene activation. It is observed that (11E, 13E)-labda-11, 13-diene-8, 15-diol, a diterpene, termed as WAF-1 (WIPK activating factor), which is responsible for activation of WIPK gene in tobacco plant against TMV. The diameter of lesion decreases with increasing concentration of WAF-1.

The study related to emission of sesquiterpenes in control plant and in damaged plant, suggested that very little amount of terpenoids are secreted in control plants but in damaged plant there is an increase in the rate of sesquiterpenes emission. ATP binding cassette transporter (ABC transporter) is a protein, having molecular weight 160 kD, which plays an important role in plant defense. The effect of antifungal terpenoid found in the plant which can induce the production of ABC transporter. The monoterpene concentration in conifer plants after attack of Bark beetles increase the concentration of monoterpene and mortality rate of Bark beetles.

It is observed that terpenoids play a major role as antioxidants. Major antioxidants found in the plants are β – carotene, α – tocopherol, zeaxanthine, carnosic acid etc. Carnosic acid, a diterpene, in mediterranean plants during water stress has an important role.

Concentration of unoxidized carnosic acid is decreased significantly with decrease in relative water content of the sage plant, which supports that during water stress carnosic acid plays a major role as antioxidants in sage plant. Various terpenes in the orchid *Ophrys sphegodes* serve as attractants for pollinators. The role of terpenoids at tissue, leaf surface, ecosystem and atmospheric level as a protectant of plant has also been established.

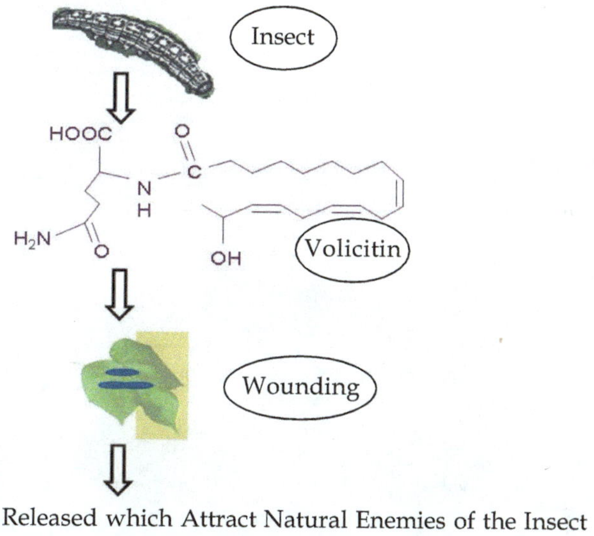

Fig 4.8 : Systemic volicitin induced volatile emission.

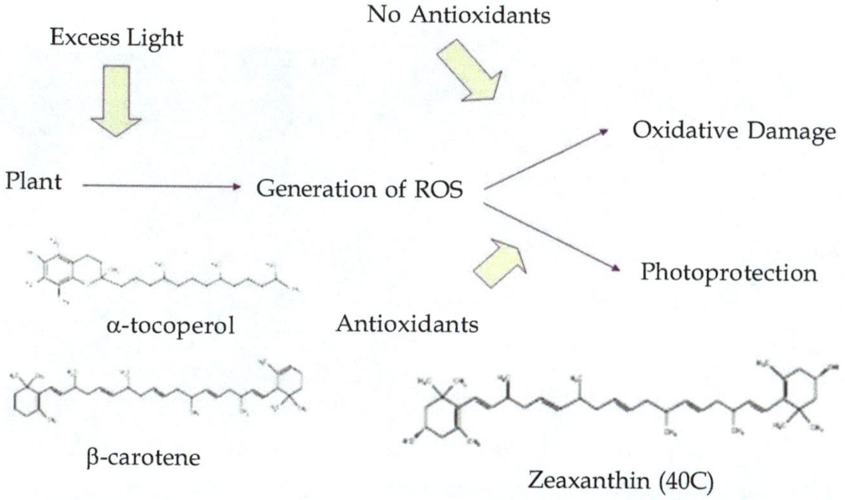

Fig. 4.9 : Role of Terpenoids as an Antioxidant in Rosemary and sage.

Table 4.3 : Diverse plant species producing terpenoids in response to herbivory

Plant	(E)-β-Ocimine	Linalool	(E)-4,8-Dimethyl-1,3,7-Nonatriene	(E,E)-α-Fernesene	(E)-β-Fernesene	(E,E)-4,8,12-Trimethyl-1,3,7,11-Trideca-teraene
Cucumber	+	-	+	+	-	+
Apple	+	-	+	+	-	+
Lima bean	+	+	+	-	+	+
Cotton	+	+	+	+	+	+
Corn	+	+	+	+	+	+
Tobacco	+	+	-	+	+	-
Potato	+	+	-	+	+	-

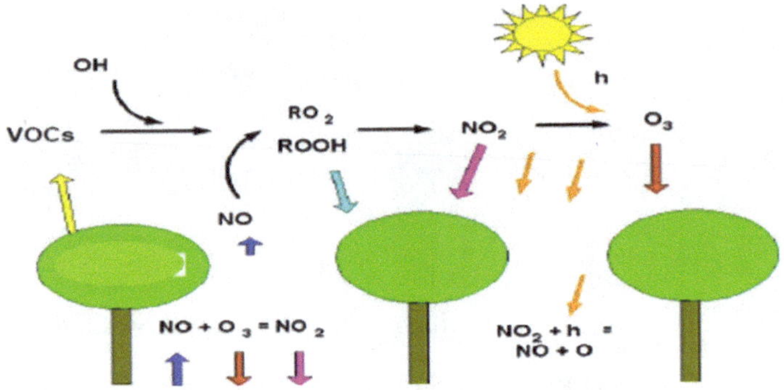

Fig. 4.10 : Formation of Tropospheric Ozone.

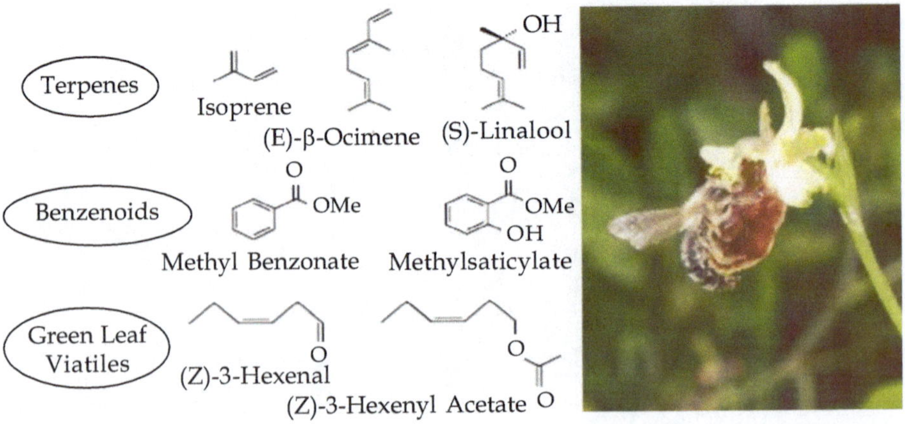

Fig 4.11 : A Flower of the Orchid *Ophrys sphegodes* with its pollinator, A male of the solitary bee species *Andrena nigroaenea*.

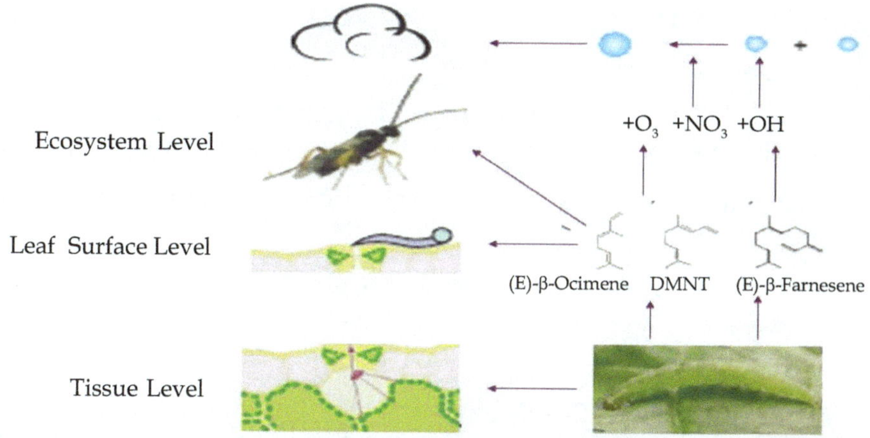

Fig 4.12 : Role of terpenoids at tissue, leaf surface, ecosystem and at atmospheric level.

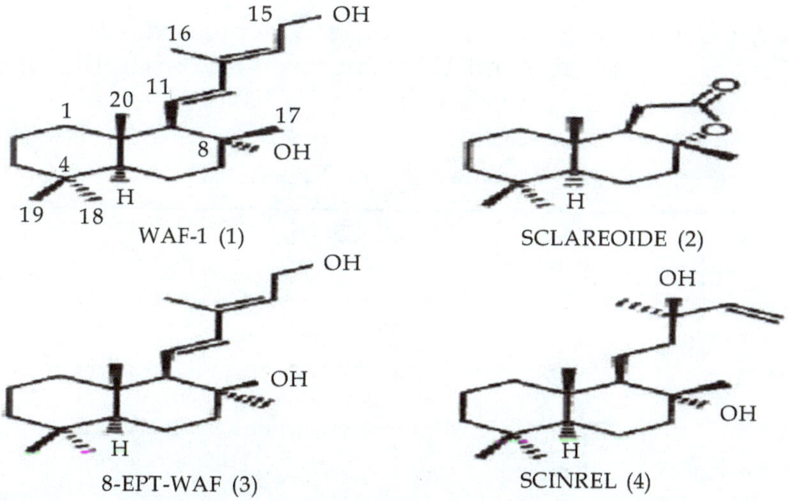

Fig. 4.13 : Structure of wound induced protein kinase activating factor.

Factor Affecting Terpenoids Concentration

Nitrogen availability, abiotic factors such as heat and light, methyl jasmonate, coculture system, inhibitors, arichidonic acid and developmental stages are various factors which affect terpenoid concentration in plants. In low nitrogen availability emission of volicitin induced sesquiterpenes is the highest. Terpenoids concentration increases with increase in concentration of methyl jasmonate. Co-culture system of plant and fungi can stimulate higher metabolic accumulation of terpenoids in plant than normal plants.

Medicinal Uses

1. Terpenes act as mild irritant.
2. It acts as bactericidal and fungicidal agent used in the preparation of ointments.
3. Volatile oils are employed for the treatment of urogenital infections.
4. It stimulates repair of tissues and assist in the removal of mucous from trachea or bronchia. Relieves the tension of the stomach and colon.
5. It acts as anthelmintic (Anti-worms) agent. e.g. Chenopodium oil is used to remove round-worms, hook-worms and intestinal amoebas (santonine which is sesqui-terpene used for this purpose).
6. When the action of heart muscle is depressed, camphor may improve cardiac conditions and remove arrhythmia (Any deviation from the normal rhythm of heart).

Table 4.4 : Medicinal uses of some common Terpenoids.

Terpenoids	Major Source	Medicinal Use
Lycopene	Tomato	Skin Protection, Reduce LDL cholesterol levels, Anti - carcinogenic
Beta Carotene	Sweet potato	Boost the activity of natural killer immune cells Stimulate DNA repair enzymes Cornea protection against UV light
Alpha Carotene	Pumpkin	Anti - carcinogenic Enhance release of immunogenic cytokines
Lutein	Corn	Protects the eye from macular degeneration and cataracts protect against colon cancer
Zeaxanthin	Corn	Protects the eye from macular degeneration and cataracts
Astaxanthin	Salmon	Antioxidants Boosts T - Cell production
Perillyl Alcohol	Cherries	Anti - Carcinogenic
Saponins	Chickpeas	Removes cholesterols Effective against colon cancer
Terpeneol	Carrot	Cause cell cycle arrest in cancer cells
Limonene	Peel	Anti - carcinogenic

2. Straight Chain Hydrocarbons and their Oxygen Derivatives

These essential oils of hydro carbons from n- haptane; which forms 90 % of oil of *Pinus sabiniana* and *Pinus jeffreyi* to compounds with 15 - 35 carbon atoms. The higher paraffin-like material may be crystallise during cooling and storage are called 'stereoptenes'. The alcohols, aldehyde and ketones are quite often contained in the low boiling fractions of the volatile oils. The typical example is leaf alcohol (cis or trans - hexen- 3 ol-1).

$$CH_3 - CH_2 - CH = CH - CH_2 - CH_2 - OH$$

This alcohol is responsible for the odour of grasses, green leaves etc.

In this group, there are also included many fatty acids which occur free or esterified with alcohol with different degree of saturation. They are present in the volatile oils of fruits.

3. Benzene Derivatives

The third major group comprise a number of flavour and perfume constituents derived from benzene specifically from n - propyl benzene. The aromatic ring may carry hydroxy, methoxy and methylene dioxy groups; the propyl side chain may contain hydroxyl or carboxyl group. e.g. Coumarin.

Structure of Coumarin

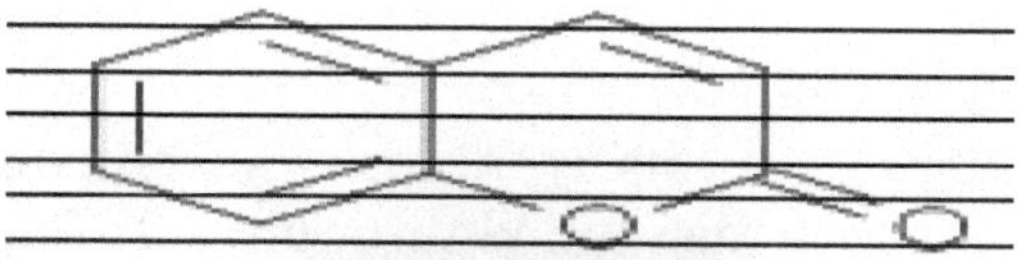

Coumarin

Many members of this group are related through chemical reaction. On isomerisation, eugenol can be converted to Vanillin, the flavouring principle of Vanilla bean.

Isomerisation of Eugenol to Vannilin

The propyl benzene derivatives take part in the synthesis of plant pigments such as anthocyanins and flavones. In view of their structural similarity, straight chain hydrocarbons are generally considered connected with fatty acid metabolism, while benzene and propyl benzene derivatives are connected with carbohydrate metabolism.

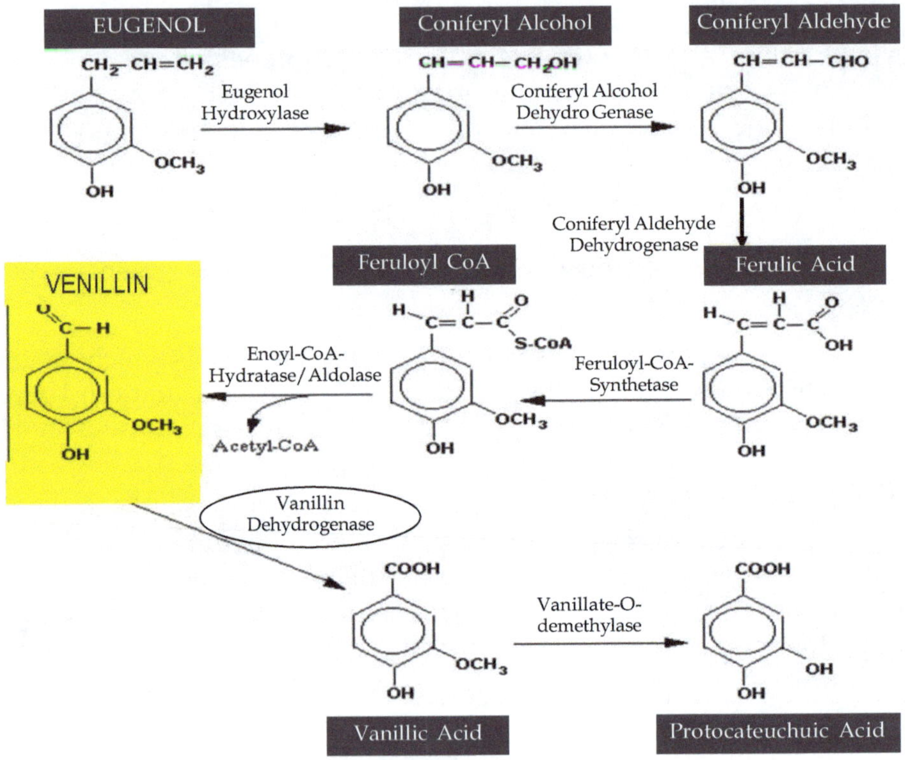

4. Miscellaneous Group

The representatives of this group are the compounds, which are not included in the above mentioned three groups. They are incidental and often rather specific for a few spp. or genera of the plants.

1. Allyl isothiocyanate : $CH_2 = CH - CH_2 - N = C = S$
   Mustard Oil
2. Di-allyl sulphide : $CH_2 = CH - CH_2 - S - CH_2 - CH = CH_2$
   Oil of Garlic
3. Butyl propenyl di-sulphide : $CH_3 - CH_2 - CH - S - S - CH = CH - CH_3$ - Asafoetida
   CH_3

- Allicin compound obtained from garlic.
- Antibacterial and anti-fungal properties that protect garlic from pathogens. Allicin is also the chemical constituent primarily responsible for the hot, burning flavor of fresh garlic.

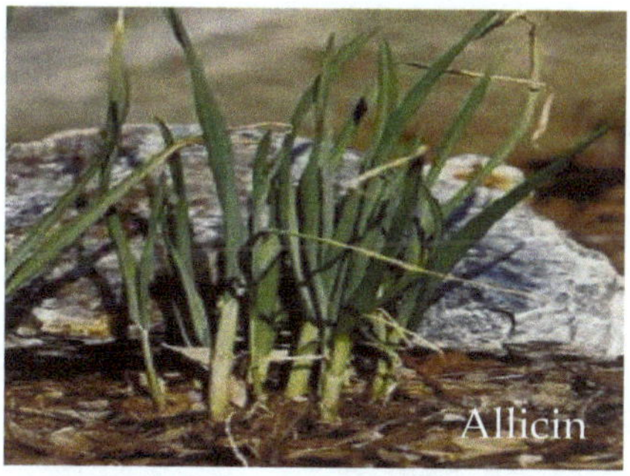

- Allicin is not present in garlic in its natural state. When garlic is chopped or otherwise damaged, the enzyme alliinase acts on the chemical alliin converting it into allicin.

Allicin is an amino acid that does not build proteins. Alliinase has been demonstrated to be irreversibly deactivated below a pH of 3; as such, allicin is generally not produced in the body from consumed fresh or powdered garlic.In light of this, Allicin is considered to be of very limited value as an oral antibiotic due to poor bioavailability.

5. Indole: Structure

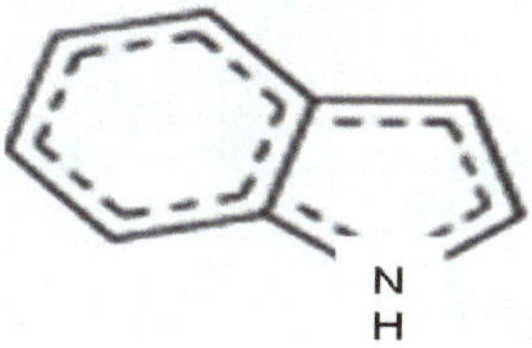

6. Methyl Anthranilate

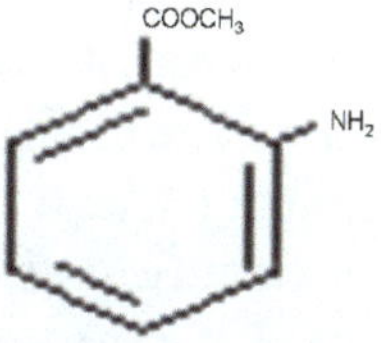

Note : No. (5) and (6) are pleasant smelling principle of orange blossom and jasmine flavour respectively.

It is clear even from this brief information of terpenoids that the evolution of function in secondary metabolites is both a complex and potentially rewarding field of study. The possibility that evolution of function can occur through insect adaptation allows for much faster and more complicated evolutionary changes in function than if changes only in plants were involved with all changes in function. Because of the myriad roles that terpenes play and the apparent speed with which those roles can change, understanding the regulation of the evolution of function is of great importance both in predicting how natural and agricultural systems will respond to large-scale environmental changes and how deliberate attempts to alter plant physiology and behaviour through genetic manipulations are likely to affect both plants and their pests.

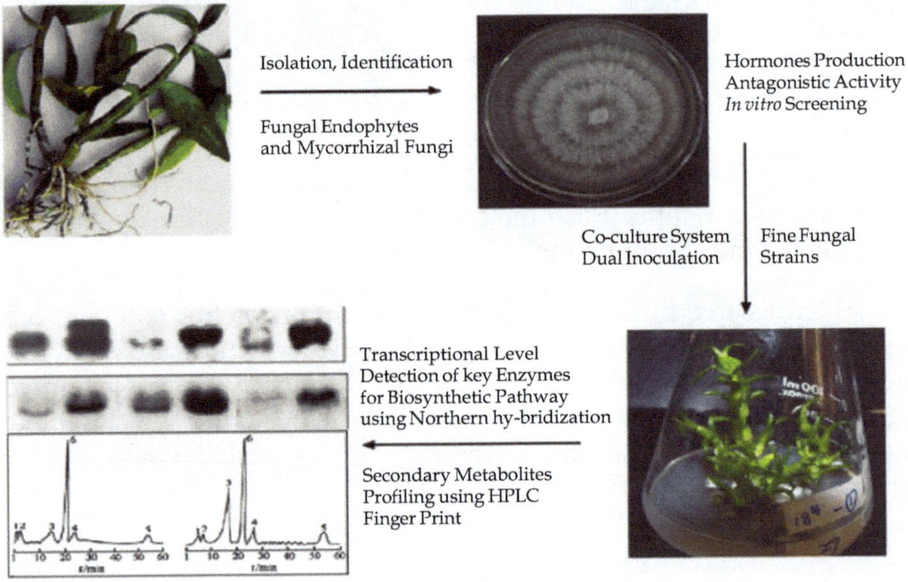

Fig 4.14 : Co culture system for secondary metabolite accumulation.

In addition, understanding the regulation of terpene (and other secondary metabolite) production opens up the possibility of manipulating the timing of gene expression and, thus, the evolution of novel function without changing the basic chemical signature of the plant. Of course, such efforts must also take into account that terpenes, as noted at the beginning of this article, play key roles in primary as well as secondary metabolism. Regulation of terpenoid metabolism, especially regulatory factors controlling enzyme genes of secondary metabolism, requires further investigation. Engineered or mutant plants with altered rates of Induced Volatile Organic Compounds (IVOCs) emission and composition will be the tools of the future to increase our understanding of the ecological impacts of IVOCs. As the largest group of natural products terpenoid provides a rich pool for exploring drug and lead compounds.

Chapter 5

Alkaloids

The alkaloids represent yet another large group of secondary plant products. Many, but not all, exhibit important pharmacological properties & some of these have been known for hundred of years. For e.g. Cinchona alkaloids, present in bark of *Cinchona* spp. have quinine as their main constituent, has been known since 1639 as an effective antimalarial agent.

An alkaloid contains nitrogen, frequently as a part of a heterocyclic ring, and most are as the general name implies, basic. Alkaloids are the naturally occurring basic, nitrogenous, organic, heterocyclic ring compounds mostly of plant origin with physiological and pharmacological properties. At present, the definition is much more pragmatic and includes all nitrogen containing natural products which are not otherwise classified as peptides, amines, non-protein amino acids, cyanogenic glycosides, glucosinolates, cofactors, phytohormones or primary metabolites (such as purines and pyrimidines bases). Even a number of antibiotics produced by bacteria or fungi are therefore included as alkaloids. Alkaloids evolved early in evolution and were already present (200 million years ago) when the angiosperms began to radiate. Today, more than 12,000 alkaloids are known to occur from more than 4000 species of Angiosperms. Ladenberg defined alkaloid as :

"Naturally occurring basic, complex, nitrogenous organic, heterocyclic ring compound of plant origin with physiological and pharmacological properties."

Occurrence

Around 5000 alkaloids of all types have been known to occur in 15% of land plants & in more than 150 families. Alkaloids are found in vascular plants. They rarely occur in *Cryptogram, gymnosperms* or mono cotyledons. They occur abundantly in di-cotyledons, *Apocynaceae, Papaveraceae, Papilonaceae, Rubiaceae,Rutaceae, Liliaceae Solanaceae,* etc. families & less common in lower plants & fungi (ergot alkaloids). *Papaveraceae* is an unusual family that all its members contain alkaloids. A few alkaloids also occur as glycosides of sugar (eg. glucose, rhamnose, galactose) e.g. alkaloids of solanum group (solanine), as amides (piperine) and as esters (atropine, cocaine) of organic acids. Alkaloids are not unique to plants. They have been isolated from numerous animal sources. Alkaloids have now been isolated from such diverse organisms as frogs, ants (pheromones), butterflies (defense), marine bacteria, sponges, fungi, spiders (venom neurotoxin), beetles (defense), and mammals, although is not yet clear whether de novo alkaloid biosynthesis occurs in each organism.

They are present in vacuoles and so do not appear in young cells until vacuolation occurs. They rarely occur in dead tissue; even in Cinchona bark, which can contain up to 12% (w/w) of alkaloids, they are present only in the parenchyma. Alkaloids are frequently stored in tissues other than their site of synthesis. The best known of this is nicotine which is synthesized in the roots of tobacco plants but is translocated to the leaves where it is stored. Secondary structural modifications often occur at sites other than that where primary synthesis took place, e.g. the basic ring system of tropane alkaloids is assembled in the roots of Datura spp. & transported to the leaves where it undergoes considerable modification. They are isolated from roots, leaves, bark of the stem or seeds of the plants. In leaves of some plants, it constitutes 0.5 to 8.0 % of dry weight. They are stored in the vacuoles or in the cytoplasm in the solid form. Their quantity depends upon the age of plant, cultivation, type of growing, place of growing and climate. Alkaloids are basic in character so they exist as salts of plant acids like oxalic, citric, malic, lactic, tannic, acetic acid etc. Most alkaloids occur in combined form with other compound however, glycosides, amides occur free (Table 5.1).

Table 5.1 : General Distribution of Alkaloids

Thallophyta	Absent except in some fungi
Bryophyta	Absent
Pteridophyta	Limited distribution e.g. *Equisetum, Lycopodium*
Spermatophyta	Limited distribution
Gymnosperms	Limited distribution
Angiosperms	
a) Monocotyledons:	Mainly in *Gramineae* & *Liliaceae*
b) Dicotyledons: mainly in	*Rubiaceae* e.g. coffee
	Papaveraceae e.g. poppy
	Solanaceae e.g. tobacco
	Leguminosae e.g. pea, bean
	Apocynaceae e.g. dogbane
	Fumariaceae
	To a lesser extent in:
	Rosaceae e.g. rose, compositae e.g. aster
	Labiatae e.g. mint
Salamandarine	Skin of salamander
Steroidal alkaloids	Frogs
Dialkylpiperidine and dialkylpyrazines	Ants
Ergot alkaloids	Fungi (*Claviceps purpurea*)

Biosynthesis

Alkaloids are a group of nitrogen-containing bases. Most of them are drugs. Only a few (like caffeine) are derived from purines or pyrimidines, while the large majority is produced from amino acids. Amino acids are the primary sources of alkaloids biosynthesis for many organisms. Most of the true alkaloids are derived from amino acids. L Lysine, ornithine, L aspartic acid, tyrosine, tryptophan and phenylalanine are the major precursor amino acids. These alkaloids are synthesized in the cytoplasm. Quinolizidine type alkaloids are synthesized in chloroplast stroma. Few alkaloids are formed ubiquitously in all plant organs, an organ or even tissue specific formation seems to be more common. Alkaloids are not formed in the extracellular spaces nor in the vacuole. Pseudoalkaloids are derived from steroids. Most recently, the first gene encoding enzymes of alkaloid biosynthesis have been isolated and cloned. In spite of their large number and great diversity of structure, it is possible to draw a few general principles applicable to the biosynthesis of many different alkaloids. The fundamental skeletons of alkaloids are derived from common acids and other small biological molecules. A few simple types of reactions suffice to form complex structures from these starting materials.

Major type of alkaloids, their amino acid precursors and examples

Alkaloid Class	Structure	Precursor	Example
Pyrrolidine	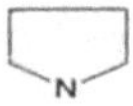	Ornithine	Nicotine
Tropane		Ornithine	Atropine, cocaine
Piperidine	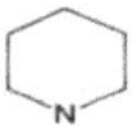	Lysine (or acetate)	Coniine
Pyrrolizidine	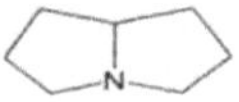	Ornithine	Retrosine
Quinolizidine	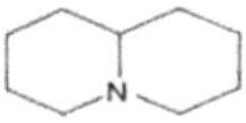	Lysine	Lupinine
Isoquinoline	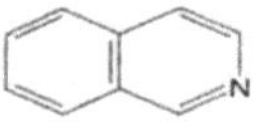	Tyrosine	Codeine, Morphine
Indole	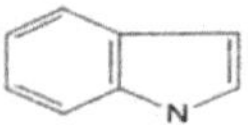	Tryptophan	Psiiocybin, Reserpine, Strychnine

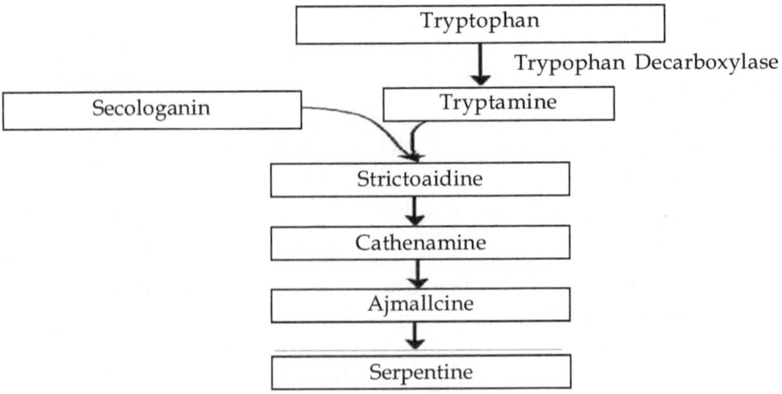

Fig. 5.1 : Key steps in the biosynthesis of Indole alkaloids in *Catharanthus roseus*

Similarities in many resembling compounds help to elucidate the nature of alkaloid biosynthetic pathway (Fig. 5.1-5.6). However, it will be difficult to reveal absolute understanding the nature of synthesis, the alkaloid, coniine, from *Conium maculatum* (hemlock) is structurally very similar to piperidine alkaloids derived from lysine, but it is a tetraketide. Conversely, divergence or elaboration of a structure from its biosynthetic origins can mask its derivation: the quinoline alkaloid, quinine, is not by inspection obviously of monoterpenoid indole-alkaloid origin. Biohemical occurrence under the influence of mild conditions of temperature and pH provide a biomimetic models. For example the alkaloid, tropinone from methylamine, acetone and succinic dialdehyde mixed together and allowed to stand at room temperature (Modifications of this reaction are still useful for the preparative synthesis of tropinone analogues). Since then it is known that none of these substances is a precursor of tropinone *in vivo* and that the nitrogen atom in this molecule derives instead from arginine or ornithine, via the diamine, putrescine (1,4-diaminobutane). Such syntheses are invariably illustrative, but area not an infallible guide to the metabolic route.

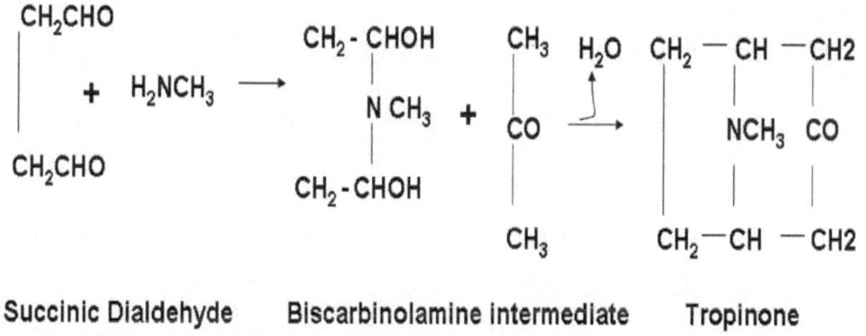

Fig. 5.2 : The classical Robinson synthesis of tropinone.

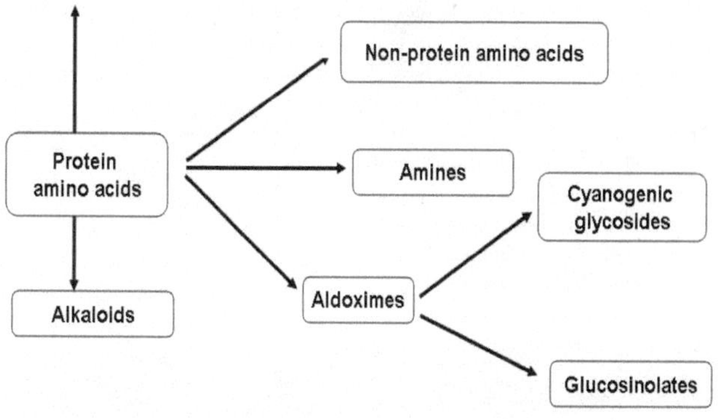

Biosynthetic relationships of nitrogen-containing plant metabolites

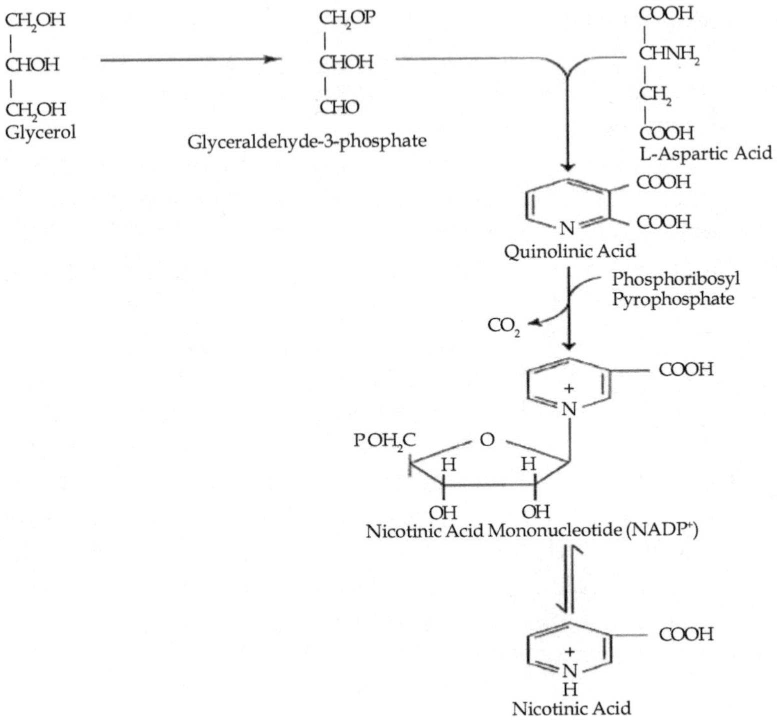

Fig. 5.3 : Biosynthesis of nicotinic acid.

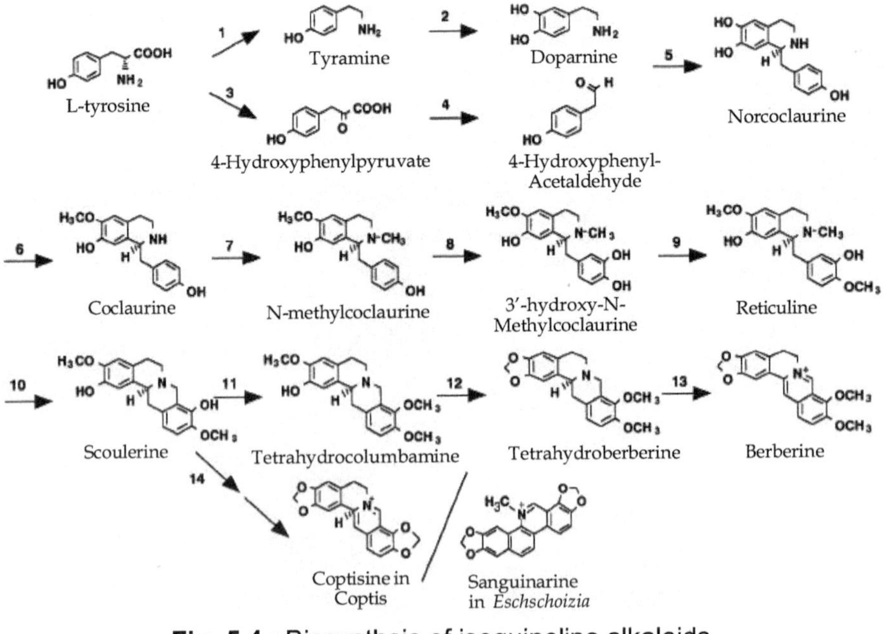

Fig. 5.4 : Biosynthsis of isoquinoline alkaloids.

1. L-tyrosine decarboxylase
2. Phenolase
3. L-tyrosine transaminase
4. Phydroxyphenylpyruvate decarboxylase
5. (S)-norcoclaurine synthase
6. (S)-adenosyl-L- methionine:norcoclaurine 6OMT
7. (S)-adenosyl-L-methionine: coclaurine N- methyltransferase
8. N-methylcoclaurine-49-hydroxylase
9. S-adenosyl-Lmethionine
   39-hydroxy -N-methylcoclaurine 49OM
10. Berberine bridge enzyme
11. S-adenosyl-L-methionine: scoulerine 9-Omethyltransferase
12. (S)-canadine synthase
13. Tetrahydroprotoberberine oxidase
14. Cheilanthifolin synthase.

Although in general alkaloids are biosynthetically derived from protein amino acids, they are usually classified into subclasses according to the carbon skeleton, e.g. quinoline, isoquinoline, etc. Nevertheless, it is clear that indole alkaloids are generally formed from the amino acid tryptophan. As will be clear from Table 5.2, most subclasses of alkaloid have quite restricted natural occurrences. Some subclasses occur in a single family (e.g. the Amaryllidaceae alkaloids), whilst others are found in only a few families (e.g. the betalains and steroids).

The tropane alkaloids, hyoscyamine and scopolamine can be derived from ornithine and arginine and nicotine from proline. Biosynthetic studies received momentum because of revolution during post world war II with the advancement of radioisotopic labeling techniques tracer studies with the principal primary metabolites, such as amino acids, acetate and mevalonate, were applied to representatives of the major classes of plant secondary products. Often, they were undertaken by wick-feeding to whole plants over a period of days, with subsequent isolation of the reaction products of interest. An illustrative example is the biosynthesis of the lysine- and nicotinic-acid-derived piperidine alkaloid, and anabasine. Studies on metabolism of alkaloids and their end products through use of precursors labeled in specific atoms with heavy isotopes, particularly ^{13}C and, later, ^{15}N. The products were then analysed by NMR or MS, which was able to give specific information on patterns of incorporation without degradation being required. Two more recent examples relate to the incorporation of acetate units during the biosynthesis of cocaine and the structurally-related *Solanaceae* tropane alkaloids. Recently, the use of specifically-labelled intermediates has led to a revision of the final stages of hyoscyamine biosynthesis. It has now been established using studies with transformed root cultures that rearrangement of the phenyllactoyl moiety to a tropoyl unit occurs after esterification with tropine.

Because new and complex secondary products are constantly being discovered and characterized, the biosynthetic map is never complete. A biosynthetic investigations may be triggered due to their importance in the pharmaceutical activity of a compound. For example, the biosynthetic origins of the diterpenoid anti-cancer drug from yew, Taxol®, continue to be investigated. More rarely, whole biosynthetic pathways may be called into question. The discovery of a new bacterial pathway to isoprenoids has caused the mevalonate pathway to be reexamined in plants. It has now been established that at least some isoprenoids may be biosynthesized by a non-mevalonate pathway involving a condensation of a triose phosphate with pyruvate, as demonstrated by NMR studies of the labeling pattern of marrubiin, a terpenoid of *Marrubium vulgare*, synthesized from [1-^{13}C]-glucose supplied as precursor. Full details of the intermediates of this new pathway and its enzymology still to be elucidated. It is possible that this pathway is widespread and explains the poor incorporation of mevalonate into some isoprenoids which has frequently been observed in the past. Non-mevalonate and mevalonate pathways may coexist in the same plant; in *Marrubium*, it was established that steroids showed a labeling pattern consistent with the established mevalonate pathway. Labeled-precursor experiments also do not prove beyond doubt that the compound is a metabolic intermediate *in vivo*. For example, labeled quinic acid is incorporated into the aromatic amino acids phenylalanine, tyrosine and tryptophan, but is not on the direct shikimate pathway. In another instance, d-N-methylornithine is incorporated into the tropane alkaloid, hyoscyamine, but is almost certainly an intermediate in a minor metabolic pathway A recent development is the use of *in vivo* NMR to study secondary metabolism. The principal advantage of this approach is that it is non-destructive;

its principal disadvantage at present is relative lack of sensitivity. Though many attempts have been made to understand the biosynthetic pathways of various classes of alkaloids, these are yet to clearly understood. More information is required about intermediates and enzymes involved in these multi step reactions. Use of plant cell cultures and radio labelled precursors proved very useful in such investigations.

Plant cell and organ cultures have made an important contribution to studies of this type since in principle a precursor can be supplied in the culture medium, at a precise concentration and under sterile conditions, over a relatively long period of time. Success obviously depends upon active expression of the biosynthetic pathway in question. When the pathway is expressed generally in the plant body, it may be expressed also in plant cell cultures; but unfortunately cell cultures as a rule do not readily express those pathways which are specific to highly-differentiated cell types. In contrast, organ cultures, such as "hairy root" cultures established by transformation with *Agrobacterium rhizogenes*, appear to express the pathways normally present in the corresponding organs of the intact plant; the obvious limitation here is that it is not possible at present to generate organ cultures of every type one might require (for example floral organ cultures).

Ornithine Derivatives

Ornithine is a precursor of the cyclic pyrrolidines that occur in the alkaloids of tobacco (nicotine, nornicotine) and other Solanaceae. Nicotine is a starting compound of numerous further tobacco alkaloids. During the biosynthesis of tropane, intermediates are produced that are at the same time starting compounds for cocaine and hyoscamine.

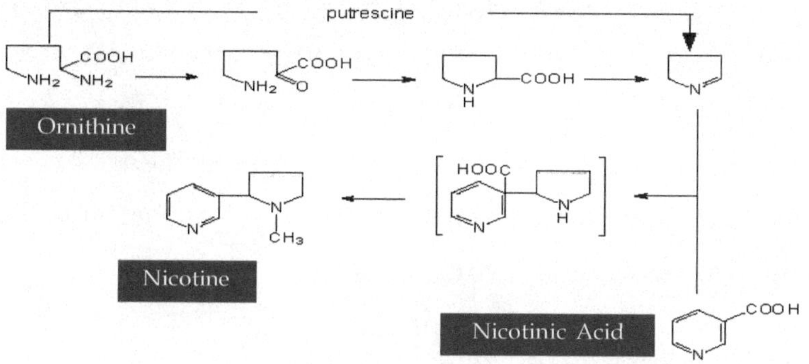

Biosynthesis of tropane: The starting compound of this synthesis is ornithine, methylornithine is the first intermediate.

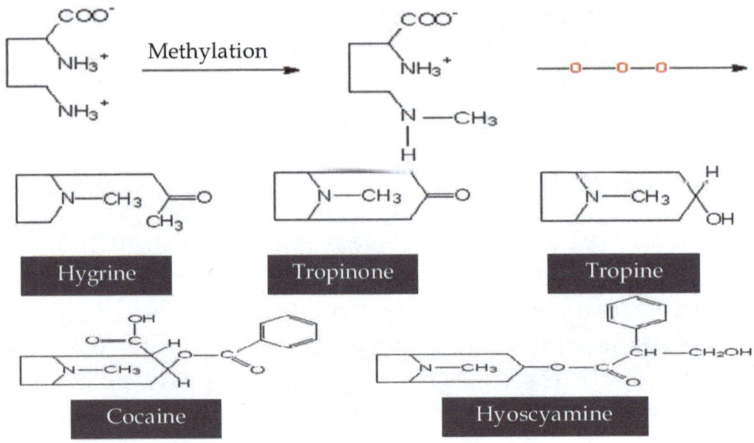

A further group is constituted by the pyrrolizidine alkaloids: Biosynthesis of The Basic Structure of Pyrrolizidine Alkaloids

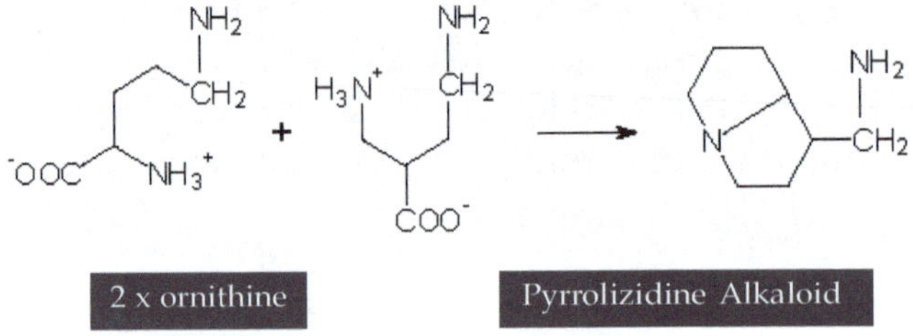

Lysine derivatives: Lysine is the precursor of piperidine that forms the skeleton of several alkaloids. Among them are the bitter principles of the lupine, lupinine and lupanine.

Lycopodine, a substance obtained from clubmoss (Lycopodium) belongs to this group, too. This is mentioned only to show how little the plants are related that are the producers of very similar substances.

Phenylalanine Derivatives : The most important are:

- *Ephedra*-alkaloids: ephedrine, pseudoephedrine,
- Alkaloids gained from micro-organisms: cytochalasine B and D,
- The *Taxus*-alkaloids: taxine,
- The *Lunaria*-alkaloids: lunarine and lunaridine,
- Alkaloids of the Lythraceae.

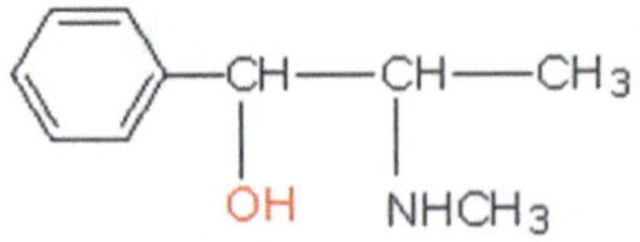

Ephedrine

Tyrosine Derivatives

Tyrosine is the starting product of a large family of alkaloids. The first important intermediate is dopamine which is the starting product of the biosyntheses of berberine, papaverine and morphine, too. Synthesis of Benzylisoquinolines, Starting with Two Mole Tyrosine

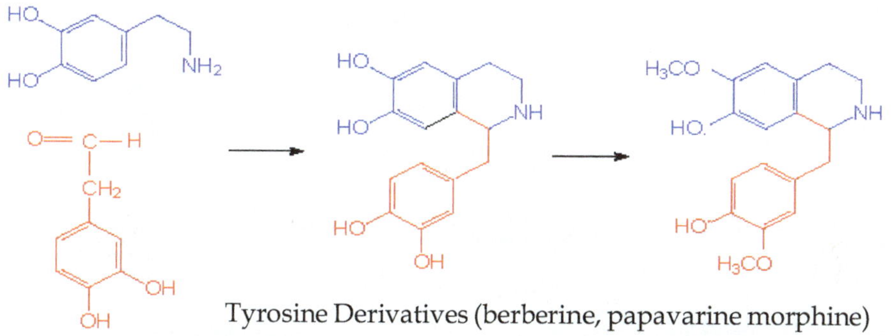

Tyrosine Derivatives (berberine, papavarine morphine)

Moreover, a number of aromatic compounds containing carboxyl-groups is incorporated into other alkaloids like, e.g., atropine, which is an alkaloid of *Atropa belladona*.

During the last years cytochalasine has gained importance in cell biology. It inhibits movements performed by microfilaments and is thus a suitable inhibitor for processes that involve actin.

Morphine synthesis

Two tyrosine rings condense and form the basic structure of morphine that is subsequently modified.

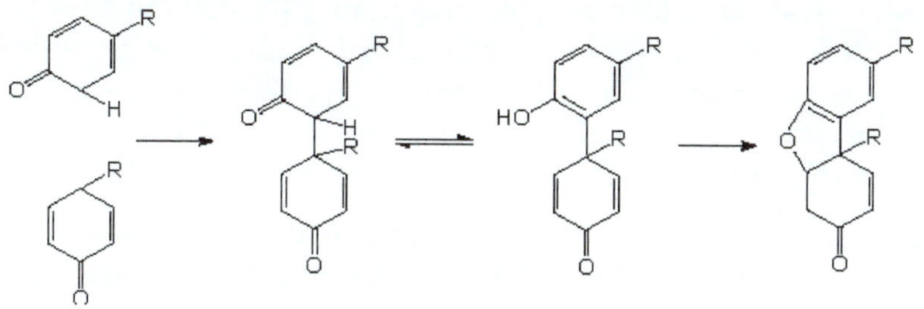

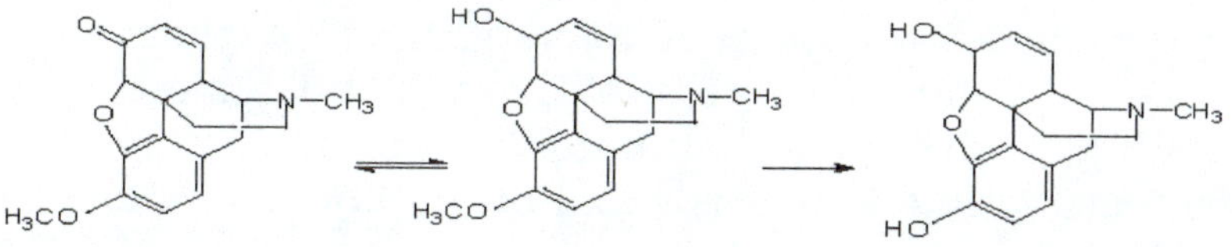

Codeinone Codeine Morphine

The formulas above represent prototypes of which a range of similar compounds (like, for example, the opium alkaloids, codeine, etc.) are derived. Colchicine, an alkaloid of the naked ladies (*Colchicum autumnale* and the related species *C. byzanthinum*) belongs also to this class. It is a poison best-known as an inhibitor of mitosis. It prevents the aggregation of tubuline dimers so that no micotubuli are formed.

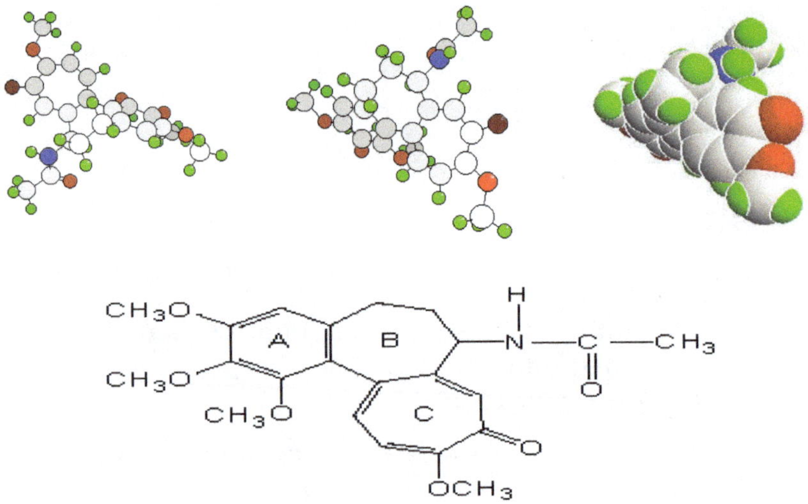

Colchicine

Indole alkaloids (Derivatives of tryptophan, etc.)

The analysis of this group has proceeded very well during the last years. Besides chromatographic techniques, especially mass spectroscopy and nuclear magnetic resonance (NMR) have been used. About 1200 different compounds all of which are tryptophane derivatives have been isolated until today. They correspond to 25 percent of all known alkaloids. Only few of them are known by a broader public although many of them are used by medicine.

Among the tryptophan-derivatives is d-tubocurarine, one of the active components of curare, the arrow poison used by South American Indians. The Apocynaceae, Loganiaceae and Rubiaceae families are characterized by a broad range of indole alkaloids of which the Vinca, Rauvolfia- and Cataranthus - alkaloids are examples a are generated by coupling iridoids, very common compounds derived from monoterpenes to indole that is based on tryptophan. A lot of well-known fungi poisons belong to this group.

In contrast to the amino acid derivatives that contain nitrogen right from the beginning, it is incorporated much later here. Gentianine as well as further toxic compounds like, for example aconitine obtained from *Aconitum* and *Delphinum* belong to this group. An important sub-group is formed by the *Solanum*- alkaloids that can be found in nearly all organs of *Solanum*- (potato) and *Lycopersicon* (tomato) - species but occur also in very different taxa (lilies and Asclepiadaceae).

Chemistry of Alkaloids

They are heterocyclic compounds having C, H, O and N in their structure (exception: Nicotine without oxygen). They are mainly composed of pyrol, pyridine, quinoline, isoquinoline and tropane structure. Morphine contains phenanthrene without nitrogen. The carbon skeleton of most of the alkaloids is derived from amino acids although moieties from other pathways such as terpenoids are often combined. In steroid alkaloid the nitrogen is derived from glutamine or other ammonical sources. All alkaloids have basic properties as well as general properties for their characterization.

Two Basic Properties

1. Heterocyclic ring structure with N in the ring structure.
2. Basic in nature.

General Properties

They are colourless and non-volatile solids. They are slightly soluble in water (Coniine and nicotine are highly soluble in water) but soluble in most organic solvent. Some are coloured substances (Barberine is yellow). Most alkaloids are optically active and are leavo rotatory but few are dextrorotatory too. While, some are optically inactive.

Almost all are bitter in taste. They are used in pharmacy. They are active at small concentration. At higher doses, they may cause death. They are basic in nature and form insoluble salts with picric acid, potassium, mercuric, iodine, etc.

Accumulation and Storage

Alkaloids accumulate mainly in four types of tissue. Vacuoles are the major compartment of alkaloid storage. Alkaloids are stored predominantly in tissue which are important for survival reproduction; i.e. growing young tissues, root and stem bark, flowers (especially seeds), seedlings and photosynthetically active tissues. Alkaloids accumulate mainly in 1) actively growing tissues, 2) epiderma and hypoderma cells, 3) vascular sheaths and 4) latex vessels. They are present in the vacuole and do not form in the young cells until vacuolation occurs. Some alkaloids are stored in special cells called as idioblast. These idioblast have been detected in *corydalis, Sanguinaria* and in *Maclea* for corydaline, sanguinarin and protopine type alkaloid respectively.

Table 5.2 : Site of biosynthesis and site of accumulation of alkaloids.

Alkaloids	**Species**	**Site of Biosynthesis**	**Site of Accumulation**
Shikonin	**Lithospermum**	Roots	Roots
Alkannine	*Echium*	Roots	Roots
Berberine	*Coptis*	Rhizomes	Rhizomes
Jatrorhizine	*Berberis*	Roots	Roots
Sanguinarine	*Papaver*	Roots	Roots
Nicotine	*Nicotiana*	Roots	Whole plant
Ajmalicine	*Catharanthus*	Roots	Roots
Harmane	*Peganum*	Roots	Roots
alkaloids	*Cassia, Morinda,*	Roots	Roots
Anthraquinones	*Rubia*	Roots	Roots
R-ginsenosides	*Panax*	Roots	Roots
Glycirrhizine	*Glycirrhiza*	Rhizomes	Rhizomes
Diosgenin	*Dioscorea*	Root	Leaf
Seneciconine		Green Tissue	
Emitine		Stem and Root	
Caffene		Bark	
Berberine		Root	Leaf
Tropane		Stem Bark	
Quinine			

Alkaloids are synthesized in one tissue and accumulate in another. For this long distance travel is needed through xylem or phloem vessels. Alkaloid passes the membrane barrier through various mechanisms such as simple diffusion, carrer mediated transport or membrane fusion.

Nomenclature

The nomenclature of alkaloids is not very exact but those with heterocyclic rings are frequently called true alkaloids & those without such rings protoalkaloids. Their distal biosynthetic precursors are almost always amino acids; other multicarbon units, e.g. acetate, are also incorporated into the final structure of some alkaloids. Alkaloids, both with & without heterocyclic rings, that are not derived from amino acids are called pseudoalkaloids. These are almost entirely represented by alkaloids in which the carbon skeleton is isoprenoid derivative.

Although, their scientific nomenclature is not possible due to their complex structures. Nomenclature can be given according to following general criteria.

1. According to their plant source. e.g. Papaverine, Berberine
2. According to their physiological actions e.g. Morphine, Narcotine, Emetine.
3. According to the name of scientist who discovered it e.g. Palatrin which was discovered by P.J.Pelletior.
4. By adding prefix or suffix in the name of plant source e.g. Cinchonine from Cinchona, quinine
5. Same isomeric alkaloids have been designated by adding prefix iso, neo, epi, α and β.
6. Some times Greek words are used in the nomenclature.

Classification : They are classified by two systems:

1. Classification based on the genera of plants in which they occur. Cinchonine from *Cinchona* spp.
2. Classification based on the nature (type) of the heterocyclic nucleus present in the structure which was given by Henry.

Alkaloids have been variously catagorized e.g. Taxonomic (solanaceous, papilionaceous alkaloids), pharmacological (analgesic, cardioactive alkaloids) & chemical. On the basis of chemical structure they are classified as under:

1. Phenyl ethyl amino group or Phenylalkyl amino group

This class of alkaloids is synthesized from phenylalanine. It includes ephedrine, pseudoephedrine, taxine tyramine & hordenine. Phenylethylamine : According to Robinson (1974), the precursors for biosynthesis of alkaloids of phenylethylamine and isoquinolide groups are the amino acids, e.g. phenylalanine, tyrosine and dihydroxyphenylalanine.

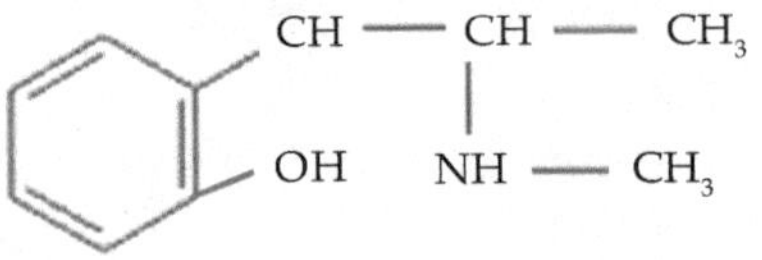

Ephridine

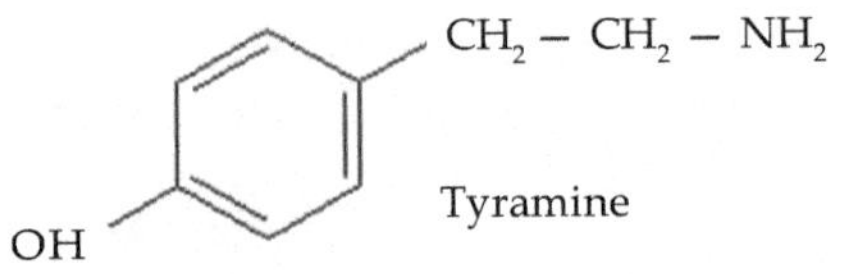

Tyramine

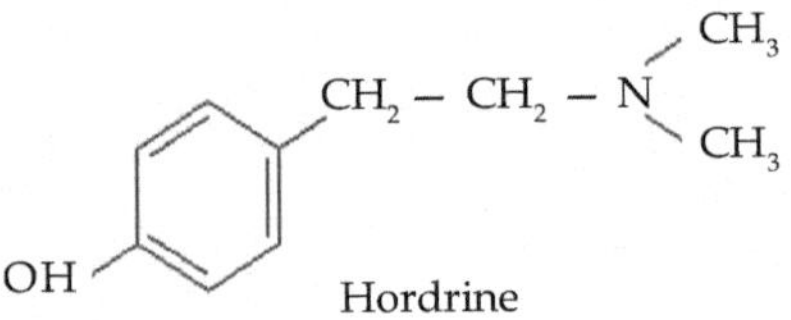

Hordrine

2 Pyrrolidine

Hygrine isolated from *Paruvian coke* in 1814. It is extremely basic and boils at 194° C.

Hygrine (C8 H15 O)

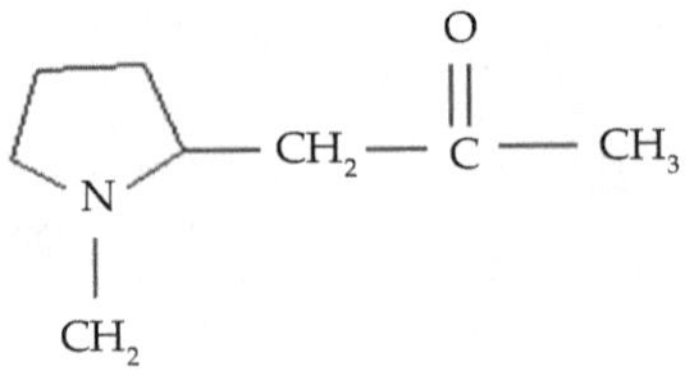

N Stachydrine (C7 H14 O N)

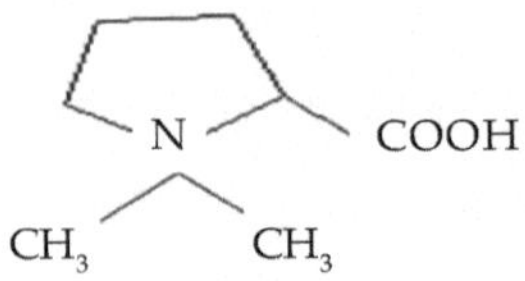

3. Pyridine: *Pyrrolidine alkaloids*

The precursors for biosynthesis of pyrrolidine alkaloids are N-methyl-Δ-pyrollinium cation and acetoacetic acid. The former is derived from ornithine and related amino acids and the latter from acetic acid. Several pathways have been reported for the biosynthesis of piperidine alkaloids in plants. However, the pathway depends on the nature of the alkaloids, e.g. the precursor for the biosynthesis of pelletierines is lysine.

They are sub- classified in three groups, which are as follows.

(a) *Hemlock alkaloid (Dhatura)* : Five alkaloids are included in this group. The main alkaloid of this group is **Coniine** was used to kill political prisoners in olden times. (Socrates was given cup of Dhatura Alkaloid)

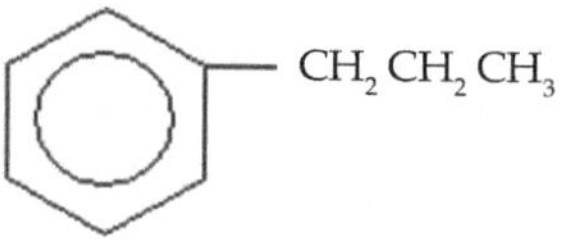

Coniine

(b) *Pepper Alkaloid* : There are two members in this group I) Piperine and-II) Chavicine. It is found with isomer Chavicine in black and white peppers (5 to 8 %). Taste is pungent. It is less toxic than other alkaloid. They are solid, optically inactive, and soluble in water. Melting Point (M.P.) = 128 ^{0} C.

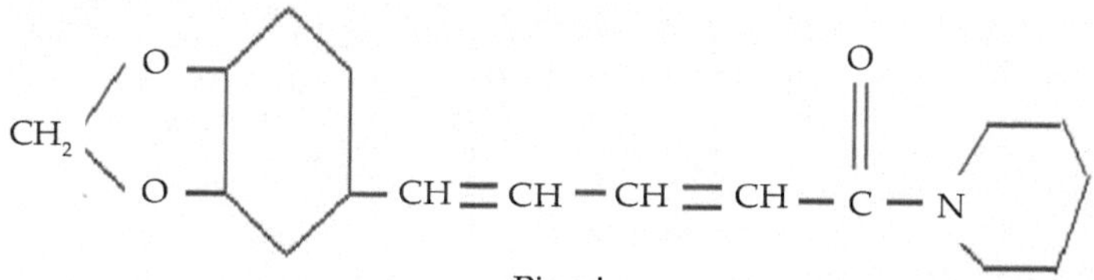

Piperine

(c) *Ricidine* : They are isolated from castor oil. They are less toxic, contain cyanide group in its structure. It is present in castor seeds, optically inactive, weak base.

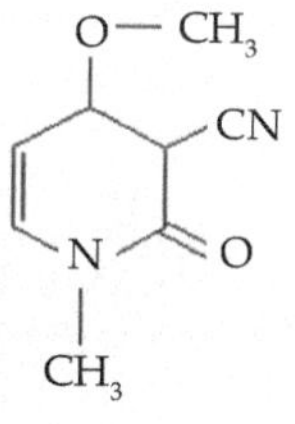

Ricidine

4 Pyrollidine- Pyridine

An example of these alkaloids is nicotine which consists of two units-pyrrolidine and pyridine (It has been shown by tracer experiments that the precursor of the pyridine ring is nicotinic acid). The latter acid is produced via quinolinic acid. It has also been proven that biosynthesis of the pyridine ring in nicotinic and that quinolinic acids involve glycerol and aspartic acid.

Nicotine

It is found in the leaves of tobacco. They occur as malic and citric acid salts. Dry leaves contain around 4 %. They are strong basic.

Optically active, found in leavo (L) form, water soluble, boiling point is 242 ^{0} C. It is most toxic alkaloid at 40mg or more, it may cause death. It can also act as good insecticide. It is also used for the manufacturing of niacin and nicotinic acid. It does not have oxygen in its structure.

Nicotine (C_{10} H_4 N_2)

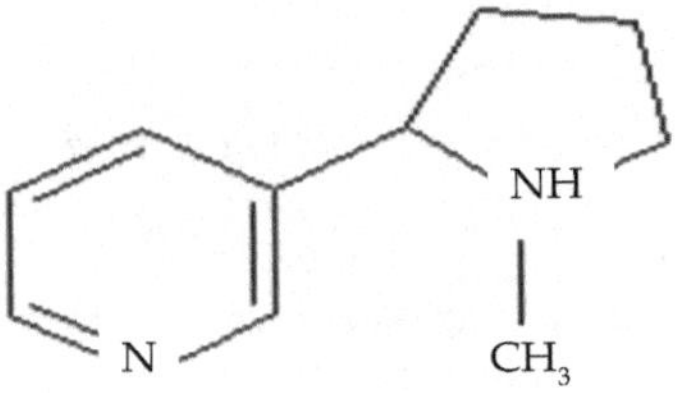

5 Tropane alkaloids

By using radiolabelled compounds such as ornithine, N-methyl putrescine, hygrine etc., it has been conclusively proven that the nitrogen atom in the alkaloid has been derived from the amino acid precursor. There are two groups. A) Solanaceous alkaloid and B) Coca alkaloids.

(a) Solanaceous alkaloids atropine (C_{17} H_{23} NO_3)

Solanaceous alkaloids: They are obtained from Solanaceae family. atropine is the main alkaloid in this group.

They are isolated from *Atropa belladonna.* They are optically inactive, alkaline, bitter in taste, having Melting Point of 115 ^{0} C. If it is taken orally, it can depress the Central Nervous System (CNS). It is used to dilate the pupils (widening of Iris) of eyes during the eye surgery.

(b) Coca alkaloids

The important member of this group is cocaine.

Cocaine : (C_{17} H_{21} NO_4) : Cocaine is extracted from leaves from coca which is grown in Java, Sri Lanka, Peru countries. It is colourless, alkaline and less soluble in H_2O. Its Melting Point is 98 ^{0} C. It is used as local anesthetic.

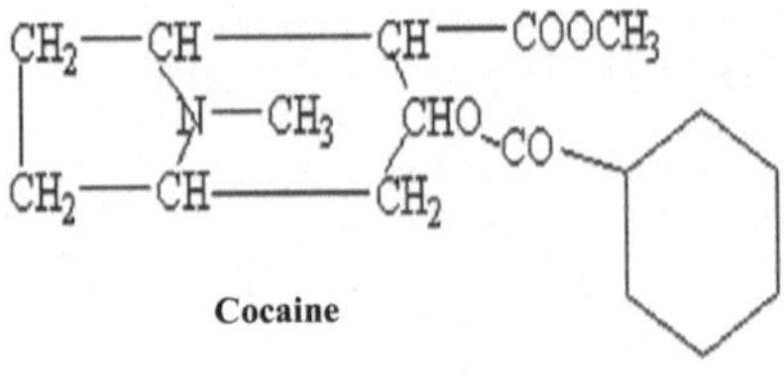

Cocaine

6 Quinoline group

Tryptophan is the precursor of biosynthesis of cinchona alkaloids. Secologanin is another precursor, which is derived from loganin, a natural terpenoid of the iridoid group. Secologanin is derived from mevalonic acid. It is also known as Cinchona alkaloid. Main alkaloids are Cinchonine and Quinine. These are isolated from the bark of Cinchona plant Spp. In middle of 17th century; the barks of Cinchona were utilized to cure fever. It was later confirmed as Quinine (for malarial fever). More than 35 alkaloids have been extracted from Cinchona. Some of them are Strychnine, cinchonine, quinine, quinidine, cuperine, epiquinine, epiquinidine etc.

a) Quinine

It is obtained from the bark of Cinchona plant. It is having bitter taste, crystalline, solid substance. Its Melting Point is 175 ^{0}C, semi soluble in ether and alcohol. It is used as quinine sulphate. The precursor for quinine synthesis is tryptophan.

Tryptophan → Corynanthrene → Cinchonamine → Quinine. It is used as anti-malarial drug.

b) Cinchonine

It is present in the bark of grey Cinchona plant. The precursor of its synthesis is tryptophan. It has bitter taste, less toxic than quinine, water soluble, optically active, dextro-rotatory, Melting Point is 265 ^{0}C.

Tryptophan → Corynanthrene → Cinchonamine → Cinchonine

Cinchonine ($C_{19} H_{22} N O_2$)

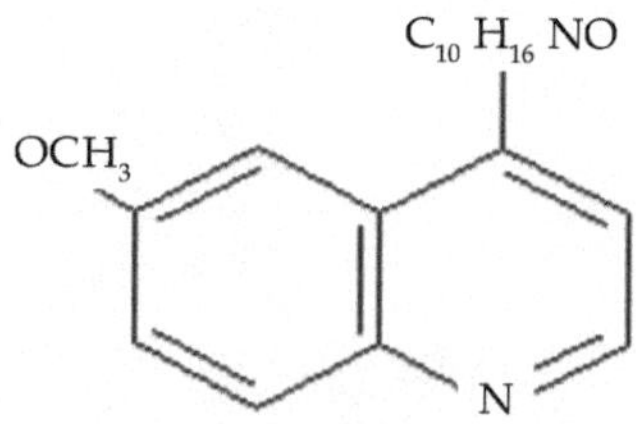

Quinine

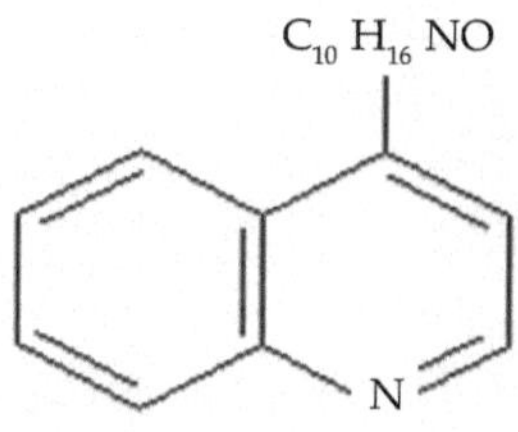

Cinchonine

7 Isoquinoline alkaloid and phenanthrene group

Papavarine is obtained from tyrosine. Tyrosine produces a mixture of dopamine and 3,4-dihydroxyphenylacetaldehyde, which by condensation yields isoquinoline alkaloid.Isoquinoline contain several alkaloids including Morphine, Thebaine, Papaverine, Narcotine, Narceine etc. Almost all these alkaloids are obtained from *Poppy* spp. (*Papaver somaniferum*).They are isolated from green capsules.

Papaverine : It is an important alkaloid of opium group. The molecular formula is $C_{20} H_{21} N O_4$

Mrphine: Opium contains 10-20 % morphine. It was isolated from *Sertüner* plants in 1806. It is insoluble in water having bitter taste, optically active, leavo - rotatory, Melting Point 255 ^{0}C. It is used as pain killer (analgesic) and sometimes as anaesthat, also used in medicine. The molecular formula is $C_{17} H_{19} N O_3$.

Berberine: Isolated from the roots of *Berberine* plants. The molecular formula is $C_{20} H_9 O_5$ N.

8 Phenanthrene alkaloid

The morphine alkaloid onstitute a separate sub-group of opium alkaloids. Phenanthrene nucleus is found in their structure. e.g. Morphine, Codeine, Thebaine (10-15 %).

9 Indole alkaloids

There are three classes on the basis of occurrence and mode of action.Tryptophan is the precursor for most of the indole alkaloids. Tryptophan decarboxylase catalyzes the first step, committing the amino acid tryptophan to secondary metabolism. Geraniol-10-hydroxylase appears to be a key enzyme in the monoterpene portion of the pathway. Strictosidine synthase catalyzes the condensation of tryptamine and secologanin. Anticancer dimeric alkaloids are synthesized from ajmalicine, serpentine and a monomeric precursors such as catharanthine in several steps. Ergot and Strychnos alkaloids are the major alkaloids of this group.

Ergot alkaloid

Their main source is ergot found on the grasses and rye isolated from fungi. There are more than 20 members.e.g. Ergotamine, Ergotaminine, Ergosine, Ergosinine. Ergot has been used is medicine as an activator in working of uterus.

Strychnos alkaloid

They are used as anti-helmentics (to kill worms and insects). It affects respiration and CNS of animals. e.g. Strychine, Bruchine.

10 Rauvolfia alkaloid

e.g. raserpine which is used in the treatment of hypertension, tension, fevers, dizziness, and insomnia.

11 Miscellaneous groups

It is also called Tropolane alkaloids. Colchicine which is present in the seeds of Colchieum is used in artificial production of polyploidy. Molecular formula is $C_{22} H_{25} NO_6$.

Biological and Medicinal Significance of Alkaloids

a) Biological Significance

1. Protect the plants against fungi, insects and animals.
2. Excretory products of plants.
3. Some scientists proposed that alkaloids serve as reservoir of N and help the protein synthesis.
4. They behave as growth regulators like hormones.
5. Colchicine is used in the multiplication of chromosome by which new varieties of crops are developed.
6. Helpful to neutralize the harmful effects of acids in plants.
7. Morphine is essential in formation of poppy seeds.
8. Alkaloids inhibit enzyme activity and seed germination. Some remove bad effects of tannins.
9. Alkaloids are known as co-product in the metabolism of protein in plants.
10. Alkaloids protect the plants from infection of plant disease.

b) Medicinal Significance

1. Alkaloids are used as medicine in several diseases.
2. Quinine is used as anti-malarial drug.
3. Morphine is used as pain killer.
4. Atropine is used to extend the size of Iris in the treatment of eye ailments.

5. Ergotine is used to stimulate the function of uterus.
6. Several alkaloids are used as insecticides and pesticides (Nicotine sulphate from tobacco and azadirachtin from neem).
7. Several compounds of opium are useful in medicines.
8. Colchicine is used to control rheumatic disease
9. Some are used to control hypertension to improve Central Nervous System.
10. Emitine is used as cough expectorant and prevent vomiting.

Alkaloids with hallucinogenic , narcotic, or analgesic properties have found medical application as pure compounds (e.g., morphine, atropine, and quinine) or served as model compounds for modern synthetic drugs, while several are abused as illegal drugs (e.g., cocaine). Other alkaloids are too toxic for any therapeutic use (e.g., coniine and strychnine), but plant constituents are still screened for new, biologically active compounds. An example is the discovery of taxol, which has cytostatic properties and is applied as an anticancer drug.

Table 5.3 : Important alkaloids of plant origin & their medicinal significance.

Alkaloid	**Source**	**Medicinal importance**
Ajmalicine	*Catharanthus roseus*	Hypotensive
Atropine	*Atropa belladona*	Anticholinergic Dilation of pupi;
Berberine	*Berberis spp*	Antispasmodic, antiprotozoal
Codeine	*Papaversomniferum*	Sedative, analgesic
Colchicine	*Colchicum autumnale*	Antimitotic
Caffeine	*Coffea arabica*	Stimulant
Camptothecine	*Camptotheca acuminata*	Antitumor
Emetine	*Cephaelis ipecacuanha*	Emetic, cough expectorant
Morphine	*Papaver somniferum*	Analgesic, sedative
Papaverine	*Papaver somniferum*	Spasmolytic
Quinine	*Cinchona ledgeriana*	Antimalaria
Reserpine	*Rauwolfia serpentina*	Reduce Hypertension
Vinblastine, vincristine	*Catharanthus roseus*	Anticancer
Colchicine	*Colchium spp*	Anti rheumatic
Ergotin	Rye grass	Stimulation of uterus muscle

Removal of alkaloid toxicity

If some one takes alkaloids orally in high concentrations, should be directed for vomiting immediately and should be given dilute tannic acid. The tannic acid precipitates out the alkaloid and thus acts as antidote. This is the reason that tea or coffee containing tannin act as antidote to alkaloid poisoning.

Chapter 6

Glycosides and Plant Pigments

Glycosides are compounds containing a carbohydrate and a non carbohydrate residue in the same molecule. They are the complex polysaccharides which are chemically heterogeneous collection of substances, which have in common one property that the molecules are linked together and contain at least one sugar unit. The term glycoside represents a group of compound containing glucose and one or more basic or acidic organic compound in chemical combination. When the sugar other than glucose is present, it is called glycoside. Each sugar is linked through a glycosidic bond to either a non sugar component, aglycones, (aglycone or aglucone is the non-sugar molecule in glycosides).

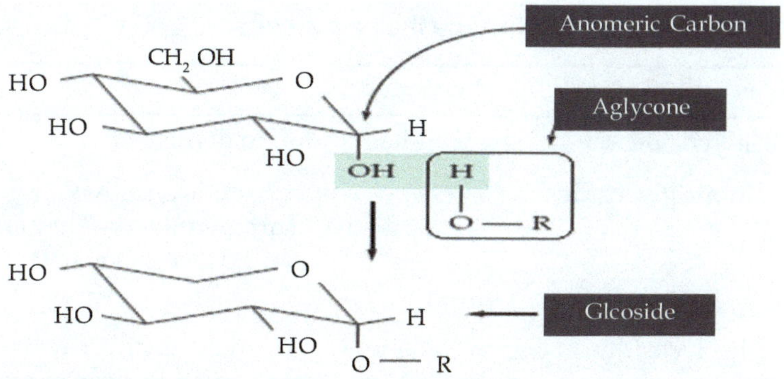

These aglycones may be methyl alcohol, glycerol, a sterol, a phenol etc. The general formula for glycoside is S-O-R where the S is the sugar and the R to be aglycones or non-sugar molecule linked with oxygen (O) to the 1st carbon of the sugar. Sometimes, even the disaccharide is also present in the glycosides. Glucosides are bound with a variety of glycosidic bonds.

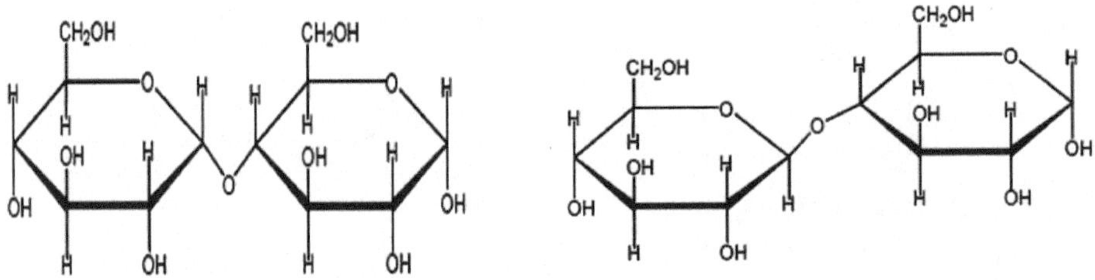

a) *Hemi-acetal:* Hemi-acetals are formed by the addition of an alcoholic component to a carbonyl function.

b) *Internal Hemi-acetal:* An alcoholic component needed to participate in the formation of a hemiacetal need not be a foreign molecule; it could be a part of same molecule (Internal hemiacetal).

c) *Acetal:* A hemi acetal, even an internal hemiacetal, can react with an additional alcohol molecule. It entails a bond formation with removal of water. The product is acetal. The bond between alcoholic component and the sugar is known as glycosidic bond.

Glycosides are widely distributed in plants especially in roots, barks, fruits and to a smaller extent in leaves.

Classification of Glycosides : They are classified on the basis of aglucone molecule (Table 6.1).

Table 6.1 : Different glycosides and their aglycones.

Glycosides	Aglycones
Alcoholic glycosides	e.g. Salicin found in genus *salix.*
Anthraquinone glycosides	These glycosides contain an aglycone group that is a derivative of anthraquinone. They are present in senna, rhubarb and aloes; they have a laxative effect
Cyanogenic glycosides	Aglycone is cynogens. E.g. dhurrin.

Flavonoid glycosides	Here the aglycone is a flavonoid. This is a large group of flavonoid glycosides
Phenolic glycosides (simple)	Here the aglycone is a simple phenolic structure. An example is arbutin found in the Common Bearberry
Saponins	Sapogenins as
Steroidal glycosides or cardiac glycosides	Terpenoids/ terpened as agycones
Steviol glycosides	e.g. stevioside and rebaudioside A found in stevia
Thioglycosides	Having sulphur compound as aglycone

Four groups of glycosides are mostly recognized which are,

1. Cyanophoric or cyanogenic glycosides.
2. Mustard oil glycosides.
3. Saponins.
4. Phenolic glycosides.

Types of Glycosides

There are two major groups of glycosides.

a) O-glycosides. and b) N-glycosides., other glycosides found are S-glycoside and Carbon C glycoside.

O-glycosides: The alcoholic component reacts with the sugar through a-OH group. In addition to true alcohols, organic acids, phenols and sugars can function as alcoholic component. The most diverse phenols occur often act as aglycones in plant.

N-glycosides: The alcoholic component react with the sugar through a -NH group. N-glycosidic linkages are found in the nucleosides and thus in the nucleotides and poly nucleotides.

Properties

1. They are widely distributed in plants especially in roots, bark, fruits and to a small extent in leaves.
2. They are white crystalline substance when in pure form.
3. They are usually bitter in taste.
4. They are soluble in water and organic solvents except in ether.

5. Glycosidic bonds can be broken by enzymes with the release of sugars. These enzymes are known as glycosidases. β-glycosidase attack β-glycosidic bonds. The reverse reaction, the synthesis of glycosides from sugars by means of glycosidases is also possible. α-glycosides and β-glycosides are distinguished by the configuration of the hemiacetal hydroxyl group.The majority of naturally-occurring glycosides are β-glycosides.

Cyanophoric Glycosides

They are distributed in over 2600 plant species belonging to 110 families. Cyanide (hydrogen cyanide, HCN) in trace amounts is widespread in the plant kingdom and occurs mainly in the form of cyanogenic glucosides (also called as cyanogens). Cyanogens are glycosides of sugar and cyanide containing aglycon. Cyanogenic glycosides are accumulated in vacuoles. As cynogenic glycosides are characterized by yielding HCN (hydrocyanic acid) on hydrolysis with mineral acids or suitable enzyme. The best known example of this group is amygdalin found in large quantities in bitter almond, kernels of apricot, peaches and plums. It is the mother substance of 'oil of bitter almond' which is largely used as flavoring agent. It yields two molecules of glucose and one molecule each of benzaldehyde and HCN. Dhurrin is a glucoside present in toxic amount in young sorghum *(jowar)* seedling hence they are unfit for the cattle feeding but as the seedling grows, the toxic glucoside disappears.

These glycosides are generally bitter in taste. The poisoning generally occurs due to consumption of new and young plants that contain higher amounts compared to the mature ones. The lethal dose of HCN taken by mouth in humans has been estimated to be between 0.5 and 3.5 mg/kg body weight. There are many economical important plants which are highly cyanogenic, e.g. white clover, linum, almond, sorghum, the rubber tree and cassava. Relatively high concentrations are found in certain grasses, pulses, root crops, and fruit kernels.

General structure of cyanogenic glycosides

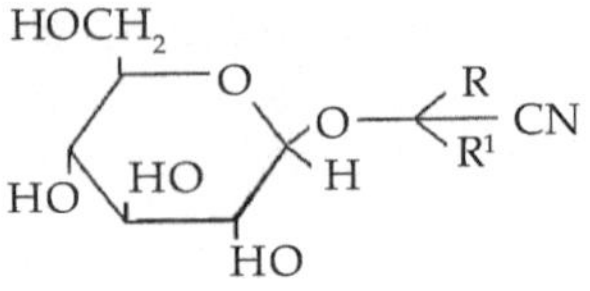

e.g. R=R′= CH_3 – linamarin

R=CH_3, R′=CH_2CH_3 – lotaustralin

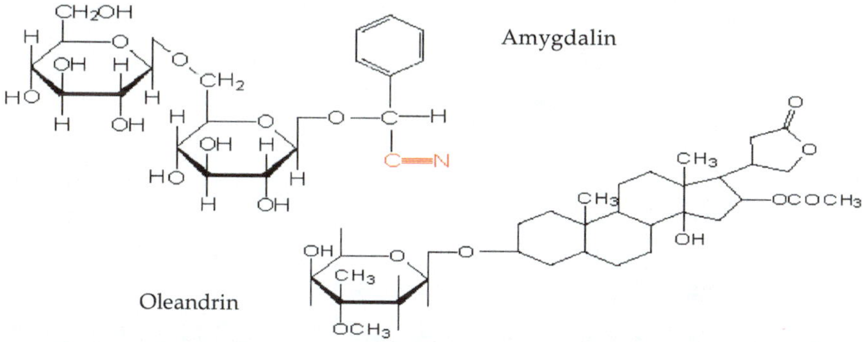

Amygdalin

Oleandrin

β-glucosidases which are located in the apoplasm, in protein bodies or in the chloroplast. β-glucosidases have varying substrate specificity. They do not hydrolyse cyanogenic glycosides that contain 2 sugar moieties. Hydroxynitrile lyases exibit no distinct substrate specificity, velocity of HCN liberation is accelerated enzymatically up to 20-folds Cyanogenesis is the process by which hydrogen cyanide is released from endogenous cyanide containing compounds, mainly cyanogenic glycosides. Cyanogenic glycosides have an important role in plant defense against herbivores due to bitter taste and release of toxic hydrogen cyanide. The effectiveness of cyanogens in deterring herbivores depends not only on morphology, physiology, and behavior of the herbivores, but also on the concentration of cyanogenic glycosides in the host plant, and the amount of toxic hydrogen cyanide, which can be released per unit time. Many plants used for human nutrition contain cyanogenic glycosides (e.g. cassava, sorghum, lima bean), so cyanide poisoning by such a food is an important problem, especially in some regions of the world.

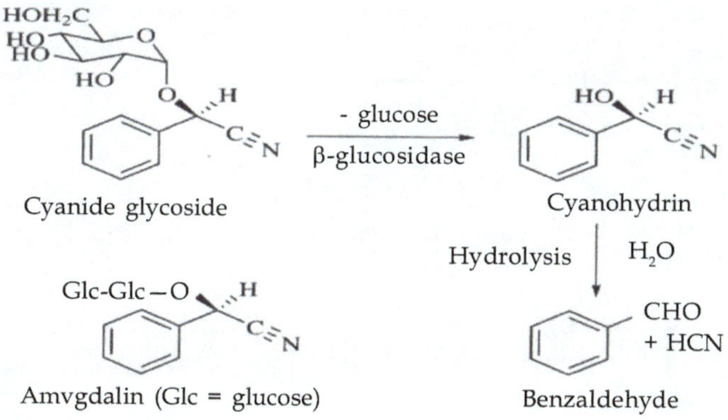

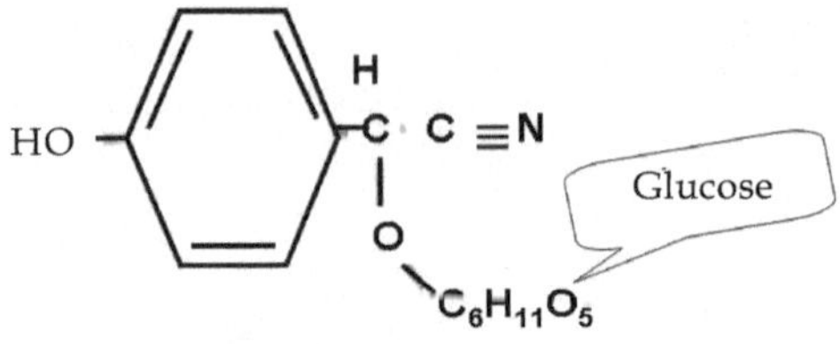

Dhurrin

Cyanogenesis is the process by which hydrogen cyanide is released from endogenous cyanide containing compounds. In cyanogenesis, the sugar moiety is cleaved from the cyanogenic glycoside in a process catalyzed by one or more β-glucosidases.

The resulting cyanohydrin is relatively unstable and degrades, either spontaneously or enzymatically, to produce HCN and an aldehyde or a ketone. Autotoxicity is prevented by spatial separation—either at the subcellular or tissue level—of the degradative enzymes and the cyanogenic glycoside.

Cyanogenesis in Plants

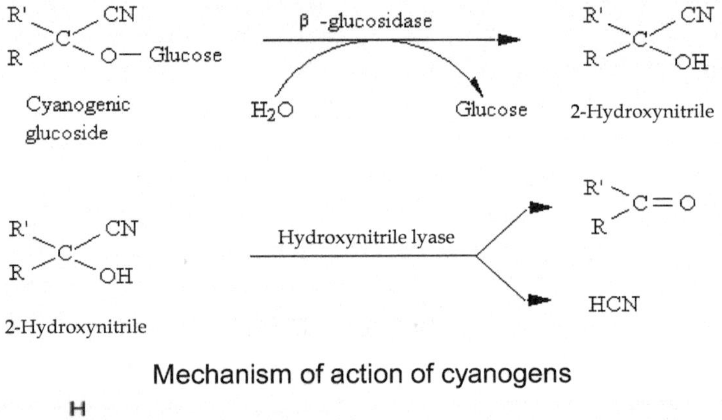

Mechanism of action of cyanogens

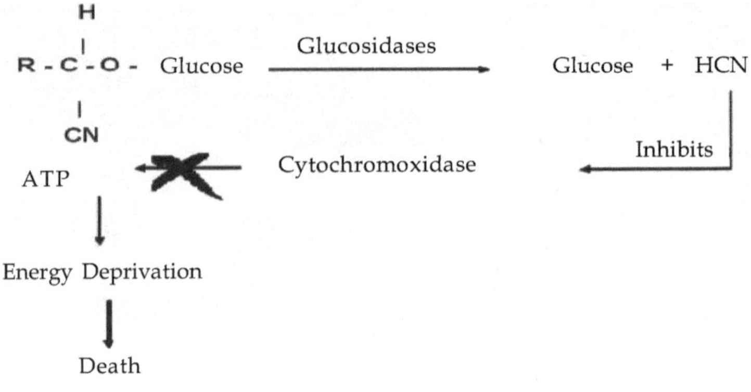

Mechanism of Action of Cyanogens

Cyanohydric acid is extremely toxic to a wide spectrum of organisms, due to its ability of linking with metals (Fe^{++}, Mn^{++} and Cu^{++}) that are functional groups of many enzymes, inhibiting processes like the reduction of oxygen in the cytochrome respiratory chain, electron transport in the photosynthesis, and the activity of enzymes like catalase and oxidases.

Biosynthesis

The biosynthesis of the aglycone is catalysed by two cytochrome P450- dependent monoxygenases.

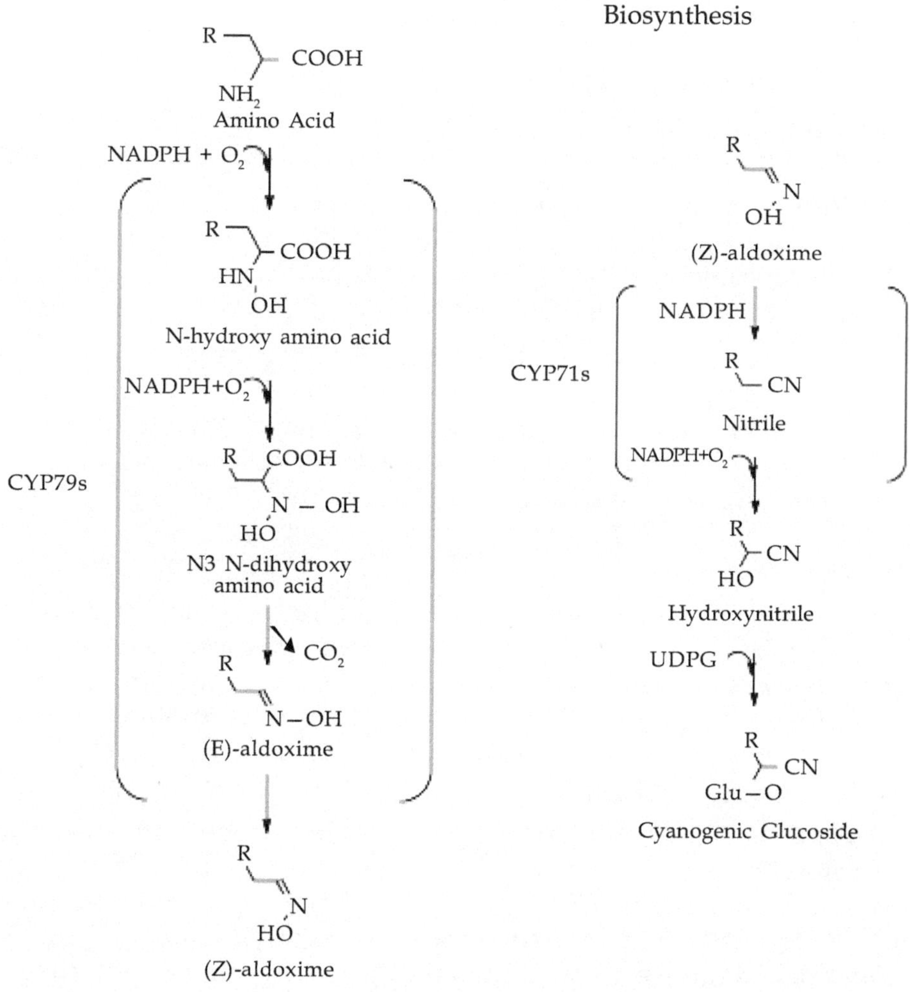

Detoxification of HCN

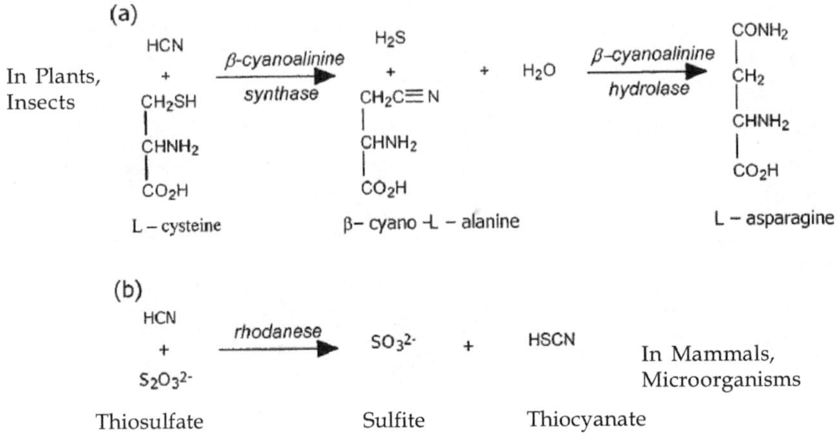

Biological effects of Cynogenic Glycosides

- Role in physiological processes: Production of HCN increased during pre germination period & preceded ethylene production.
- Effects on human organisms: Intake of larger amounts of plants having cynogenic glycosides leads to enhanced S-CN concentrations in blood. S-CN interferes with iodine metabolism and cause iodine deficiency disorders like goitre and cretinism.
- Role in plant defence: In defence mechanisms against various phytopathogens and also act as feeding deterrents or phagostimulants, e.g. dhurrin acts as oviposition activator for the pests. They are also associated with metabolism and transport of nitrogen and the control of germination.

Removal of toxicity

Cyanogens can be removed by drying; for example, hay-making removes cyanogens by volatizing the cyanide released. Soaking and fermentation of cassava and discarding the water containing cyanide makes the cassava safe for human or livestock consumption.

Mustard Oil Glycosides

These are sulphur containing glycosidic compounds e.g. glucosinolate found in *Cruciferae*. Glucosinolates are polar molecules, found in cytoplasm & stored in vacuoles. They are anions that occur only in the cells of a limited number of dicotyledonous families. Glucosinolates are very common in the order Capparales (best-known family: *Brassicaceae*) where they occur in every species hitherto examined. Among the best-known representatives are the active ingredients of horse-radish, radish and mustard. The elimination of aliphatic glucosinolates in rape (isothiocyanate or oxaziolin-2-thione, for example from glucorapiferin; or rhodaninion from glucobrassicines) achieved by cultivation resulted in so-called double zero varieties (00-varieties). The cultivation of simple zero varieties (0-varieties) is based on the elimination of erucic acid, a long-chained unsaturated fatty acid. These glycosides are stable at neutral pH, can occur as salts with cations such as K+ or sinapine to balance the negative charge. They are generally found in seeds & roots in good amount. Concentrations are in the range 0.1-0.2% fresh weight in leaves, up to 0.8% in roots & up to 8% in seeds.

On hydrolysis, they yield organic compounds containing isothiocyanate (-NCS) and possess a peculiar characteristic odour. An endogenic enzyme myrosinase accompanies in the mustard seed act as hydrolyzing agent when seeds are ruptured. All plants containing glucosinolates also contain enzymes that are capable of decomposing these compounds. These β-glucosidases are generally called myrosinases. Nitrile formation is favored by low pH values & also promoted by ferrous ions. After tissue disruption, isothiocyanates are normally the predominant products.

Allyl isothiocyanate is responsible for pungent taste of mustard and horseradish. It is a colorless to pale yellow liquid that is slightly soluble in water, but well soluble in most organic solvents.

Allyl isothiocyanate itself does not occur in the mustard seed. when ground mustard seeds are mixed with water, vinegar, or other liquids or when they are chewed, a chemical reaction between the enzyme myrosinase and a glucosinolate known as sinigrin from the seeds of black mustard (*Brassica nigra*) or brown Indian mustard (*Brassica juncea*) leads to the production of allyl isothiocyanate. Allyl isothiocyanate can also be produced synthetically, synthetic mustard oil, reaction of allyl iodide and potassium thiocyanate. Synthetic allyl isothiocyanate is used as an insecticide, as an animal repellent, to denature alcohol, and as a topical anesthetic. It is also highly antibacterial, and can also help combat mold growth. Glucosinolates are hydrolysed by the enzyme commonly known as myrosinase to a variety of compounds (isothiocyanates, nitriles, thiocyanates, epithionitriles, oxazolidines), the composition of which depends on pH, metal ions and other protein elements. Mustard oil glycosides are present in *Armoracia lapathifolia, Brassica campestris, B. napus, B. oleracea, B. carinata,B. juncea, B. hirta, Carica papaya, Rhaphanus sativus, Capparis spinosa,Cranbe abyssinica, Lepidium sativum, Camelina sativa,* and *Moringa oleifera.*

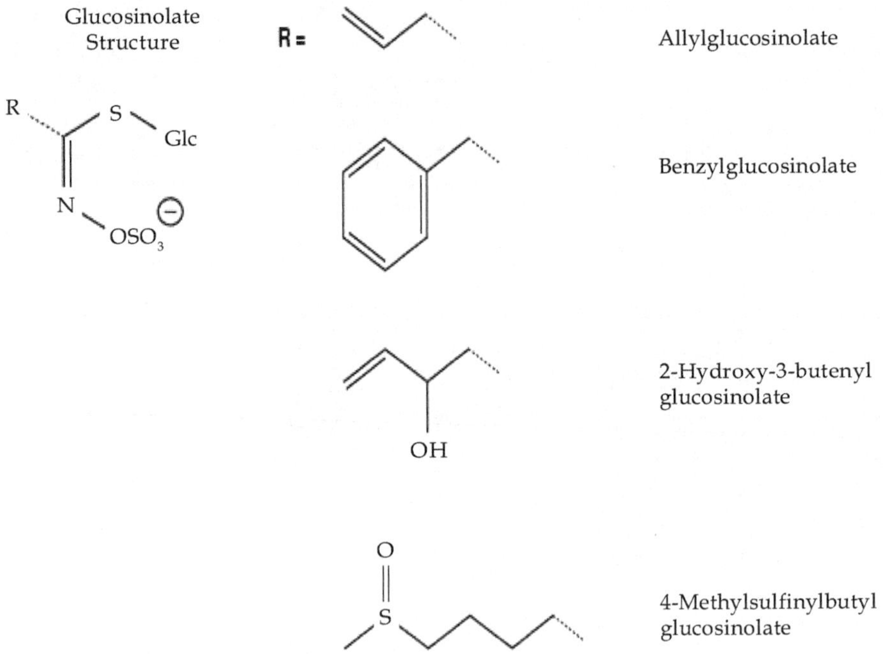

Mechanism of action

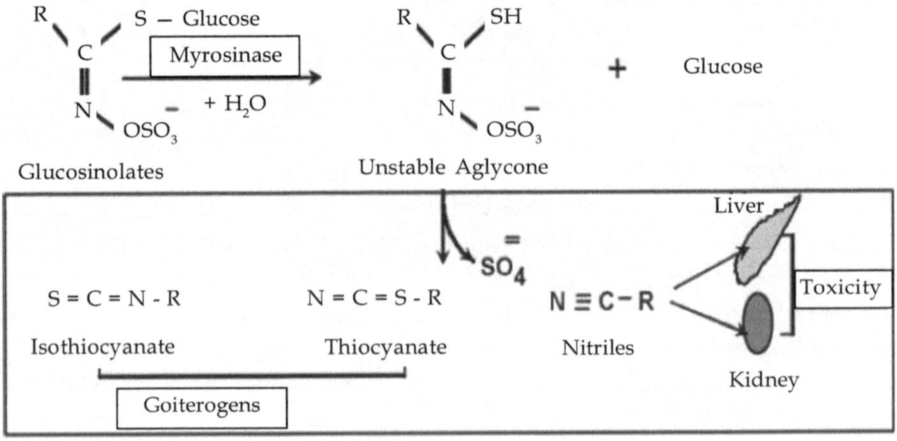

Sinigrin

The molecular formula of sinigrin is $C_{10}\ H_{16}\ O_9\ N\ S_2\ K$ which is a simplest mustard oil glycoside. It occurs not only in black mustard seed but also in other spp. of Brassica. A related compound allyl sulphide is responsible for the flavor of onion and garlic.

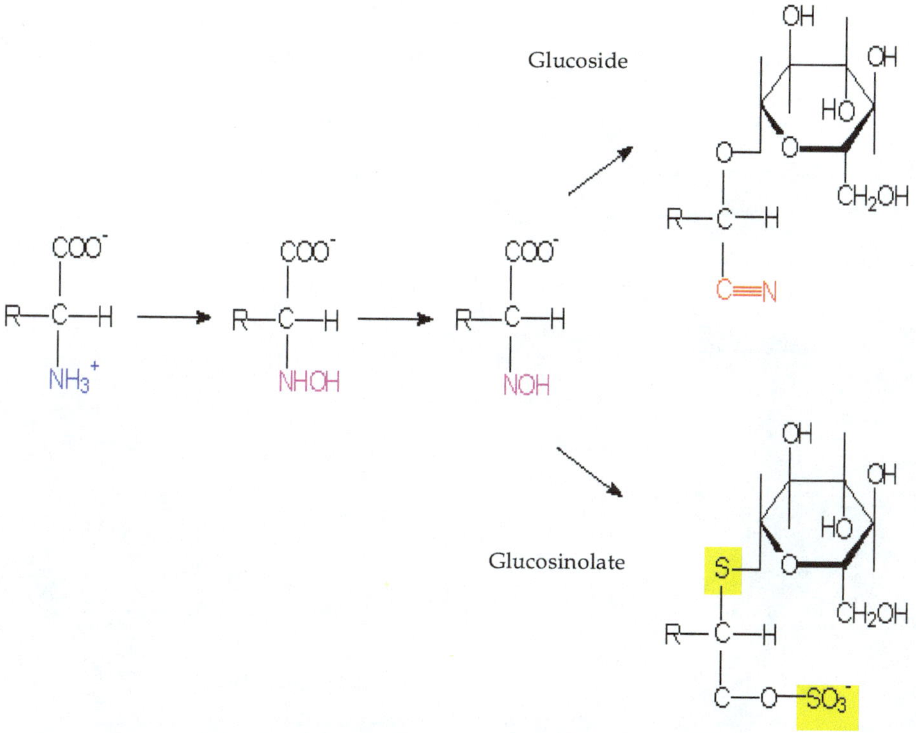

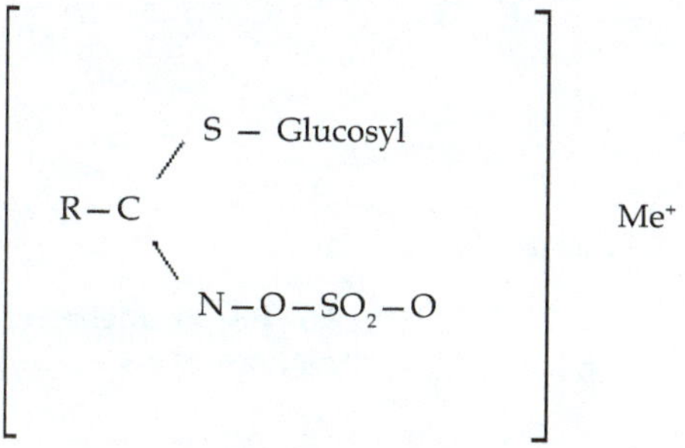

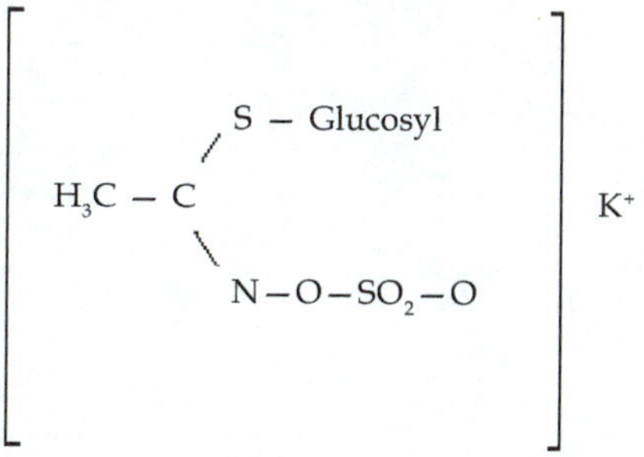

Mustard Oil Glucoside

Glucocapparine

Mustard Oil
$R-N=C=S$

Biosynthesis of mustard glycosides

a. Side chain elongation of precursor amino acids: Through transamination, the aminoacid is converted to the corresponding ketoacid, followed by incorporation of an acetyl residue from acetyl coenzyme A. After isomerization the compounds are oxidized. The keto-acid produced is transaminated to yield aminoacid that is elongated by a methylene group.

b. Biosynthesis of basic glucosinolates: It involves the conversion of aminoacids to oximes which is followed by addition of sulfhydryl group & glycosylation of thiohydroximates.

c. Side chain modification of basic glucosinolates.

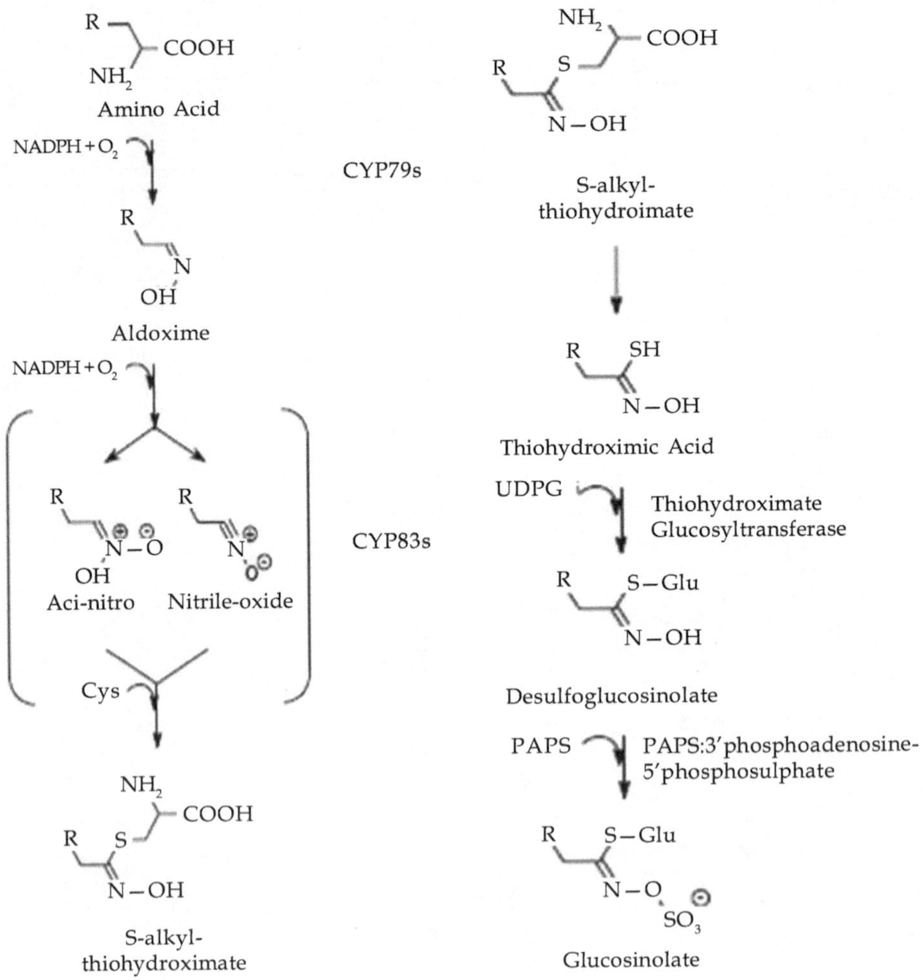

Biological Significance

- Interactions with herbivores and microorganisms: Deterrents by rendering plant unpallatable. However, interactions with microorganisms show little effect on them.
- Glucosinolates & Nutrition: Isothiocyanates stimulate anticarcinogenic process.

Saponins

Saponins are generally known as non-volatile, surface active compounds that are widely distributed in nature, occurring primarily in the plant kingdom. The name 'saponin' was derived from the Latin word sapo, which means 'soap', because saponin molecules form soap-like foams when shaken with water .Chemically referred to as triterpene and steroid glycosides.They consist of nonpolar aglycones coupled with one or more monosaccharide moieties. These combinations of polar and non-polar structural elements in their molecules explain their soap like behaviour in aqueous solutions. The main Dietary sources of saponins are legumes (soybeans, chickpeas, mungbeans, peanuts, broad beans, kidney beans, lentils), they are also present in oats, allium species (leek, garlic), asparagus, tea, spinach, sugarbeet, and yam.

Soap bark tree (*Quillaja saponaria*), fenugreek *(Trigonella foenum-graceum)*, alfalfa (*Medicago sativa*), horse chestnut (*Aesculus hippocastanum*), licorice (Glycyrrhiza species such as *Glycyrrhiza glabra*), soapwort (*Saponaria officinalis)*, Mojave yucca (*Yucca schidigera*), gypsophila genus (such as *Gypsophila paniculata*), sarsaparilla (*Smilax regelii* and other closely related species of Smilax genus) and ginseng (Panax genus) are the main non-food sources of saponins used in health and industrial applications.

They are widely distributed in plants especially in the roots, leaves and seeds. An outstanding property of this glycoside is their ability to form colloidal solution in water which gives soapy foam and forms stable emulsion with oils, fats and resins. The soapwort and soapnut (Aritha) owes their names to this property which gives them the power to occlude the gases. The non-toxic saponin Sarsaparilla is used commercially in the manufacturing of carbonated beverages. Saponin glycosides are divided into two types based on the chemical structure of their aglycones (sapogenin).

Saponins = Sugar + Sapogenin

Saponins are glycosides containing one or more sugar chains on a triterpene or steroid aglycone backbone also called a sapogenin. They are categorized according to the number of sugar chains in their structure as mono, di-, or tridesmosidic. The most common monosaccharides include: D-glucose (Glc), D-galactose (Gal), D-glucuronic acid (GlcA), D-galacturonic acid (GalA), L-rhamnose (Rha), L-arabinose (Ara), D-xylose (Xyl), and D-fucose (Fuc).

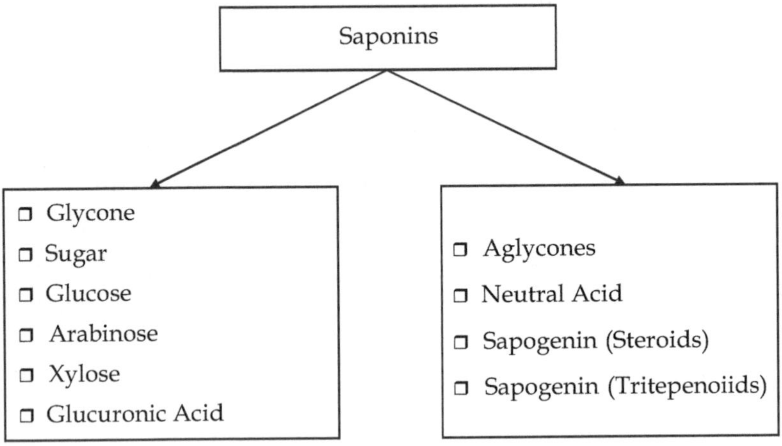

The so called neutral saponins are derivatives of steroids with spiroketal side chains. The acid saponins possess triterpenoid structures. The main pathway leading to both types of sapogenins is similar and involves the head - to - tail coupling of acetate units. However, a branch occurs after the formation of the triterpenoid hydrocarbons, squlene that leads to steroids in one direction and to cyclic triterpenoids in the other direction.

Glycyrrhiza is the dried rhizome and roots of *Glycyrrhiza glabra.* Glycyrrhiza contains a saponin glycosides called Glycyrrhizin (Glycyrrhizinic acid) glycyrrhizin is fifty times more sweeter than common sugar sucrose. Upon hydrolysis, the glycoside losses its sweet taste and is converted to the aglycone glycyrrhetinic acid is a penta cyclic triterpenod derivative of the beta-amyrin type. It has expectorant and antitussive properties. Expectorants are used to decrease the viscosity of tenacious mucus, or to increase the secretion of mucus in the dry irritant unproductive cough, thereby lubricating the air passages and making coughing more productive. It is used considerably as a flavoring agent and is frequently employed to mask the taste of bitter drugs such as aloe, quinine etc.

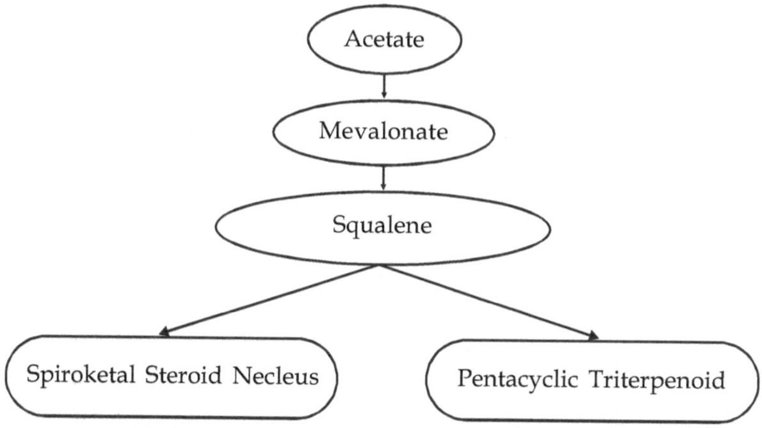

The saponins are usually light colored powder and few are crystalline. On hydrolysis, they yield variety of sugars such as glucose, galactose, arabinose and some unique pentoses together with sapogenin substances which are physiologically active. Saponins form colloidal solution in water (hydrophilic colloids) which froths upon shaking. These substances lower the surface tension and hence foam when shaken. This has led to their use to increase the foaming of beer. Due to the presence of a lipid-soluble aglycone and watersoluble sugar chain(s) in their structure (amphiphilic nature), saponins are surface active compounds with detergent, wetting, emulsifying, and foaming properties. In aqueous solutions surfactants form micelles. They are generally bitter.

Industrial applications of saponins include their use in cleaning industrial equipment and fine fabrics and as powerful emulsifiers of certain resins, fats and fixed oils. When taken by mouth, Saponins are comparatively harmless, being not absorbed from the intestinal tract. Sarsaparilla, for example, is rich in saponins but is widely used in the preparation of nonalcoholic beverages. Saponins are toxic especially to cold-blooded animals e.g. frogs. Many are used as fish-poisons.

Biological Activity

Saponins hemolyze red blood cells by nonspecific interactions with membrane proteins, phospholipids, and cholesterol of erythrocytes.

Saponins can impact the immune system through their adjuvant activity, their ability to improve effectiveness of orally administered vaccines by facilitating the absorption of large molecules, and their immuno stimulatory effects. Saponins lower cholesterol due to inhibition of the absorption of cholesterol from the small intestine, or the reabsorption of bile acids.

Anticancer Activity

The toxicity of saponins to insects (insecticidal activity), parasite worms (anthelmintic activity), molluscs (molluscicidal), and fish (piscidal activity) and their antifungal, antiviral, and antibacterial activity.

Low oral toxicity to humans due to low absorption rate from intestine.

Commercial Applications

Food Applications

Licorice and licorice derivatives are used in foods such as baked foods, beverages, chewing gum, candy, herbs and seasonings, plant protein products, and vitamin and mineral dietary supplements as a flavoring agent. Quillaja extract is used in foods and beverages mainly for its foaming properties.

Cosmetics

Saponins are being utilized as natural surfactants in cleansing products in the personal care sector such as shower gels, shampoos, foam baths, hair conditioners and lotions, bath/shower detergents, liquid soaps, baby care products, mouth washes, and toothpastes. (Due to surface active property).

Pharmaceutical /Health Applications

Raw materials for the production of steroid hormones and drugs, e.g. the synthesis of progesterone from the sapogenin diosgenin. Saponin-containing plants such as ginseng, yucca, horse chestnut, sarsaparilla, and licorice have been used in traditional medicine. Ouabaine glycoside from *Strophanthus* sps. inhibits active transport of Na^+ in cardiac muscle.

Phenolic Glycosides

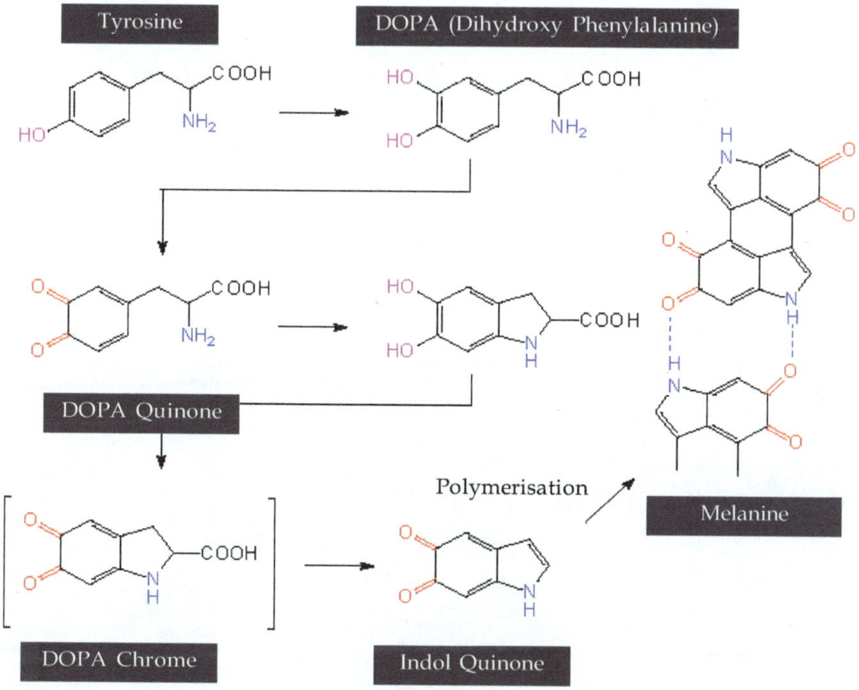

Most phenolic compounds belong to the flavonoids. Lignin, the primary substance of wood, is the most common member of this group. The following table outlines the most important groups of plant phenolic compounds.

The starting product of the biosynthesis of most phenolic compounds is shikimate. Phenols are acidic due to the dissociability of their -OH group. They are rather reactive compounds and as long as no steric inhibition due to additional side chains occurs, they form hydrogen bonds. Consequently, many flavonoids have intra molecular bonds. Another important feature is their ability to form chelate complexes with metals. Also, they are easily oxidized and, if so, form polymers (dark aggregates). The darkening of cut or dying plant parts is caused by this reaction. They have usually an inhibiting effect on plant growth. Among the phenylpropanol derivatives of lower molecular weight are a number of scents like the coumarins, cinnamic acid, sinapinic acid, the coniferyl alcohols and others. These substances and their derivatives are at the same time intermediates of the biosynthesis of lignin.

The Most Important Classes of Phenolic Compounds in Plants

Number of C-atoms	Basic skeleton	Class
6	C_6	simple phenols, benzoquinones
7	$C_6 - C_1$	phenolic acids
8	$C_6 - C_2$	acetophenone, phenylacetic acid
9	$C_6 - C_3$	hydroxycinnamic acid, polypropene, coumarin, isocoumarin
10	$C_6 - C_4$	naphtoquinone
13	$C_6 - C_1 - C_6$	xanthone
14	$C_6 - C_2 - C_6$	stilbene, anthrachinone
15	$C_6 - C_3 - C_6$	flavonoids, isoflavonoids
18	$(C_6 - C_3)_2$	lignans, neolignans
30	$(C_6 - C_3 - C_6)_2$	biflavonoids
n	$(C_6 - C_3)_n$	lignins
	$(C_6)_n$	catecholmelanine
	$(C_6 - C_3 - C_6)_n$	(condensed tannins)

The aglucones of these glycosides are all aromatic compounds containing phenolics group to which sugar is attached. The aglucone may be a simple phenol or may in addition be alcohol, aldehyde, ketone etc. Arbutin, gein, phloridzin, saicin and populin are the important members of this group.

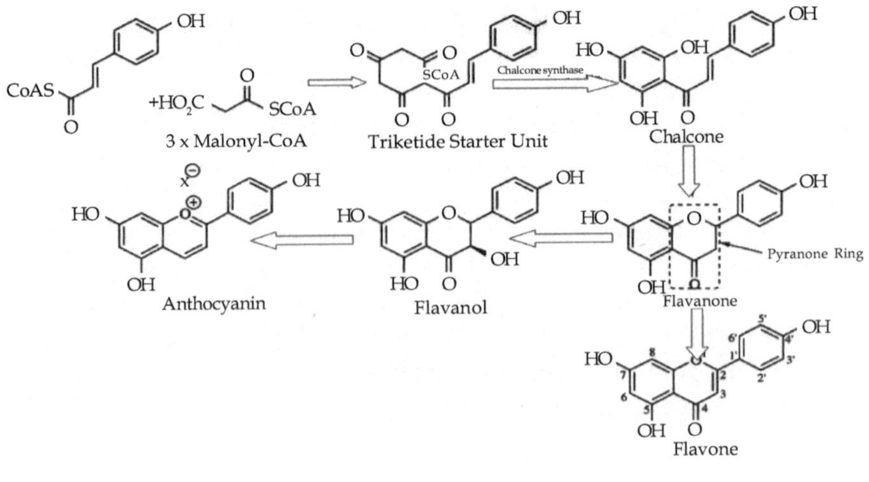

Tannins

Chemically tannins are either free phenol acids or more commonly glucosides of these acids. A part of tannin is hydrolysable with acids to yield phenolic derivative and in some cases sugars, usually D-glucose. Tannin is general name of group of substances distributed widely in higher plants. They are found in leaves, stems, bark and particularly in unripe seeds. Plant galls are especially rich, to the extent of 75 % of tannin. They are absent in animal body.

Tannin and tannin like compound are wide spread in nature and are probably present in all plant materials. Those are polyphenolic compounds divided in to two main group hydrolysable and condensed. Hydrolysable tannin contain a polyhydric alcohol usually if not always glucose esterified with gallic acid or with hexahydroxy diphenic acid. Condensed tannin are mostly flavanols and are probably polymer of flavan 3-ol and these can not be hydrolyse to simple component. Among the cereal sorghum has been found to contain higher amount of polyphenols, even though high polyhenol seed are imune to attach by bird and disease they display impaired nutrition quality lower digestibility and reduction of food consumption.

Tannins can be broadly classified in two categories.

1. Pyragallol tannins and
2. Catechol tannins.

Properties of Tannins

- They are amorphous and rarely crystalline
- They have astringent taste.
- They yield characteristic (inks) with ferric salts.
- They are precipitated from solution by potassium dichromate, lead acetate and by alkaloids.
- They precipitate gelatin from solution, a property that is used in conversion of hide into leather.
- Readily soluble in hot water to form colloidal solution.
- Tannins are astringent, bitter-tasting plant polyphenols that bind and precipitate proteins.
- The term tannin refers to the use of tannins in tanning animal hides into leather; Tannins have molecular weights ranging from 500 to over 3,000.

- The tea plant (*Camellia saneness*) high tannin content. When any type of tea leaf is steeped in hot water it brews a "tart" (astringent) flavor that is characteristic of tannins. This is due to the catechins and other flavonoids. Tea "tannins" are chemically distinct from other types of plant tannins such as tannic acid and tea extracts have been reported to contain no tannic acid.

Functions of tannins

Because of wide distribution of tannins in plant kingdom, they have different roles to play.

1. It is suggested that plant builds up tannins as a means of neutralising acids by esterification. Tannins are accumulated wherever intense metabolism is in progress. e.g. leaves, young tissues, galls, germinating seeds etc. Thus tannins serve as safe accumulation or excessive synthetic or metabolic products.
2. On ripening of fruits, fruits attain different colours, attributing a role of tannins in the pigment formation.
3. Certain tannins are believed to serve as protective agents to prevent the growth of parasitic fungi on fruits.
4. The presence of tannins in unripe fruits impart an astringent taste is a special protection against the damage by animals.

Uses

Tannins are an important ingredient in the process of tanning leather. Tannins may be employed medicinally antidiarrheal, hemostatic, and antihemorrhoidal compounds. Tannin is a component in a type of industrial particleboard adhesive. Tannins, including gallo and ellagic acid (epigallitannins), are inhibitors of HIV replication. Inhibited HIV replication in infected H9 lymphocytes with little cytotoxicity. Two compounds, punicalin and punicacortein C, inhibited purified HIV reverse transcriptase.

Cardenolides (Cardiac glycosides)

Cardenolides are C23 steroid derivatives which have cardiac activity & hence called Cardiac glycosides. Digitalin is the cardiac glycoside in *Digitalis* species. In low doses, cardenolides are widely used as a medicine against heart disease. The closely related cardiac glycoside, strophanthin, is found in the Apocynaceae. They occur in several plant families & some insects.

Plant Pigments

Pigments are heterogeneous group of chemicals found both in plants and animals. They are coloured substances and absorb light in visible range. We will study only the pigments of plant origin as their relation with agriculture.

Plant pigments are of two types, which are as under.

1. Plastid pigments (Chlorophyll, Carotenoids, Phycobillins)
2. Cell sap or soluble pigments (Anthocyanins and Anthoxanthins).

Chlorophylls

They are green plant pigments that absorb light for photosynthesis. There are four types of chlorophylls *viz.*, chlorophyll a, b, c and d. The chlorophyll a and b are more prominent of all. Chlorophyll a is present in all green plants including some bacteria while chlorophyll b is present in higher plants and green algae. While chlorophyll c is observed in diatoms and chlorophyll d in some red algae. Chlorophylls in higher plants are found in chloroplast. They are soluble in organic solvents such as ether, acetone, benzene etc. They can be separated by Thin Layer Chromatography.

Chlorophylls have a porphyrin structure or a tetra pyrrole nucleus with Mg atom in the centre. A phytol tail and a methyl group are attached to the nucleus. Both chlorophyll work in close co - operation for the conversion of light into chemical energy. The differences between chlorophyll a and b lies in methyl group attachment in ring two of chlorophyll a whereas an aldehyde group in chlorophyll b. The Mg atom of chlorophyll remained attached with four pyrrole group.

Properities of Chlorophylls

- Ash present is 4.5 % as MgO
- Phytol a mono atomic alcohols forms 1/3 of the molecule.
- Associated yellow pigments are not a part of chlorophyll.
- Chlorophyll when saponified with KOH, the colour changes to brown.
- There is no change in absorption of crude chlorophyll with the pure chlorophyll preparations.

Carotenoids

It is a principle pigment of carrot roots. Carotene ($C_{40}H_{56}$) is a mixture of two isomers α and β carotene. They do not have oxygen molecule. β carotene is a precursor of Vitamin A synthesis. It is yellow in colour situated in chloroplast lamella. They absorb light in the region of 430 - 480 nm. It is a isoprenoid hydrocarbon.

Phycobilins

Phycobilins are algal pigments, which absorb light. The light absorbed by these pigments is transferred to chlorophyll where it can be used for photosynthesis. Thus they help chlorophyll in photosynthesis so they are called "Accessory pigments". There are two types of phycobillins:

1. Phycoerythrobillins (A red phycobillin) are found in red algae.
2. Phycocyanobillins (A blue phycobillin) are found in blue green algae. They do not contain Mg atom in the structure. They do not have phytyl side chain unlike chlorophyll. They have linear tetra - pyrrole structure.

Cell Sap (Soluble Pigments)

Only the cell sap pigments such as anthocyanins and anthoxanthins are having the properties of glycosides.

Anthocyanin

These are the red, violet and blue pigments which occur in the cell sap of flowers, many fruits, stems and leaves of some plants.

They are the derivatives of 2-phenyl-benzopyrrilium salt. The principal differences between various anthocyanins are due to following reasons:

1. The degree of hydroxylation of the phenyl ring and
2. Presence or absence of methyl ester.

Structurally these are glycosides having glucose, galactose or mannose sugars. These sugars are always attached to carbon No.3. Hydrolysis of anthocyanins yields sugars + anthocyanidin and sometimes other residues such as para amino hydroxy benzoic acid (PHBA), para hydroxy cinnamic acid etc. They are amphoteric and forms salts with acids.

Their solutions give three distinct colors at different pH.

Red Colour	→	Acidic pH
Violet Colour	→	Neutral pH
Blue Colour	→	Alkaline pH

Anthoxanthines

Among the water soluble pigments, these are glucosides which occur as amorphous or crystalline form. Glycosides of anthoxanthins are almost colourless but free anthoxanthins and potassium salts are yellow. Anthoxanthins include phenolic derivatives of 5 modifications of benzo pyrone structures.

Flavones : Found in yellow Dahlia. Flavones are a class of flavonoids based on the backbone of 2-phenylchromen-4-one (2-phenyl-1-benzopyran-4-one).Natural flavones include Apigenin (4',5,7-trihydroxyflavone), Luteolin (3',4',5,7-tetrahydroxyflavone) and Tangeritin (4',5,6,7,8-pentamethoxyflavone). Synthetic flavones are Diosmin and Flavoxate.

Flavanols : Found in tea leaves

Flavanones : Found in Flowers and shaddock

Xanthones : Found in gentianaceae

Flavonoids :

In 1975, the number of identified flavonoids was estimated to be larger than 2000. Some important representatives and their biological significance are listed in the table below.

The Most Important Classes of Flavonoids and their Biological Significance

Class	**Number of known members**	**Biological significance (so far as known)**
anthocyanin(s)	250	red and blue pigments
chalcons	60	yellow pigments
aurones	20	yellow pigments
flavones	350	cream-coloured pigments of flowers
flavonols	350	feeding repellents (?) in leaves
dihydrochalcons	10	some taste bitter
proanthocyanidins	50	astringent substances
catechins	40	some have properties like those of tannins
biflavonoids	65	pigments of flowers, leaves and seeds
isoflavonoids	15	oestrogen effect, toxic for fungi

Isoflavones

They are a class of organic compounds and biomolecules related to the flavonoids. They act as phytoestrogens in mammals. They are also very strong antioxidants. Isoflavones are thought of by many as useful in treating cancer. Isoflavone found in orange fruit. Isoflavones chemical structure of it backbone (3-phenyl-4*H*-1-benzopyr-4-one differs from flavone in the following: in isoflavones, the position of the phenyl group on the 4*H*-1-benzopyr-4-one skeleton is in position 3 relative to the oxygen of the ring, whereas in flavones it is in position 2. Isoflavones are polyphenolic compounds produced almost exclusively by the members of the *Fabaceae/Leguminosae* (bean) family. They have significant in cholesterol-reducing effects and protection against certain types of cancers, as well as other benefits. Critics claim that isoflavones increase the incidence of epithelial hyperplasia, which precedes cancerous tumors, and that they cause goitre and hyperthyroidism. Early evidence that plants produced estrogen-like compounds was observed in the infertility among sheep eating large amounts of clover.

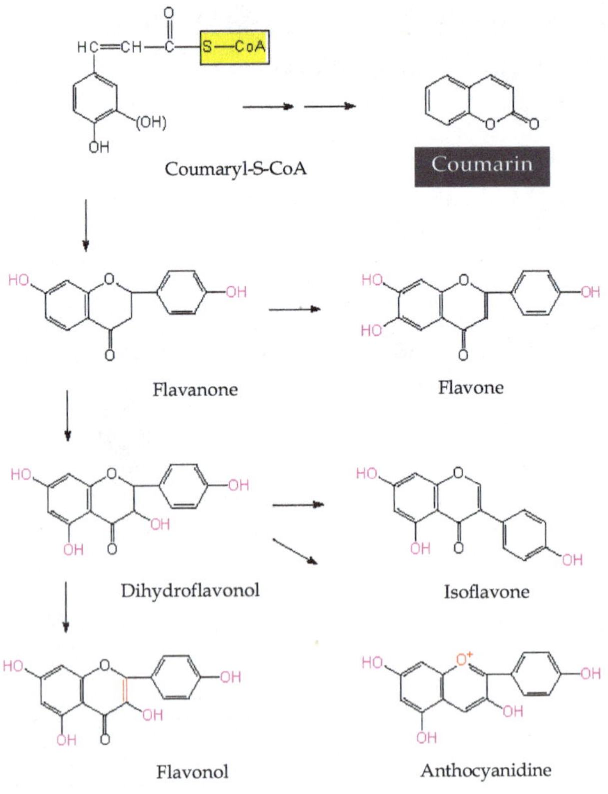

The basic structure of flavonoids is derived from the C_{15} body of flavone. They differ from other phenolic substances in the degree of oxidation of their central pyran ring. and very fundamentally, also in their biological properties. While some classes (e.g., the flavonones,) are colourless, the members of other classes (e.g., the anthocyanes) are always coloured and known as pigments of flowers or other plant parts. Anthocyanes are normally red or yellow, their colour is pH-dependent. Blue pigments are achieved by chelate formation with certain metal ions (Fe^{III} or Al^{III}, for example).

The variability of the flavonoids is largely based on the hydroxylation and/or methylation pattern of the three ring systems. A correlation between two flavonoids points often to a relationship between the producing plant species. They have therefore proven to be suitable traits for the study of the phylogenetic relations between higher plants. The quinones are another group of phenolic compounds. As has been mentioned before, phenolic compounds occur usually not unbound within plant tissues. They are mostly coupled to other molecules, often to glucosyl residues, but to sulphate- or acetyl-residues, too. One of the reasons may be that they are toxic when in a free state and are detoxified, at least partially, if coupled. Many low molecular weight compounds, for example thymol, are used in medicine as antiseptics due to their toxicity. Different types of bonds between flavonoids (for example anthocyanes) and a glycosyl residue lead to different derivatives that increase the range of flower colours (and colour shades). The glycosylation of flavonoids has an additional, ecologically not less important function. It has been brought into connection with pest protection and protection against other animals.

Physiological role and biological significance of glycosides

With such a wide variety of glucosides, whose only similarity is that they contain a sugar residue, it would be strange to expect that they will have same functions in the plants but their functions are varied in nature.

1. They act as reserve food materials.
2. As a means of removal of injurious compounds.
3. Act as antiseptics or hormone.

Biological importance of anthocyanins/athoxanthins

- Due to anthocyanins, various natural colors are imparted to the flowers to which attract the insect for the cross pollination.
- Isoflavones as genistein, present in clover and other legume forage crops are weak estrogen and when consumed in sufficient quantities reduce the fertility of sheep.
- On the other hand, the ingestion of clover isoflavones may be beneficial in the cow as they contribute to the well known 'Spring-flush' of milk i.e. higher milk production in cows.

Uses

- Used as a stabilizer in such dairy products as ice creams, sherbets, chocolate milk, yogurt and whipped cream
- Used in lotions to soften the skin & prevent premature wrinkling
- Used to thicken cosmetics
- Used as a binding agent in toothpastes etc.
- Used in brewing as a fining
- It has also been used to treat bronchitis, goiter, thyroid problems, and to tone and strengthen the body's glands.
- It have mild anticoagulant effect on the blood; treats chronic lung diseases, dysentery, diarrhoea and disorders of kidney and bladder.

Chapter 7

Gums and Mucilages

The plant gums are the neutral salts and complex polysaccharide acids which contain methyl pentose, pentose, hexose and uronic acid residues joined glycosidically by linkages involving various carbon atoms within one molecule to form branched chain structure. Uronic acid is generally present in all cases. The sugars include L-fructose, D-xylose, L-arabinose, D-rhamnose, and D-galactose.

General Properties of Gums

They have high molecular weight. Some are linear while some are branched. They are generally viscous in nature. Some forms a gel also. They have tremendous commercial application in food industry. Gums may be an exudates gum produced by the plant or may be a seed gum, which is accumulated during the seed maturity. Gums of polysaccharide origin are obtained from *Acacia spp.* (gum Arabic), *Cymopsis tetragonolobus* (guar gum), *Guggle gum, Ficus indica,* chia gum etc (Table 7.1).

Table 7.1 : Sugar components of some gums and mucilage.

Gums	**Plant spp**	**Sugars present**
Gum Arabic	*Acacia* spp.	D-galactose, L-arabinose, L-rhamnose D-glucuronic acid
Cherry Gum	*Prunus* spp.	D-arabinose, D-xylose, D-mannose, D-galactose, D-glucuronic acid
Mucilage	**Plant spp.**	**Sugars present**
Flax Seeds	*Linum* spp.	D-xylose, D-galactose, D-rhamnose, D-galacturonic acid
Blond Psyllum	*Plantago* spp.	D-xylose, L-arabinose, L-rhamnose, D-galacturonic acid

Gums and mucilage are either soluble in water or strongly hydrophilic but not soluble in organic solvents. The solutions are leavo-rotatory. Glucuronic acid occur as Na, Ca or K salts but enough free carboxyl groups remain to produce slightly acidic solution. Gums generally harden upon drying. Gums generally differ from mucilages based on following criteria.

Gums	**Mucilage**
Produced in response to injury	Normal plant constituent
Found as exudates on various trees.	They are found in xerophytes, seeds and young buds
Sometimes, associated with triterpenoid compounds as gum-resin	Associated with sugars only
Contain glucuronic acid in the structure.	Contain galacturonic acid
Examples: gum-arabic, guar-gum cherry gum etc	*Examples:* Mucilage of Isabgol and okra seeds

Exudate Gum

They may be exuded in small quantity or in large amount depending upon the plant species. These gums are produced by either shrub type or low growing type trees. The examples are gum Arabic, gum, karaya, gum ghatti. Acacia trees are useful for preventing the desert encroachment.

Acacia Gum

It has lowest molecular weight and lowest viscosity. It is used in food industry, confectionary as an anti-crystallizing agent for sugars, thickening agent. It has varied uses in chewing gum, cough drops and a stabilizer for the ice-cream and *'sharbat'*. These gums are also used in baking industry as flavor fixative as well as in cosmetic, paint, ink, lithography and textile industry.

Seed Gums

It is a well known fact that the seeds store starch as reserve food material, but many plant seeds such as *Psyllum (*Isabgol), flax, guar and locust seeds produce a non-starch food reserve polysaccharide.

Gum Arabic (Gum Acacia)

It is exuded from African spp. of *Acacia* is a well known example of a gum. This compound is a salt in which Ca, Mg and K have replaced some of the hydrogens on the carboxyl group. The plant mucilage are water soluble polysaccharide that contain d-galacturonic acid and the same general gluco sugars of gums.

Guar Gum (*Cymopsis tetragonolobus*)

The gum produced by *Cymopsis tetragonolobus*, which is a legume crop is called guar gum. This gum finds wide industrial applications. The endosperm of the seed has 35-42% gum which is a galactomannan. The pure form is called **Guaran**. The seed hull contains 14-17 % while seed germ has 43-47 % gum. The gum produced by endosperm has commercial value.

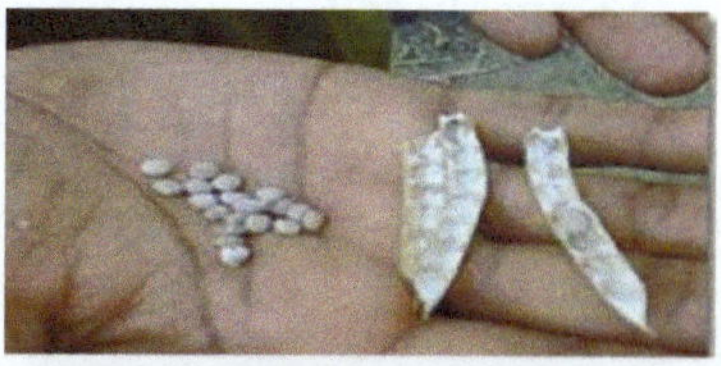

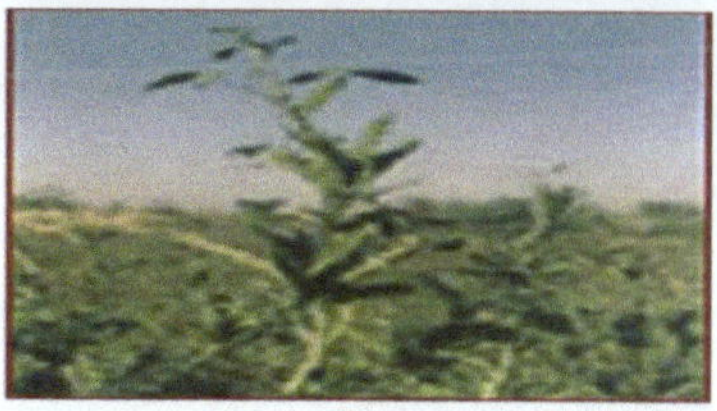

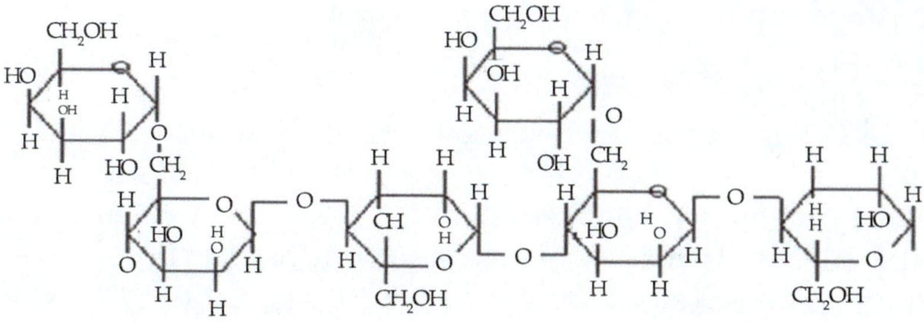

The structure of guaran suggest a linear chain of ($1 \rightarrow 4$) linked β-D-mannopyranosyl units with a single α-D-galactopyranosyl unit attached to every second unit by a $1 \rightarrow 6$ linkage. It has linear structure and highly viscous even at low concentrations. Solution of guaran is highly stable. The galactose units of the chain can be broken down enzymatically to make it only mannose residues. This composition has a capacity to form gel which can be used in the food industry. Guar seeds are excellent source of proteins and trypsin inhibitors.

Uses

- It is used as thickening agent in food industry.
- It has applications in sizing of paper and textile industry.
- Control physical properties: suspending agent, dispersant, emulsifier, stabilizer.
- It can form gel by modifying the gum enzymatically to be used as gel forming agent and as coagulant.
- It can be used as binder, lubricant and film former too.

Guggle Gum (*Commiphora Spp.*)

Guggle is a medicinally important plant which produces a unique type of gum that is called oleo-gum-resin of guggle.

Locust Bean Gum
Carob Gum

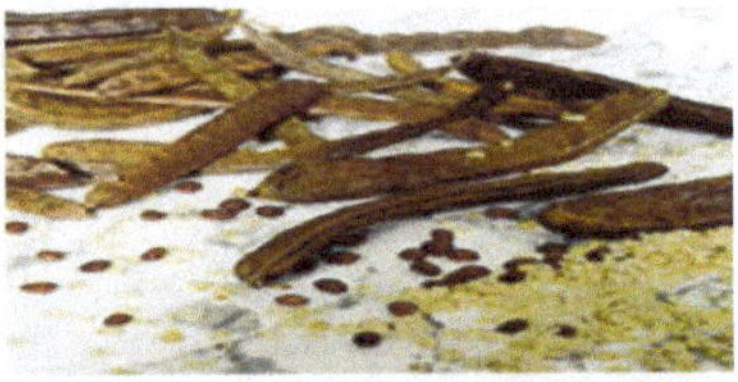

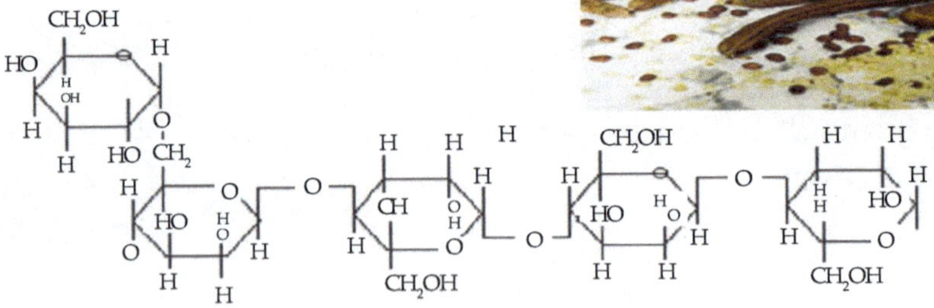

Oleo-Gum-Resin of Guggle

The oleo-gum-resins are the mixtures of resin, gum, volatile oils and occasionally combined with small amount of other substances. It is yellowish in colour, which solidifies to an agglomerate of tears of stalactitic pieces. It has insoluble and soluble portions in equal proportions. It has ketonic and non-ketonic fractions. The ketonic fraction has 12 % of ethyl acetate soluble neutral part. This is a steroidal part having two compounds namely z-gugglesterone and e-gugglesterone. This has a lipid lowering activity. The non-ketonic fraction exert synergistic action on the biological activity of ketonic fraction.

Uses

This guggle gum has many medicinal uses. It is used for the treatment of rheumatism, for reducing the obesity and arthritis. It has a property of reducing the cholesterol of the blood.

- It contains polysaccharide Galactomannan D-Mannose (1-4) with Galactose (1-6) every 4th mannose
- Its molecular weight 330,000 ± 30,000
- Its neutral - relatively unaffected by ions, pH.
- Its not soluble in cold water
- Fully hydrated if heated 10 minutes at 80° C
- Solutions are cloudy, off-white
- Modify properties of
  - Carrageenan
  - Xanthan Gum

Mucilage Producing Plants

1. Aloe vera
2. Cactus
3. Chondrus crispus (Irish moss)
4. Drosera(sundews)
5. Fenugreek
6. Flax seeds
7. Kelp
8. Liquorice root
9. Marshmallow
10. Mullein
11. Okra
12. Parthenium
13. Pinguicula (butterwort)

Mucilages of *Aloe vera*

Aloe vera Gel is the colourless mucilaginous gel obtained from the parenchymatous cells in the fresh leaves of *Aloe vera*. They are Viscous, colourless, odourless, taste slightly bitter. It consists primarily of water and polysaccharides (pectins, hemicelluloses, glucomannan, and mannose derivatives). It also contains amino acids, lipids, sterols (lupeol, campesterol, and -sitosterol), tannins, and enzymes. Mannose 6-phosphate is a major sugar component.

Uses

Aloe vera Gel is widely used for the external treatment of minor wounds and inflammatory skin disorders.

Chondrus cripus (Irish moss)

- It is composed of polysaccharides (carrageenans), sulphur compounds, protein, iodine, bromine, iron, other mineral salts, vitamins A and B1.
- Irish Moss is not a moss it is a seaweed. It varies in colour from a greenish-yellow to a dark purple or purplish-brown; but when preserved it turns a yellowish and translucent.
- The principal constituent of Irish moss is a mucilagienous body, made of the polysaccharide about 55%; the plant also has nearly 10% of protein and about 15% of mineral matter.

Uses

- Used as a stabilizer in such dairy products as ice creams, *sharbets*, chocolate milk, yogurt and whipped cream
- Used in lotions to soften the skin & prevent premature wrinkling
- Used to thicken cosmetics
- Used as a binding agent in toothpastes etc.
- Used in brewing as a fining
- It has also been used to treat bronchitis, goiter, thyroid problems, and to tone and strengthen the body's glands.
- It have mild anticoagulant effect on the blood; treats chronic lung diseases, dysentery, diarrhoea and disorders of kidney and bladder.

There are many plants which produces a hetero-polysaccharide, viscous material in the seeds which is called mucilage. The mucilage producing plants are *Plantago ovata* (Isabgol), *Hibiscus esculentus* (Okra mucilage), *Fenugreek {methi} mucilage (Trigonella foenum), Actinidia spp., Jew's mellow leaves mucilage* etc. The all mucilage contain methyl pentose, glucose, galactose, fructose and galacturonic or glucuronic acid. The okra and Isabgol mucilage are acidic in nature, while the fenugreek mucilage is neutral. Mucilage is synthesized in specialized cells which upon death become mucilage containers. They play important role in water and calcium economy of plant.

Mucilage of Isabgol (*Plantago ovata)*

Isabgol seed is encased in rosy white layer of husk. When soaked in water, the whole seed appears swollen because of expansion of mucilage in the husk. The mucilage of husk consists mainly of xylose, arabinose, and galacturonic acid. It also contains rhamnose and galactose. The mucilage constitutes over 30 % of the whole seed weight.

The mucilage of *P. ovata* seeds consists of two types of polysaccharides I and II. The polysaccharide I from seed is extracted with cold water which has 20 % uronic anhydride, 52 % pentosan and 18 % of methyl pentosan. Polysaccharide I , upon hydrolysis gives large amount of xylose. After extraction with cold water, further extraction with hot water (90-95° C) gives polysaccharide II. Polysaccharide II has 3 % uronic anhydride, 90 % pentosan and no methyl pentosan. They have 80 % xylose, 14 % arabinose and trace of galactose. The major sugar of Isabgol mucilage is xylose.

Uses

- Seed coat (husk) of Isabgol is used as a bulk laxative.
- Seeds after removal of husk are by-products of Isabgol used as ice-cream stabilizer.
- It is also used as cattle feed having a cooling demulcent effect.
- It has been reported to be effective in curing inflammation of mucus membrane of gastro-intestinal and genito-urinary tract.
- It has been used for termination of pregnancy.
- It has been found effective for curing piles.

Mucilage of Okra (*Hibiscus esculentus*)

The mucilage of immature okra fruit is obtained when fruits are placed in water. When the pod is boiled, fruit becomes highly mucilagenous. It is an acidic polysaccharide which is associated with minerals and protein. The polysaccharide is composed of galacturonic acid, rhamnose, galactose, xylose and glucose. It also contains methyl pentose and fructose. The maximum, viscosity is at neutral pH. It is unstable when heated. The concentration of glucuronic acid is higher than galacturonic acid.

Uses

Mucilage of okra is used in the sizing operation of paper. It is useful as a serum albumin and egg white extender. It is a good thickening agent for gravy preparation.

Fenugreek Seed (*Methi*) Mucilage (*Trigonella foenum*)

It is neutral mucilage having mannogalactan polysaccharide. It contains D- galactose and D- mannose. It also constitutes 25 % arabinose, 15 % methyl pentose, 11 % galactose, 22 % mannose and some fructose (6 %). There is absence of galacturonic and glucuronic acid residue suggesting their neutral nature.

Uses

It has many medicinal properties to be used as medicine.

Agar-Agar

The word agar comes from the *Malay* word agar-agar (meaning jelly). Agar or agar agar is a gelatinous substance chiefly used as a culture medium for microbiological work.

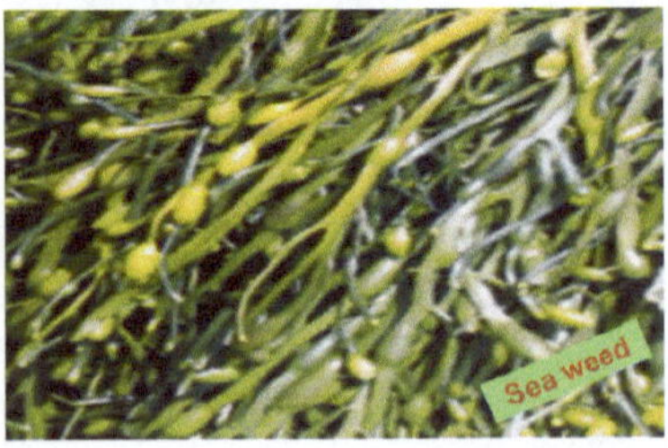

It is an unbranched polysaccharide obtained from the cell membranes of some species of red algae or seaweed. Seaweeds are any of a large number of marine benthic algae. They are macroscopic and multicellular, in contrast with most other algae. Seaweeds are often found in the seashore. Seaweeds consist of several groups of multicellular algae: the red algae, green algae, and brown algae.

Chemically, agar is a polymer made up of subunits of the sugar galactose. It can be used as a laxative, a vegetarian gelatin substitute, a thickener for soups, in jellies, ice cream and Japanese desserts such as *anmitsu*, as a clarifying agent in brewing, and for paper sizing fabrics. One of the best example of mucilage is agar-agar which is obtained from sea weed, *Gracilaria spp.*. About 30 % of the compound is made up of polysaccharide which galactose on hydrolysis. The polysaccharide is combined with H_2SO_4 in ester linkage with hydroxyl group. If Ca in the structure is removed, an acid known as Agar acid is produced. Solution of agar acid will not gel, but solution of agar salt will gel. This compound is useful to all the microbiologists because of its use in the preparation of semi-solid culture media for cultivating bacteria, fungi and actinomycete in the laboratory Petri dishes.

At the temperature of boiling water, it forms a solution but changes to gel on cooling at 45° C. There are no enzymes in bacteria or digestive tract capable of hydrolyzing agar. This becomes an added advantage of its use in preparation of laxative for constipation in animals.

Uses

- Agar agar is extensively used as solidifying agent the culture media preparations.
- It is used in the preparation of laxative for the constipation.

Chapter 8

Oleoresins

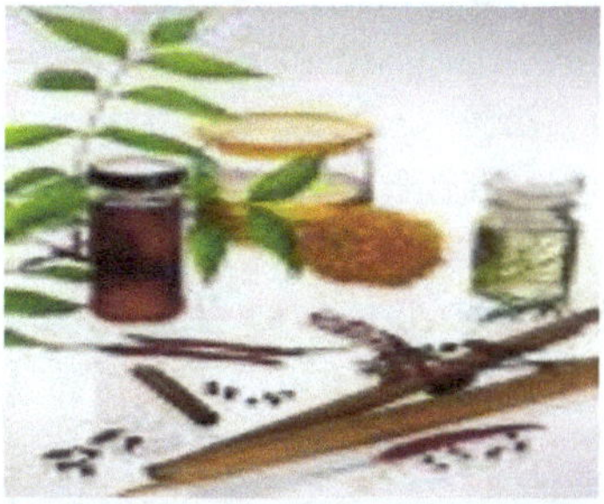

Plant oleoresins, often referred to as resins, are sticky plant secretions synthesized in large quantities by about 10 % of plant families. Resin is secreted when a plant is disturbed and the sticky substances produced contain many toxic compounds used to defend the plant from herbivores and pathogens. A major component of resin is the terpenoid compounds. Although terpenoid compounds can be quite complex, they are all composed of five-carbon units, with an isoprene unit as the base. The simplest of these terpenes are the monoterpenes that possess 10- carbon atoms derived from two fused isoprene units. Monoterpenes are an important component of the volatile portion of terpenes and often emit very strong odors.

Plant resin is a complex chemically diverse mixture of terpenoids that serve many functions. All living organisms contain terpenoids, but plants contain the highest diversity of terpenoids. Many terpenoids are considered secondary metabolites because they appear to lack direct function in basic growth and defense. These secondary metabolites of terpenes contain insect and microbial toxins and other agents that act to deter insect herbivory. Terpenes also act as band aids by sealing a plant wound. Once plant tissue is exposed to the air, the volatile terpene portion evaporates leaving a semi- hardened mass. Even though terpenoids are chemically diverse and perform many functions they are all made up of fusion of a five-carbon unit, known as isoprene. Production of terpenes takes place via similar chemical pathways and terpenes are then stored for defense. The amount of terpenes produced and released depends on several factors, such as drought and fire. Furthermore, the same terpenes that are produced for defense can be used by plant herbivores in host location and selection.Fossils from the carboniferous tropical forests demonstrate the earliest evidence of resin synthesis as well as the internal storage of resin in secretary canals. During this period resin was not produced in large amounts like current species. Based on phylogenetic analysis it seems that all plant terpene synthases share a common evolutionary origin and it has been suggested that the gene for multiple monoterpene synthase arose by gene duplication.

Primary terpenes are produced by the secretary epithelial cells and accumulate in resin cells. The complexity of the resin cells depends on the plant species. In conifers, resin cells can be isolated, as in cedars (*Thuga* sp.), or they can form blisters, as in true firs (*Abies* sp.). The most complex systems are those of pines (*Pinus* sp.) that form a highly complex network of branched canals capable of transporting resin many meters. When this network is severed, resin ducts will exude large amounts of resin. In addition to primary terpene production, conifers also possess an inducible terpene defense system that is produced by the parenchyma cells when injury occurs. This defense system leads to the formation of new traumatic resin ducts and increased resin flow in the area surrounding the injury.

The oleoresins represent the complete flavour which is non-volatile, resinous fraction present in spices and many medicinally important crops. The oleoresins have tremendous commercial and industrial value in the international markets.

It comprises of heat component, fixative, natural anti-oxidant and pigments. Hence, oleoresins can be designated as " true essence " of spices. The best-known example of oleoresin is the *capsicum* oleoresin from the chillies. Chilli contains an average of 8-16 % oleoresins in the fruits.

In food and beverage industries, chilli has acquired a great importance in the form of oleoresins, which permits better distribution of colour, and flavour in food as compared to chilli powder. The food industry prefers to use highly coloured and less pungent chillies for preparation of oleoresins.

Oleoresins in chillies offer many advantages over straight spices *viz.* cleanliness and uniform flavour. Oleoresin is used in preparation of processes products and also incorporated into number of pharmaceutical preparations. Demand for high quality oleoresin in chilli is preferred in international market.

For production of oleoresins, the clean, dry, graded spices are commuted and subjected to distillation to obtain the volatile essential oils which represents the aroma of spices. The de-oiled spice is dried, ground finer and extracted with suitable food grade solvents like hexane, ethylene dichloride etc. to recover the non-volatile taste principles. The aroma and taste fractions are proportionally blended and the 'true essence'. The oleoresins can be obtained in a single step by elimination of the steam distillation process. The oleoresins represent the flavour profile of spices.

Oleoresins can also be converted to powder form by dispersing on dry carriers such as flour, starch and dextrose. Conventionally, spice oils and oleoresins are extracted from dry spices. Oleoresins from fresh spice retain the wholesome flavour, matching with the parent spice. Such compounds are called 'green spice oleoresins'. In delicate flavour and seasoning formulations, such green spice oleoresins are preferred.

Advantages of Oleoresins / Spice Oils Compared to Whole Spice

a) Economy : Lower dose of oleoresin is required as compared to whole spice leading to economical use and saving.

b) Flavour Consistency : The flavour profile of a spice is influenced by variety, agro-climatic conditions, maturity of harvest, post-harvest conditions etc. which affect the flavour principle. Oleoresins provide consistent flavour in the food.

c) Hygiene : Oleoresins are free from dirt, dust, fungus and other contaminants associated with raw spice / spice powder. Oleoresins are sterile, with anti-microbial activity due to essential oils present in it.

d) Stability:Raw spice, on storage, gradually loses aroma compounds. Carotenoids present, undergo oxidative degradation. Even microbial contaminant reduces shelf life. Oleoresins are stable over long storage period.

Oleoresins contain non-volatile principles contributing to their taste. Piperine in black pepper, capsaicin in capsicum and gingerols in ginger, turmerin in turmeric are the examples of oleoresins.

Oleoresins of spice like capsicum and turmeric contain natural pigments hence find applications in food colouring. The consistency of flavour, colour and viscosity are maintained over repeated batches of extraction by various organic solvents used and minimal residual levels present there-of ; acetone, hexane, ethylene chloride, etc. which are commonly used. Commonly used oleoresins present in different spices have been discussed.

1. **Oleoresins of Ajwain** (Bishop's Weed)

It is pale green oily liquid (33-60 %) with a characteristic aroma and sharp taste.

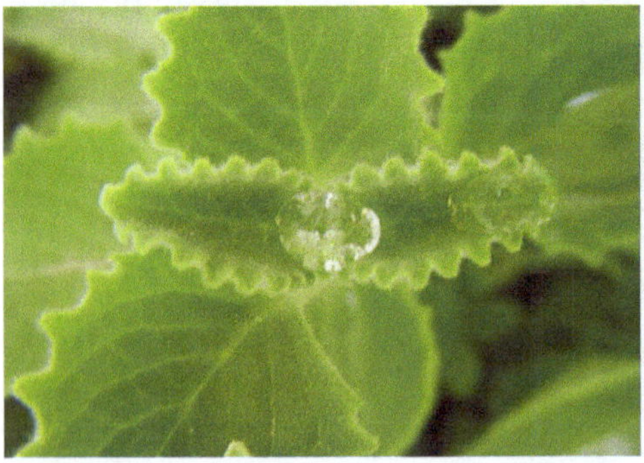

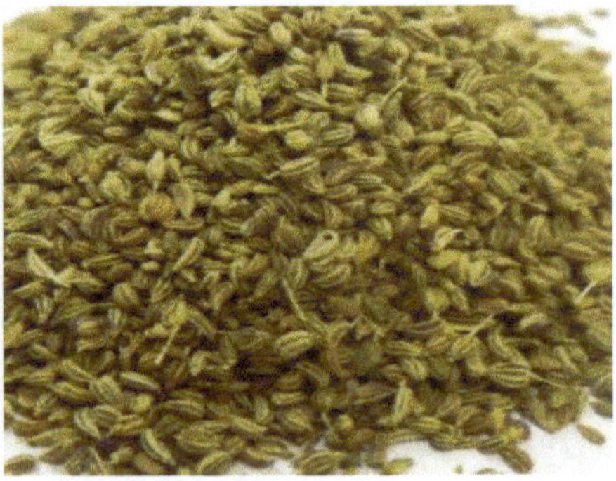

Uses

It is used as expectorant in respiratory ailments. It is used in perfumery, disinfectant soaps and as an insecticide. Thymol is an antiseptic used no. of skin ointment, deodorant, mouth wash, tooth paste and gargles.

2. **Caraway Seed Oleoresins** (*Shah Jira*)

It is greenish yellow in colour having the flavour of essential oil but with a bitter astringent after taste.

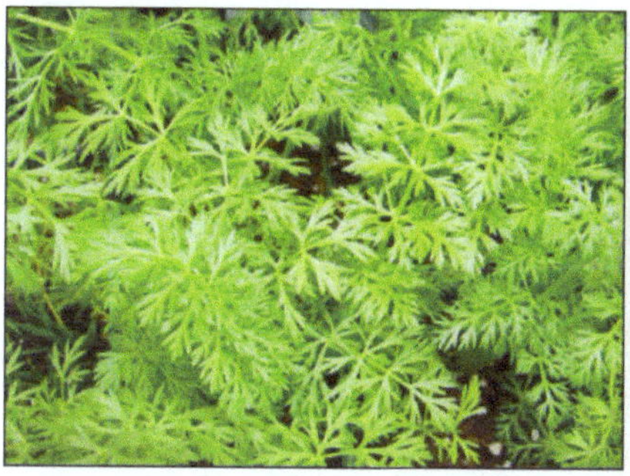

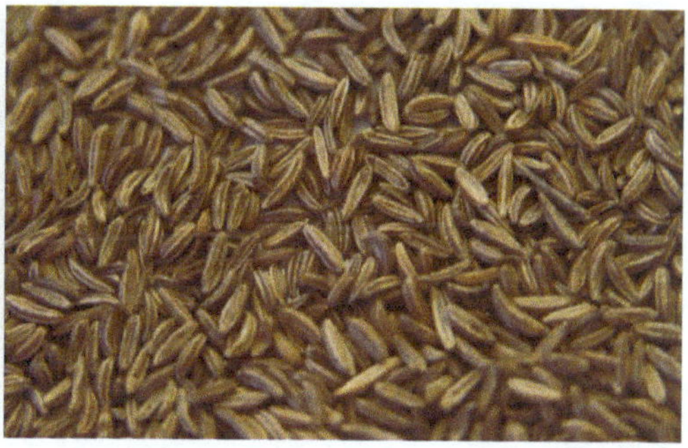

Uses

It is used in seasoning of processed meat, non-alcoholic beverages, baked goods, sauces etc. The oil and caravone of celery has pharmaceutical use to over come bad odour and taste as mouth wash and chewing gums.

3. Cinnamon Oleoresins (*Ilaichi*) (*Cinnamomumverum*)

The term cinnamon oleoresin is a general one which, is a mixture of volatile oils with other organic constituent ranging from 16-60 %. Different parts of Cinnamon give oils such as bark oil, leaf oil, chip oil etc. The bark oil contain cinnamaldehyde (62-65 %), phenols (eugenol) which is 16-18 % while leaf oil contain higher amount of. Coumarin is a non-volatile component of cinnamon.

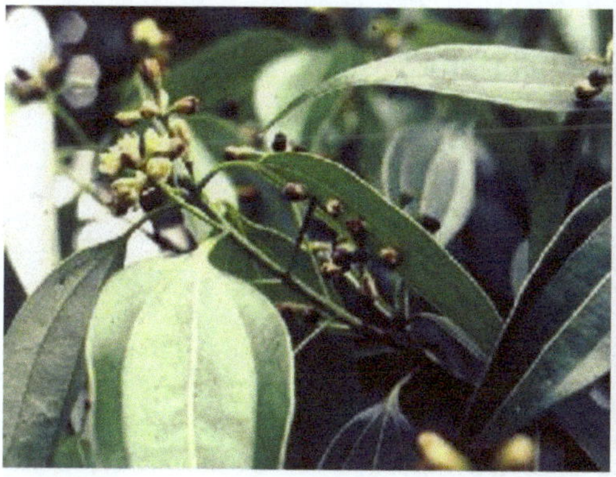

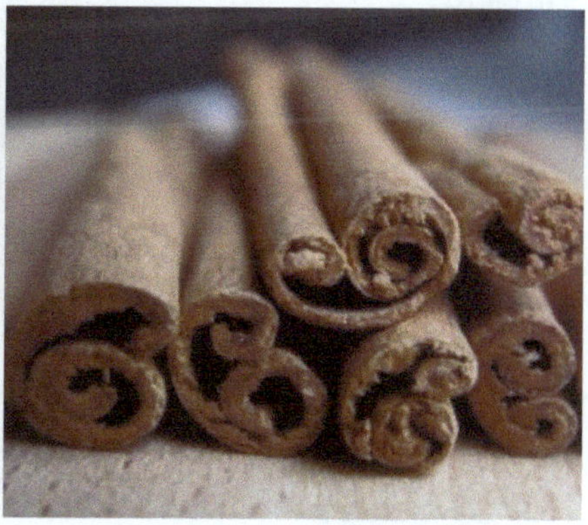

Uses

The oleoresins have commercial value as food additive for flavour and taste. They have medicinal value in digestive disorders such as flatulence.

4. Coriander Oleoresins (*Dhania)*

It is brownish yellow liquid having fruity aromatic smell.

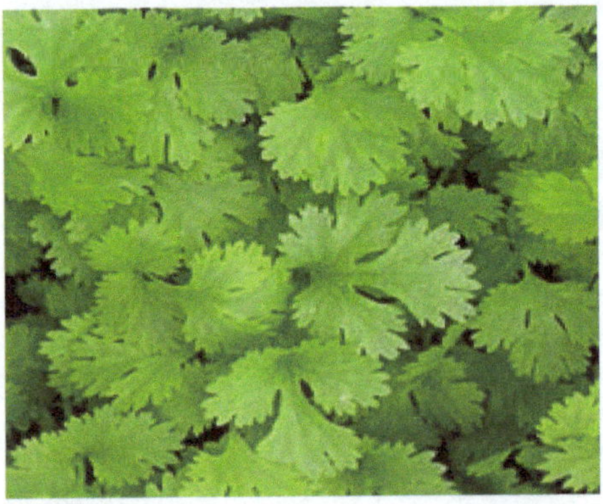

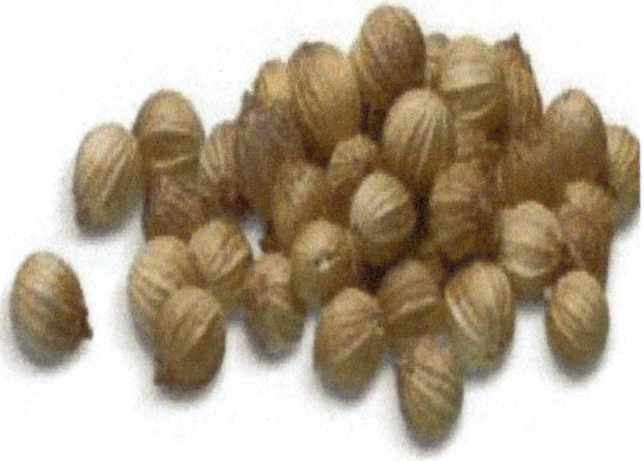

Botanical Name	*Coriandrum sativum* L. (Fam. Umbelliferae)
Preparation	Obtained by solvent extraction of the fruit with the subsequent removal of the solvent.
Appearance and odour	Caramel colour liquid with the characteristic odour and flavour of Coriander
Volatile Oil Content	7-8 ml / 100g
Residual solvent	<15 ppm
Solubility	Soluble in vegetable oil.
Equivalence	1 Kg of Coriander Oleoresin is of equal value to 10-15 Kg of seeds.
Storage	In tight full container in a cool, dark and dry place

Uses

- Coriander use has a medicinal plant has been reported since 1500 B.C. both as a spice and as a medicine.
- It has now spread well beyond its native Mediterranean and Caucasian regions.
- It aids digestion, reduce flatulence and improves appetite.
- It helps relieving spasms within the gut and counters the effects of nervous tension.

- Coriander is also chewed to sweeten the breath, especially after consumption of garlic (*Allium sativum*).
- It is applied externally as a lotion for rheumatic pain. Coriander essential oil is used in the manufacture of perfumes, cosmetics and dentifrices. Main Properties: Digestive, antispasmodic, anti-rheumatic.
- It is used as seasoning agent for sausages and meat products, baked goods, condiments, chewing gums, alcoholic and non-alcoholic beverages.
- It is also used in curry mix.

5. Cumin Oleoresins (*Jira)*

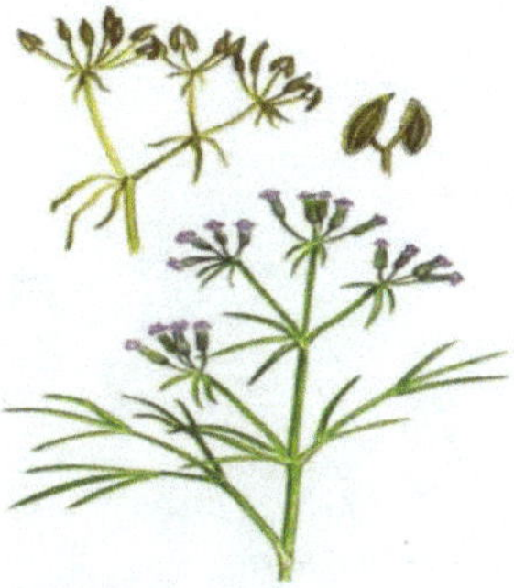

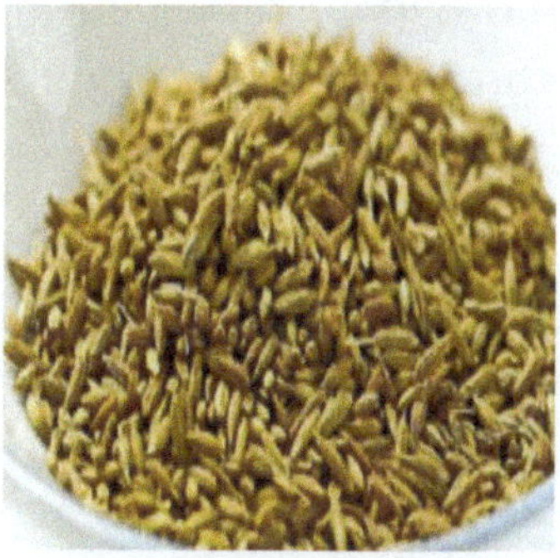

Botanical Name	*Cuminum cyminum* L. (Fam. Umbelliferae)
Preparation	Obtained by solvent extraction of the seeds with the subsequent removal of the solvent
Appearance & odour	Dark colour liquid with the characteristic odour and flavour of Cumin
Volatile Oil Content	30 - 35 ml/100g
Residual solvent	<15 ppm
Solubility	Soluble in vegetable oil.
Equivalence	1 Kg of Cumin Oleoresin is of equal value to 15-20 Kg of seeds
Storage	In tight full container in a cool, dark and dry place.

Uses

- The smell is very exotic.

- It is extremely powerful, green spicy, but not sharps, more of a soft and mellow scent.
- If used in a blend a drop of this scent goes a long way.
- This oil is wonderful for digestive disorders and colic too.
- It is good for exhaustion and works well in blends for that purpose, It helps to build the immune system; it is known to help with allergies to a degree. It helps with poor circulation and lymphatic congestion. It is a yellowish brown liquid.
- It is a seasoning agent used in snacks, soups, cheese, pickles and meat products.

6. Fennel Oleoresins (*Variali*)

It is brownish green liquid with volatile oil content.

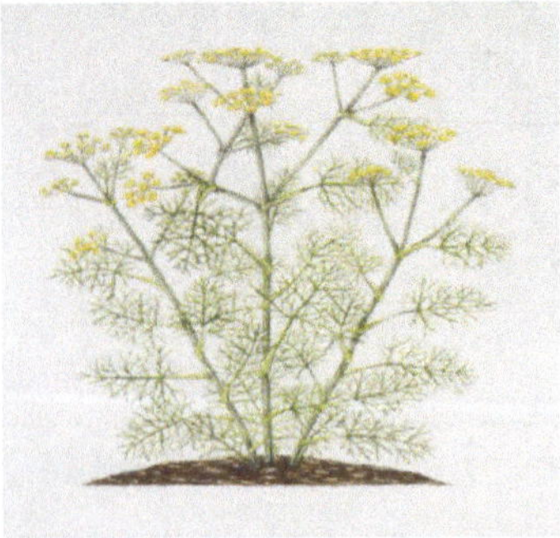

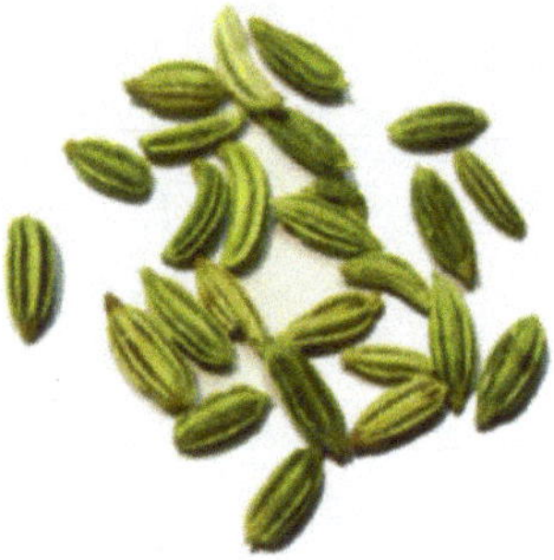

Botanical Name	*Foeniculum vulgare* (Fam. Umbelliferae)
Preparation	Obtained by solvent extraction of the seeds with the subsequent removal of the solvent
Appearance & odour	Dark brown liquid with the characteristic odour and flavour of Sweet Fennel
Volatile Oil Content	16-21 ml / 100g
Residual solvent	<15 ppm
Solubility	Soluble in vegetable oil
Equivalence	1 Kg of Fennel Oleoresin is of equal value to 10-15 Kg of seeds
Storage	In tight full container in a cool, dark and dry place

Uses

Fennel (Sweet) *Foeniculumvulgare*

- This essential oil has an anise scent and flavor. One of the most important facts about Fennel is that it is anti-toxic oil.
- According to Patricia Davis its most valuable application is in counterbalancing alcoholic poisoning, and it has played an important part in the treatment and rehabilitation of alcoholics.
- It also helps with gout, arthritis etc, to prevent the build-up of toxic waste in the body which precedes the inflammatory condition of the joints.
- It is helpful to regularize the menstrual cycle, particularly where periods are scanty and painful with cramping pains.
- Use of Fennel a lot for quick relief of indigestion and nausea. And it also helps to decrease the appetite.
- It is used in pizza sauces, sauces, toppings, non-alcoholic beverages, baked good, ice-cream, seasoning of processed meat.

7. Fenugreek Oleoresins (*Methi*)

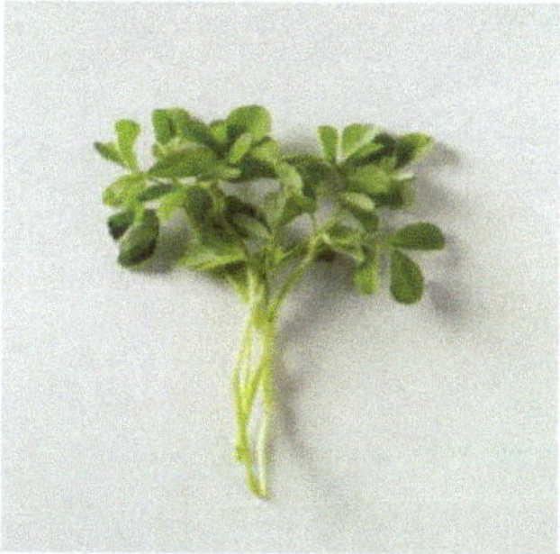

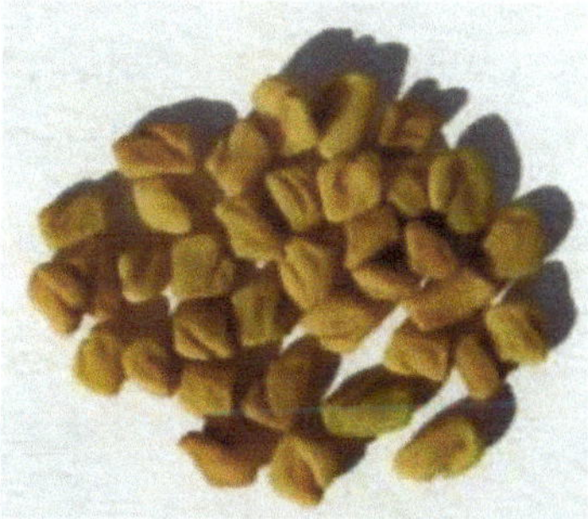

Botanical Name	*Trigonella foenumgraecum*
Family Name	Fabaceae
Name in some international Languages	Spanish - Alholya, Arabic- Hulba, and Chinese - k'u -Tou
Flavour Characteristics	Bitter Pungent, Flavour
Usage Profile	Foods, Cosmetics, Medicines etc.
Commercial Part	Fruit or seed
Harvesting Season	February to May

Specifications

Product	Brown Thick Paste. Fenugreek Oleoresin
Description	Characteristics Odour & Bitter in taste. Fenugreek Oleoresin is obtained by the solvent extraction of the dried seeds of *Trigonella foenum graceum*
Extraction	By 90% Methanol
Additive	Max 8% Glycerine
Water Solubility	Note less than 40%
Alcohol Solubility	Not less than 70% (50% v/v)
Total Ash	Note more than 8%
Heavy metals as Pb	Note more than 30 ppm
Colour & appearance	Brownish yellow in colour and thick viscous liquid
Odour	Characteristic aromatic odour of Fenugreek
Volatile oil content	0.4%
Residual solvent	<10 ppm
Solubility	Water soluble
Yeast & Mould	Absent
Pathogenic micro-organisms and their toxins	Absent
Purity Pure	Fenugreek oleoresin (no other additives)
Storage	Store preferably in air tight Containers and keep in a cool & dry place protected from light.

Uses

- It is oleoresin derived from the dried ripe seeds of *Trigonella foenum-graccum* commonly known as Fenugreek.
- The seeds of the fenugreek contain 50% fiber from which 20 % is mucilagenous fiber.

- The Oleoresin of the spice contains proteins, saponins and possess nutritive and restorative properties. Oleoresin does not contain fiber
- Fenugreek has grown widly in India, the Mediterranean, North Africa, and Southern Africa for centuries. In India, it is grown in the states of Rajasthan, Gujarat, Uttar Pradesh and Tamil Nadu. It is mainly used in spices or curry powder and excellent for fish and sea food dishes, candy, baked goods, ice cream, chewing gum and soft drinks.
- It also has medicinal benefits like it is used in reducing the blood sugar level and blood pressure; it is rich in vitamins, minerals and proteins. Green Earth Products has the reputation of exporting this spice in its whole and powdered form all across the globe.
- It is light yellowish green in colour with a typical smell.
- It is used in preparation of flavouring agent in pharmaceuticals, It is also used in seasoning of meat products and curry mix.

8. Pepper Oleoresins (*Kala Mari*) (*Piper nigrum L*)

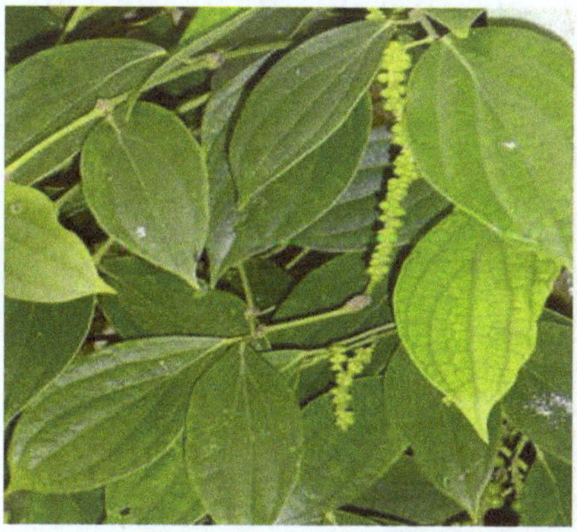

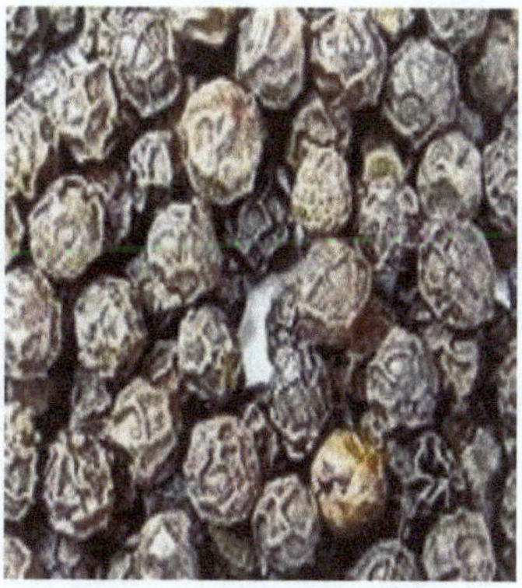

Extraction of black pepper with organic solvents provides oleoresins possessing odour, flavour and pungent principles. Piperine is a major constituent (35-55 %). Pepper oleoresins are dark green, viscous, heavy liquid with strong aroma which, on standing, crystallises the piperine. Oleoresins of pepper may be dissolved in edible solvents, emulsified with gum Arabic and dry powder is prepared.

Botanical Name	*Piper nigrum,*
Family Name	Piperaceae
Name in some International Languages	Spanish-Pimienta, Arabic-Filfil Aswad, Chinese-Hu- Chiao
Flavour Characteristics	Highly aromatic and hot,
Usage Profile	Foods, Preservatives and Medicines
Commercial part	Fruit
Harvesting Season	December to March
Oleoresin Black Pepper Specifications	
Description	Oleoresin Black Pepper is the natural extract of dried tender berries of Piper Nigrum Linn of family Piperaceae.
Manufacturing Process	It is obtained by the solvent extraction of Black Pepper and the solvent traces are removed by distilling it in vacua at controlled temperature.
Physical Appearance	It is a yellowish brown viscous liquid with pungent slightly biting aroma of Black Pepper.
Spice Equivalent	About 5-10 kgs of Oleoresin replaces 100 Kgs of dried black Pepper
Technical Specifications	
Residual Solvent (By gas chromotography)	< 10 ppm
Volatile Oil content v/w	20 ml/100gm
Piperine content	40%
Microbiology	Free from Microbial contaminants
Preparation	By solubilization of the in ethanol
Appearance	Dark-brown
Storage	In tight full container in a cool, dark and dry place

Uses

- *Piper nigrum* Linn or Black peppercorns is produced through steam distillation to get the aromatic, odorous constituent of the spice i.e., the volatile oil.
- The pungent, non volatile principles for which the pepper is so highly esteemed as a condiment is present in its oleoresin, which is obtained by the extraction of berries with volatile solvents and concentrating to remove the solvent.
- The crushed black pepper generally yields 1 to 2.5 percent of volatile oil which contains mainly Terpenes, Sesquitenpenes and Oxygenated compounds, and is used for flavouring and perfumery.
- The oleoresin of pepper contains Alkaloids, Piperine (4-10 percent) and Chavicine, which contributes for its pungent taste
- The oleoresins has commercial value as food additive for flavour and taste.
- They have medicinal value in digestive disorders such as flatulence.

9. Chilli (*Capsicum* spp)

a. Oleoresin Capsicum (African Capsicum Oleoresin) : It is highly pungent, contains 4 - 14 % capsaicin. It contains considerable amount of fixed oils.

b. Red Pepper Oleoresins : The capsaicin content is around 0.6-3.9% only. It is moderately pungent. It is prepared from different variety of Capsicum.

c. Paprika Oleoresins : It is prepared from *Capsicum annum*. It has a high colouring value. It has little capsaicin but is used for giving the colour). Paprika oleoresins (Natural Food Color).

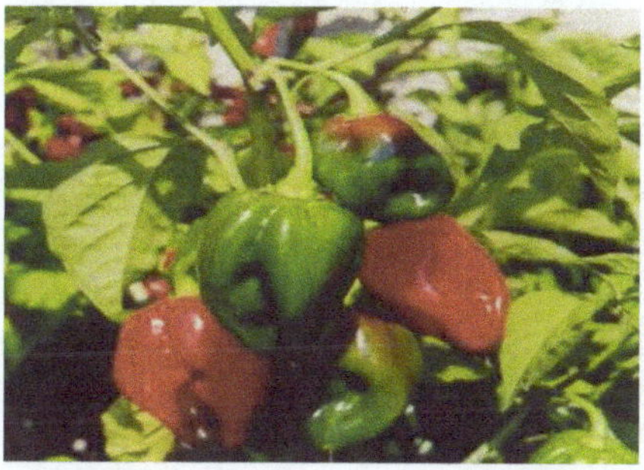

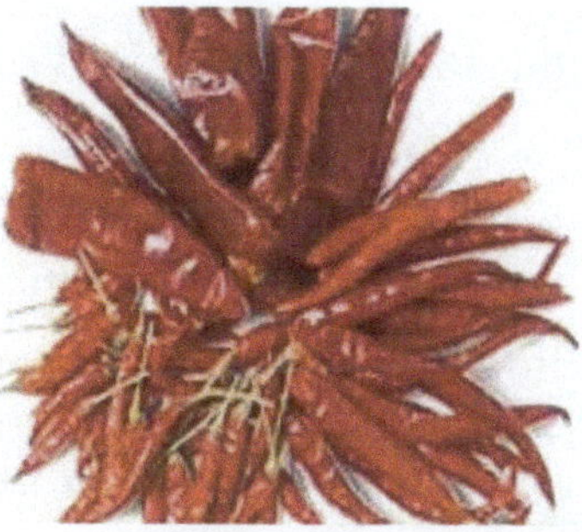

Botanical Name	*Capsicum annum*
Family Name	Solanaceae
Name in some International Languages	Spanish - Pimento , Arabic - Filfil Ahmar, Chinese - Hesiung Yali Chiao
Flavour Characteristics	Lightly Bitter Pungent, Flavoursome
Usage Profile	Foods, and some Medicines
Commercial part	Green as well as ripe & dried pod (fruit)
Harvesting Season	January to August, September to December
Capsicum Oleoresin Specifications	
Description	Extract of Indian red chillies, *Capsicum annum* L. or capsicum frutescens L.
Storage	Store in full, tight containers in a cool dry place, protected from sun light.
Appearance	Dark red viscous liquid parameters
Odour	Characteristic pungent odour of Chillies
Additives	Permitted additives to standardise the product
Dispersibility/ solubility	No preservative or antioxidants used.
Spice Equivalent	Can be dispersed in dry/liquid carriers such as salt, dextrose, edible oils, lecithin, benzyl alcohol etc.
Capsaicin	One kg replaces 100 kg raw chillies. 10% - UV spectrometric difference
Colour Value	15000 CU (max) - MSD –10
Residual solvent	20 ppm (max) EOA
Microbiology	Free from microbial contaminants
Shelf Life	12 months under the specified storage conditions
Handling	Avoid contact with skin and eyes. Warm slightly and stir well before drawing the product from the container.

Caution	Use only additives/diluents compatible with this product; use of non-compatible diluents/ additives can lead to sedimentation. Add the proposed diluent/additive to a sample of the product in the same proportion and confirm absence of sedimentation prior.

Uses

- Capsicum Oleoresin is prepared by extracting the crushed capsicum (Capsicum Annum Linn) with volatile solvents by percolation method.
- It contains the pungent principles, capsicin not less that 8 percent.
- It also contains the red colouring matter called Capsanthin. This product is a powerful irritant and a carminative, which is also used as a counter irritant in lumbago and neuralgia.
- It can also be used to treat stomach ache that involves poorly functioning stomach muscles and as an antibacterial agents.

a. Organoleptic, Physical, Chemical and Microbiological Characteristics

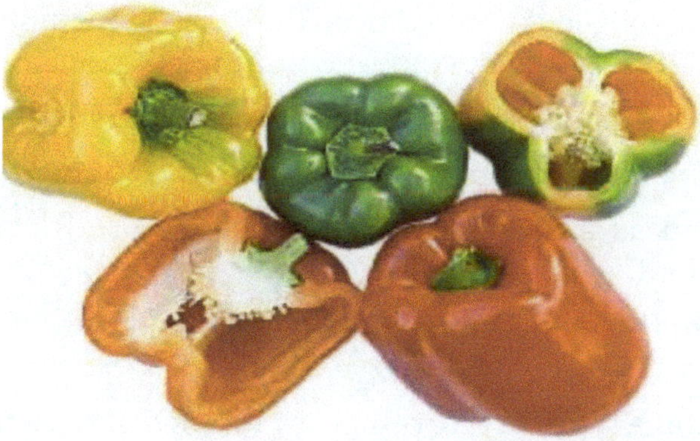

Description	Oleoresin Paprika is the pungency-free colour concentrate of the dried fruit of Indian red chillies
Specifications	Appearance: Dark red viscous liquid
Odour	Characteristic mild aroma of red chillies

Shelf life and Storage	10 ppm 12 months under the specified storage conditions. Store preferably in full, tight containers in a cool, dry, place protected from light.
Additives	Permitted additives to standardize the product. No preservatives or antioxidants added.
Handling	Avoid contact with skin and eyes. Stir well before drawing the product from the container.
Dispersibility/solubility	Can be dispersed in dry/liquid carriers such as salt, dextrose, edible oil, lecithin, benzyl alcohol etc. Soluble in edible oils.
Spice Equivalent	One Kg replaces 70 kg of Paprika Powder.
Technical Specifications	
Colour value	100000 CU-MSD-10- SIC/Q.M/202
Residual solvent	10 ppm-EOA
Microbiology	Free from Microbial contaminants.

Uses

- Paprika oleoresin is derived from the dried ripe fruits of Capsicum annum Linn, and is devoid of any pungent principles.
- It chiefly contains pigments namely capsanthin and carotenes.
- The pigments are responsible for the red colour.
- It is used as a colouring agent in food products and as an antioxidant.
- There are three types of oleoresins prepared from dried fruits of capsicum
- All the three types of oleoresins are supplied as free flowing form or dispersed in suitable carrier in the commercial preparation.

Capsaicin

Capsaicin is the pungent principle, which possess hydroxyl and methoxy group having a structural relationship with vanillin. Capsaicin is the amide of Vinillyl amine and isodecenoic acid. The complex group of compounds are present in the form of capsaicinoid which include capsaicin, dihydro capsaicin, nordihydro capsaicin, homo capsaicin , homodihydro capsaicin etc. The pungency principles are located in seeds (10 %), dissepiments and the pericalp (skin). As the fruit matures, the concentration of pungency principle increases.

Colour Principles of Chilli

Colour is imparted by Carotenoids. Over 30 carotenoids have been detected. The major pigment is capsainthin which is a keto-carotenoid containing a cyclo-pentane ring. Paprika powder contains 70-80 % capsainthin, which impart colour. Other pigments present in capsicum are capsorbulin, zeaxanthin, violaxanthin, leutein, neoxanthin etc.

10. Saffron Oleoresin

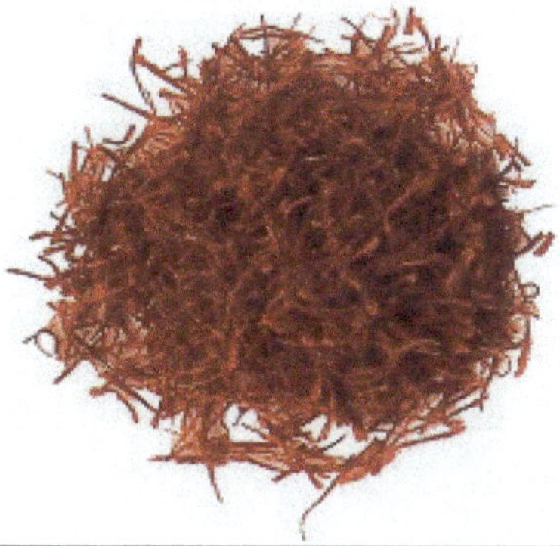

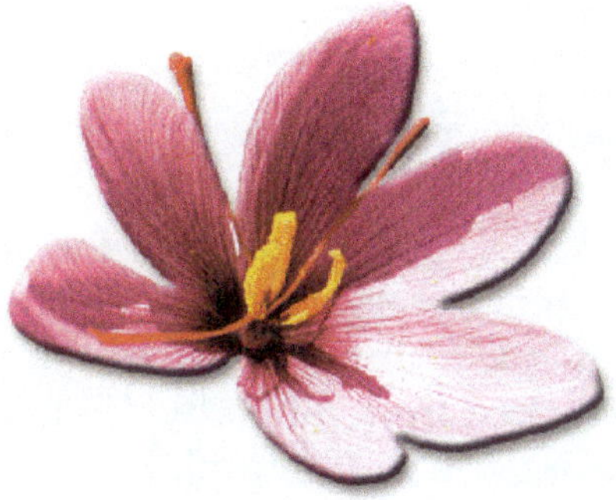

Appearance	Dried dark red filaments, with a small percentage of yellow or white stamens and styles.
Aroma & flavour	Characteristic of the product, aromatic.
Size of filaments	15 - 40 mm in length
Moisture	< 12.0 %
Ash Content	< 8.0 %
Acid Insoluble Ash	< 1.0 %
Extraneous Matter	< 0.5 %
Storage	For best results, saffron should be stored in an ambient temperature and protected from exposure to light. The product is normally good for at least 3 years from the date of packing.

Extraction	Oleoresin of saffron obtained from stigmas of Crocus sativus L., extracted with different solvents, i.e. methanol, ethanol, propanol, acetone, ethyl acetate and petroleum ether. The variables studied were nature of extracting solvent, extraction temperature, extraction yield, solvent stripping. The quality of oleoresin extract was evaluated using high performance liquid chromatographic and spectrophotometric methods. This study attempts to get the best condition for the extraction process that gives the best yield and quality of oleoresin from dried saffron.

Uses

- Saffron is a very costly spice, used to flavor and color food.
- A flower's stigma accepts the pollen that is produced by the stamen, which becomes the seeds of the next generation. Each stigma is very small, and tens of thousands of individual strands go into a single ounce of the spice; since the stigmas are hand-plucked from the individual flowers, saffron's high cost becomes more understandable. It is thought that saffron is the most expensive spice in the world.
- Saffron originated in the Middle East, but is now also associated with Greek, Indian and Spanish cuisines.
- A very little saffron goes a long way – it is a spice to be added one thread at a time. Just a thread or two can flavor and color an entire pot of rice. The flavor is distinctive and pungent.
- It is widely used in Ayurvedic medicine, India's traditional system of health that relies on natural products, prevention and balance.
- It is used in remedies for everything from arthritis and asthma to infertility and impotence.
- Ancient Egyptians used saffron to treat kidney problems, and there are now research results that might suggest that one of the ingredients in saffron lowers (or assists in lowering) high cholesterol.
- There are even suggestions that saffron may have been used against cancer in the Middle Ages, although with what success is unknown.

11 Onion Oleoresin

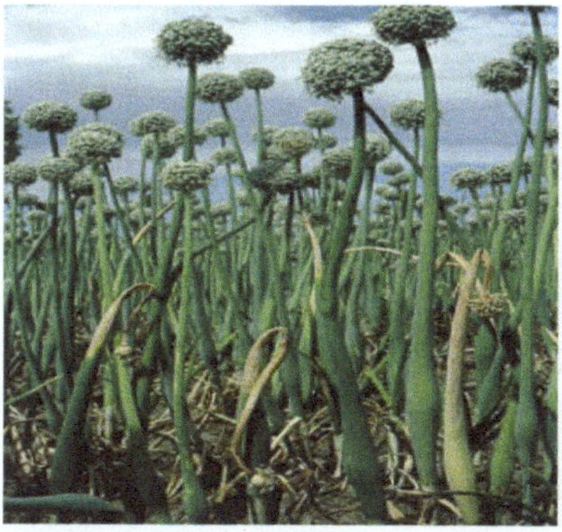

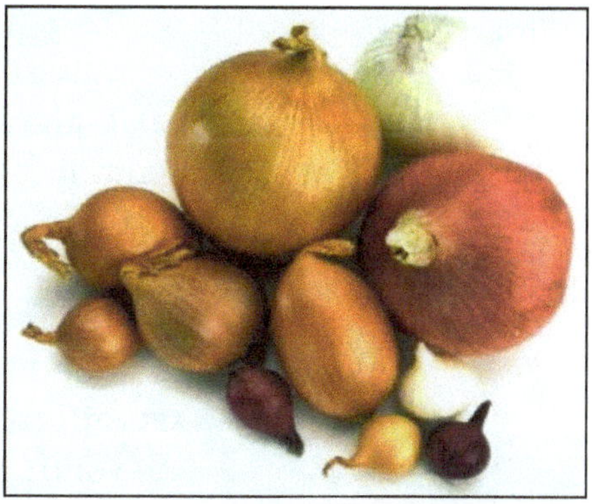

Family	Liliaceae,
Synonyms	Common onion, Strasburg onion
Product	Onion Oleoresin
Appearance	Dark brown to lack colour, free flowing liquid with the Characteristic aroma of fresh Onion.
Description	Reddish Brown to Brown thick paste
Organoleptic Test	Slightly sweet & characteristic Flavours of Onion
Total Ash	Not more than 3%
Technical Specifications	
In Water	Not less than 70%
In 50% Alcohol	Not less than 65%
Matter Insoluble	Not more than 2%
Additive	5% Glycerine will be added by Wt.
Distribution	Native of Western Asia and the Middle East; it has a long history of cultivation all over the world, mainly for culinary use. The essential oil is produced mainly in France, Germany and Egypt from the red onion.
Extraction	Essential oil by steam distillation from the bulb.
Characteristics	A pale yellow or brownish-yellow mobile liquid with strong, unpleasant, sulfur odor with a tear producing effect.

Uses

Herbal/ folk tradition	Onion has an ancient reputation as a curative agent, highly extolled by the schools of Galen and Hippocrates. It is high in vitamins A, B and C and shares many of the properties of garlic, to which it is closely related. Raw onion helps keep colds and infections at bay, promotes strong bones and a good blood supply to all tissues. It acts as an effective blood cleanser that, along with the sulfur it contains, helps to keep the skin clear and in good condition. It has a sound reputation for correcting glandular imbalance and weight problems; it also improves lymphatic drainage, which is often responsible for edema and puffiness. It has long been used as a home simple for a wide range of conditions.
Aromatherapy/home use	None, due to its offensive smell
Other uses	Used in some pharmaceutical preparations for cold, coughs. The oil is used extensively in most major food categories, especially meats, savories, salad dressings, as well as alcoholic and soft drinks. It is not used in perfumery work
Actions	Anathematic, anti-microbial, antirheumatic, antiseptic, antisclerotic, antispasmodic, antiviral, antibacterial, carminative, depurative, digestive, diuretic, expectorant, fungicidal, hypocholesterolemic, hypoglycemic, hypotensive, stomachic, tonic, vermifuge
Safety data	Specific safety data on a bed of the present – probably similar to garlic i.e. generally non-toxic, non irritant, possible sensitization

12 Cardamom Oleoresin

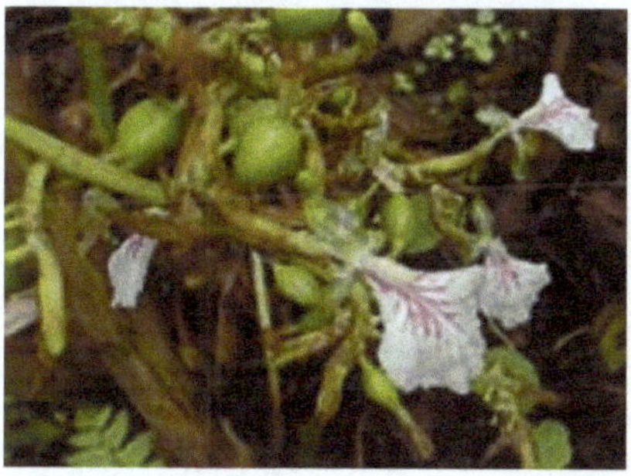
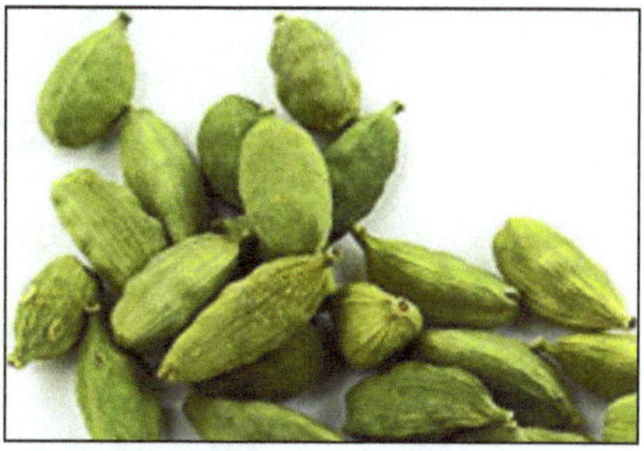

Botanical Name	*Elettaria cardamomum*
Family	Zingiberaceae
Hindi Name	Chhoti Elaichi
Part Used	Fruit

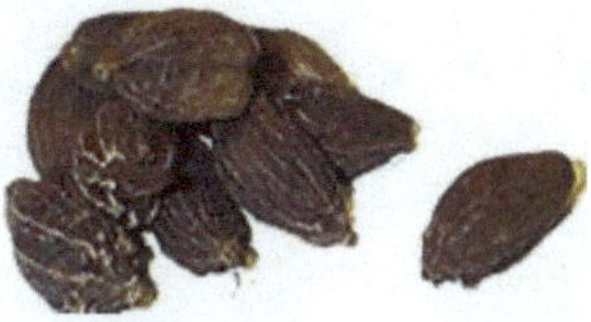

Botanical Name	*Amomum subulatum* Roxb
Family	Zingiberaceae
Hindi Name	Badi Elaichi
Part Used	Fruit
Synonyms	Cardamom, Cardomomi, Musore
Safety data	Non-toxic, known irritant, non-sensitizing
Distribution	Native to tropical Asia especially Southern India; cultivated extensively in India, Sri Lanka, Guatemala and El Salvador. The oil is produced principally in India, Europe, Sri Lanka and Guatemala.
Extraction	Essential oil by steam distillation from the dried ripe fruit. An oleo resin is also produced in small quantities
Characteristics	A colorless to pale yellow liquid with a sweet-spicy, warming fragrance and a woody-balsamic undertone. It blends well with rose, olibanum, orange, bergamot, cinnamon, cloves, caraway, ylang ylang, labdanum, cedarwood, orange blossom, and oriental bases in general.

Uses

Herbal/folk tradition	Used extensively as a domestic spice, especially in India, Europe, Latin America and Middle Eastern countries. It has been used in traditional Chinese and Indian medicine for over 3000 years, especially for pulmonary disease, fever, digestive & urinary complaints. Hippocrates recommended it for sciatica, coughs, abdominal pain, spasms, nervous disorders, retention of urine and also for bites of venomous creatures. Current in the British herbal Pharmocopoeia as a specific for flatulent dyspepsia.
Aromatherapy/home use	Digestive system - anorexia, colic, cramp, dyspepsia, flatulence, griping pains, halitosis, heartburn, indigestion, vomiting. Nervous system - mental fatigue, nervous strain.
Other uses	Employed in some carminative, stomachic and laxative preparations; also in the form of compound cardamom spirit to flavor pharmaceuticals. Extensively used as a fragrance component in soaps, cosmetics and perfumes especially oriental types. Important flavor ingredient particularly in curry and spice products.
Actions	Antiseptic, antispasmodic, aphrodisiac, carminative, cephalic, digestive, diuretic, stimulant, stomachache, tonic (nerve).

13 Anise Oleoresin

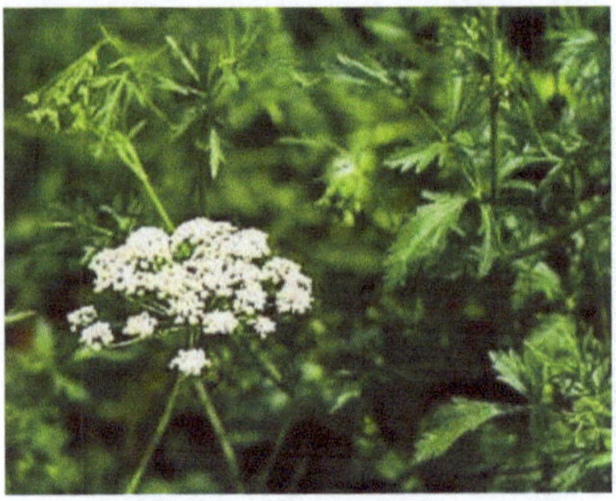

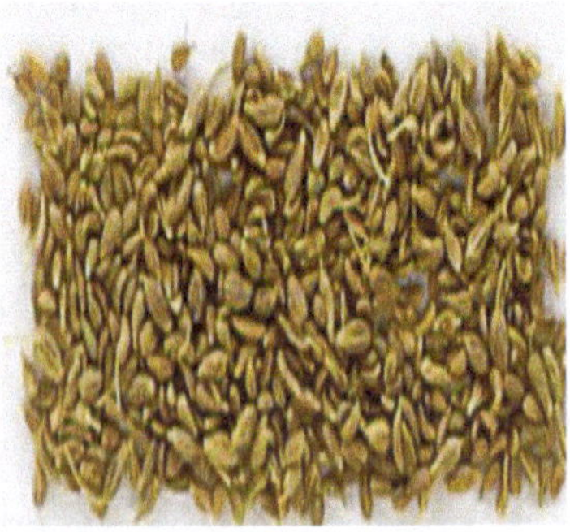

Specifications

Botanical Name	*Pimpinella anisum* L. (Fam. Umbelliferae)
Preparation	Obtained by solvent extraction of the seeds with the subsequent removal of the solvent
Appearance and odour	Dark brown liquid with the characteristic odour and flavour of Anise
Volatile Oil Content	6 - 8 ml / 100g (EOA No.: 57-G)
Residual solvent	<15 ppm
Solubility	Soluble in vegetable oil
Equivalence	1 Kg of Anise Oleoresin is of equal value to 6 - 8 Kg of seeds.
Storage	In tight full container in a cool, dark and dry place.
Spice Description	Though the roots and leaves are also edible, it is the seeds that are concerned with. The seeds are grey-green to brownish, ribbed and ovate, measuring 2-4 mm (.08 -.16 in) long. Some seeds retain the fine stalk that passes through the centre of the fruit.Bouquet: sweet and fragrant, Flavour: similar to fennel with a mild licorice taste.

Uses

- Anise is native to the eastern Mediterranean region, the Levant, and Egypt.
- Anise bears a strong family resemblance to the members of the carrot family, that includes dill, fennel, coriander, cumin and caraway.
- Many of these relatives have been described as having a licorice flavour, to some extent, but anise is the true taste of licorice— its oils are distilled into the flavouring for licorice candy (not from the herb licorice, which has a different taste).
- The early Arabic name was anysum from which was derived the Greek anison and the Latin anisun. It is one of the oldest

known spice plants used both for culinary and medicinal purposes since ancient times.

- There is evidence that anise was used in Egypt as early as 1500 B.C. Anise is used in the manufacture of many commercial cough syrups and sore throat medications, used to flavour other medicines and to scent soaps and perfumes.

14 Clove Oleoresin

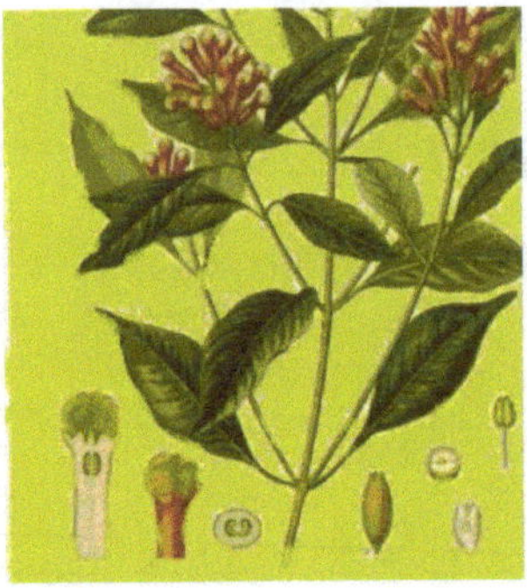

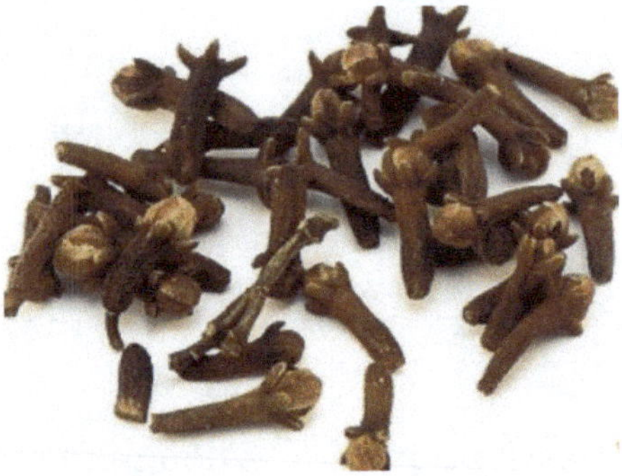

Family	**Myrtaceae**
Distribution	Believed to be native to Indonesia now cultivated worldwide, especially in the Philippines, and Madagascar. The main oil-producing countries are Madagascar and Indonesia.
Extraction	Essential oil by water distillation from the buds and leaves, and by steam distillation from the stalks or stems. A concrete, absolute and oleoresin are also produced by the buds in small quantities.
Characteristics	Clove bud is a pale yellow liquid with a warm, sweet-spicy odor and a fresh, fruity top note. The bud oil is flavored in perfumery work. It blends well with rose, lavender, vanilla, clary sage, bergamot, bay leaf, all spice, ylang. Clove leaf is dark brown oil with a crude, burnt-woody earned odor. Clove stem oil is a pale yellow liquid with a strong spicy-woody odor.

Safety data	All clove oil can cause skin and mucous membrane irritations; clove bud and stem oil may cause dermatitis. Clove bud is the least toxic of the tree oils because of the lower eugenol percentage. Use in moderation only, and low dilution (< 1 percent).

Uses

Herbal/folk tradition	Extensively used as a domestic spice worldwide.Tincture of cloves has been used for skin infections (scabies, athlete's foot); for digestive upset; to dress the umbilical cord; for intestinal parasites; to ease the pain of child birth (steeped in wine); and notably for toothache. The tea is used to relieve nausea. In Chinese medicine the oil is used for diarrhoea, hernia, bad breath and bronchitis as well as for those conditions mentioned above.
Aromatherapy/home use —Only use clove bud oil, not the leaf or stem oil.	Skin care-acne, athlete's foot, bruises, burns, cuts, insect repellent (mosquito), toothache, ulcers, wounds. Circulation, muscles and joints -arthritis, rheumatism, sprains. Respiratory system-asthma, bronchitis. Digestive system-colic, dyspepsia, nausea. Immune system-colds, flu, minor infections.
Other uses	Used in dental preparations, and as a fragrance component in toothpaste, soaps, toiletries, cosmetics & perfumes. Extensively employed as a flavor ingredient in major food categories, alcoholic and soft drinks. Used in the production of printing ink, glue and varnish; clove leaf oil is used as the starting material for the isolation of eugenol.
Actions	Anthelmintic, antibiotic, anti-emetic, antihistaminic, antirheumatic, antineuralgic, antioxidant, antiseptic, antiviral, aphrodisiac, carminative, counter irritant, expectorant, larvicidal, spasmolytic, stimulant, stomachic, vermifuge

15 Garlic Oleoresin

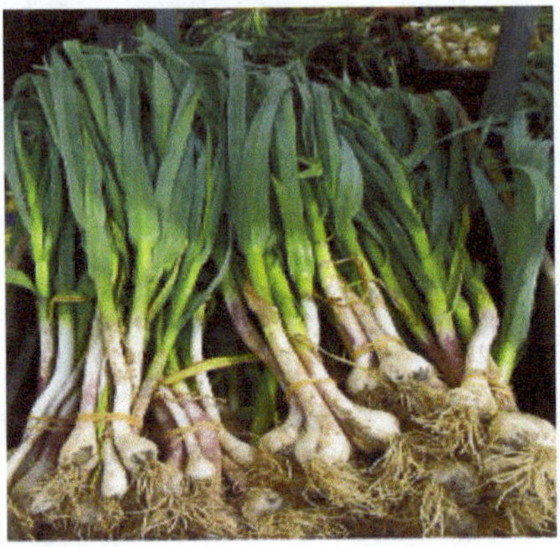

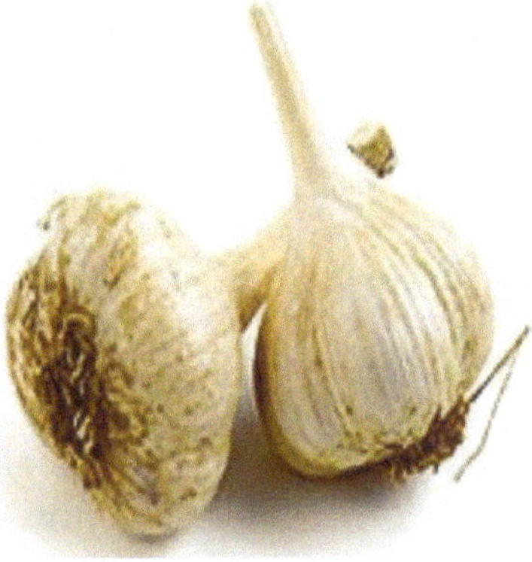

Botanical name	*Allium sativum*
Family Name	Liliaceae
Name in some International Languages	Spanish-Ajo, Arabic-Thum, Chinese-Suan
Flavour Characteristics	Pungent, Sulfurous and strong odour
Usage Profile	Foods, and Medicines
Commercial part	Bulb
Harvesting Season	December to January
Garlic Oleoresin	
Product	Garlic Oleoresin
Appearance	Dark brown to lack colour, free flowing liquid with the Characteristic aroma of fresh Garlic.
Description: Brown	Thick Paste with characteristic odour
Organoleptic Test	Characteristic Flavour
Extraction	By 80% Methanol
Additive	Max.8% Glycyrine
Water Solubility	Not less than 70%
Alcohol Solubility	Not less than 60% (50% v/v)
Total Ash	Not more than 3%
Heavy metals as Pb	Not more than 30 ppm
Volatile Oil content	Not less than 1%

Uses

- Garlic Oil is derived from the crushed bulbs of garlic, *Allium sativum* Linn.
- They have a powerful and obnoxious odour due to the presence of disulphides.
- The bulbs contain 0.06% to 0.1% of volatile oil whose active constituents are propyl /-disulphide, alliin and allicin.
- The yellow oil of garlic is a valuable flavouring agent in perfumery, as insect repellant. Allicin present in volatile oil is a powerful antibacterial.

16 Ginger Oleoresin

a) Organoleptic, Physical, Chemical and Microbiological Characteristics

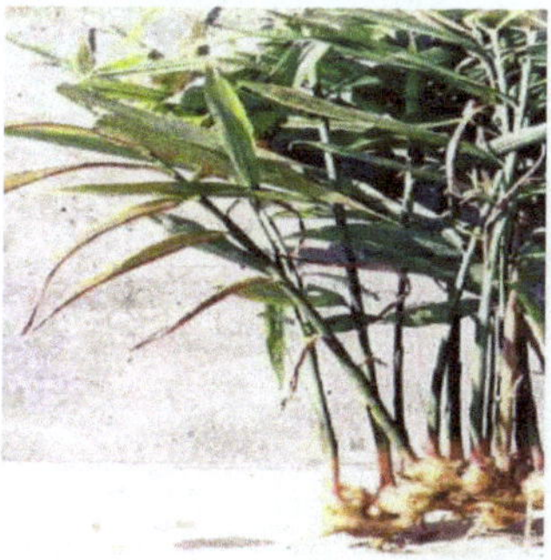

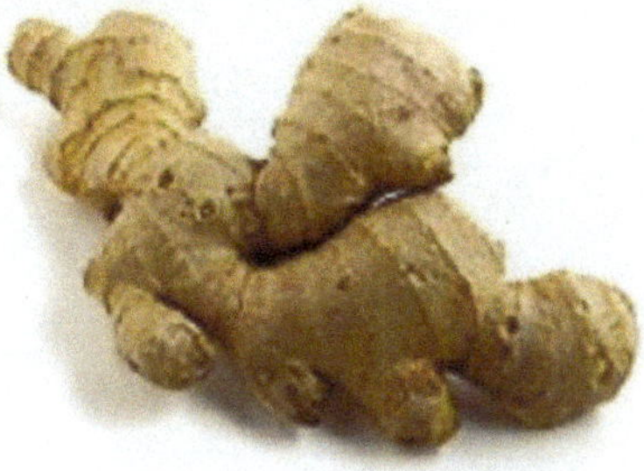

Botanical Name	*Zingiber officinale*
Family Name	Zingiberaceae
Name in some International Languages	Spanish - Jengibre, Arabic - Zanjabil, Chinese - Chiang
Flavour Characteristics	Hot and Pungent
Usage Profile	Foods, Preservatives and Medicines
Commercial part	The rhizome
Harvesting Season	December to February in plains, February to March in higher elevations.
Product	Ginger Oleoresin

Description	Ginger Oleoresin is obtained by solvent extraction of the dried seeds of rhizomes of *Zingeber officianalis*
Colour & appearance	Dark brown in colour & viscous liquid
Odour	Characteristic odour of ginger
Volatile oil content	35%
Residual solvent	<10 ppm
Solubility	Soluble in Oil
Yeast & Mould	Absent
Homogeneity	Ensured by uniform emulsification
Pathogenic micro-organisms and their toxins	Absent
Purity	Pure Ginger oleoresin (no other additives)
Storage	Store preferably in air tight containers and keep in a cool & dry place protected from light.

Uses

- Ginger oil, Oleoresins are the volatile oil derived by steam distillation of ginger and oleoresin is obtained by percolating the powdered rhizomes of Ginger, *Zingiber officinale* with volatile solvents.
- Ginger contains 1 to 2% of volatile oil 5-8% of pungent acrid oleoresin and starch.
- Zingiberene is the chief constituent of oil of ginger.
- Oil is employed for flavoring of all kinds of food products and confectionary and finds limited use in perfumery.
- Oleoresin, commercially called Gingering contains pungent principles viz. gingerol and shogaol apart from the volatile oil of ginger and is used as an aromatic, carminative, stomachic and stimulant.

17 Nutmeg Oleoresin

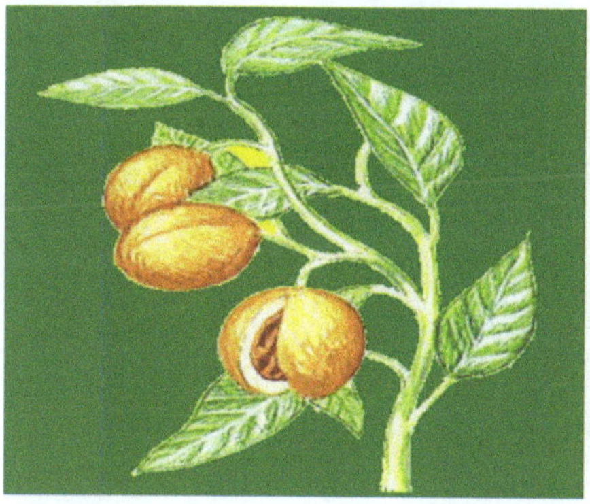 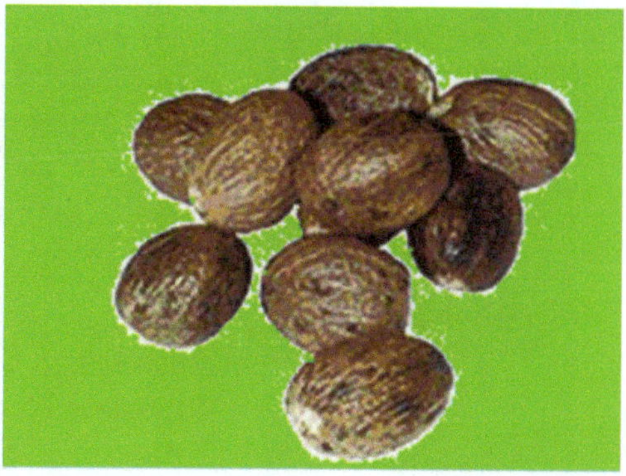

Family	Myristicaceae
Synonyms	Myristica (oil), Mace (husk), Macis (oil)
Distribution	Native to the Moluccas cultivated in Sri Lanka, West Indies, and Granada.
Extraction	Essential oil by steam (or water) from: 1. dried worm-eaten nutmeg seed; 2. dried orange-brown aril or husk - mace 3. Oleoresin by solvent extraction from mace
Characteristics	• Water-white or pale yellow, mobile liquid with a sweet, warm-spicy odor and a terpeney top note. • Water-white or pale yellow mobile liquid with a sweet, warm-spicy scent. • Orange-brown viscous liquid with a fresh, spicy-warm, balsamic fragrance. Has good masking power. Blend well with oakmoss, lavandin, bay leaf, Peru balsam, orange, geranium, clary sage, rosemary, lime, petigrain, mandarin, coriander and other spice oils.
Safety Data	Nutmeg and mace are generally non toxic, non irritant and non-sensitizing. However, used in large doses they show signs of toxicity such as nausea, stupor and tachycardia.

Uses

Herbal/Folk Tradition	Widely used as domestic spices and have been used for centuries as a remedy mainly for digestive and kidney problems. Current in the British Herbal Pharmacopeia for flatulent dyspepsia, nausea, diarrhoea, dysentery, rheumatism
Aromatherapy/Home Use	Large quantities are hallucinogenic and excitant to the motor cortex. Nutmeg is probably safer to use than mace. Use in moderation and with care in pregnancy. Circulation, muscles and joints - arthritis, gout, muscular aches and pains, poor circulation, rheumatism.Digestive System - flatulence, indigestion, nausea, sluggish digestion. Immune System - bacterial infection. Nervous System - frigidity, impotence, neuralgia, nervous fatigue
Other Uses	Flavoring agent especially analgesic and tonic preparations. Soaps, lotions, detergents, cosmetics, perfumes. Mace oleoresin used in colognes, perfumes, both oils and oleoresin are used in most major food categories.
Actions	Analgesic, anti-emetic, antiseptic, antirheumatic, antiseptic, antispasmodic, aphrodisiac, carminative, digestive, emmenagogue, gastric secretory stimulant, larvicidal, prostglandin.

18 Rosemary Oleoresin

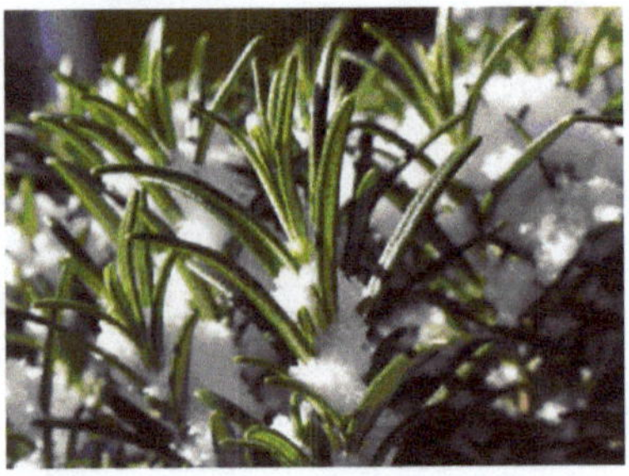

Botanical Name	*Rosemarinus officinalis*
Family Name	Lamiaceaee
Name in some International Languages	Spanish-Romero, Arabic-Iklil Aj, Chinese-Hu-Chiao
Flavour Characteristics	Highly aromatic and hot
Usage Profile	Foods, preservatives and medicines
Commercial part	Fruit
Harvesting Season	December to March.
Rosemary oleoresin	
Synonyms	Rosemary oleoresin
Odor Description	Fresh Leaf Fragrance of Rosemary
Appearance	Dark Brownish Yellow Semi-solid.

Uses

- It is oleoresin obtained from Rosemary *Rosemarinus officinalis.*
- It is prepared by soaking the leaves in volatile solvent using the percolation process.
- They chiefly contain volatile oil, resin and bitter principles.
- The volatile oil is composed of Borneol, Camphor and Tupenes.
- They also contain Phenolic Acids like Carnosic Acid, which is used as antioxidant.

Besides it is used for flavoring cosmetics, liniments and hair lotions. The Oil is used as Carminaline.

19. Turmeric Oleoresin

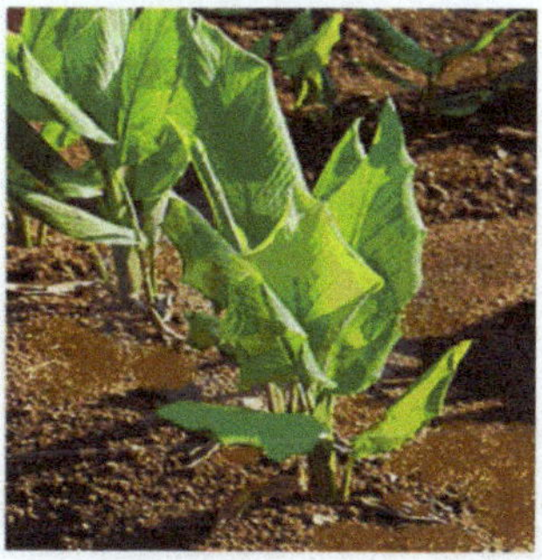
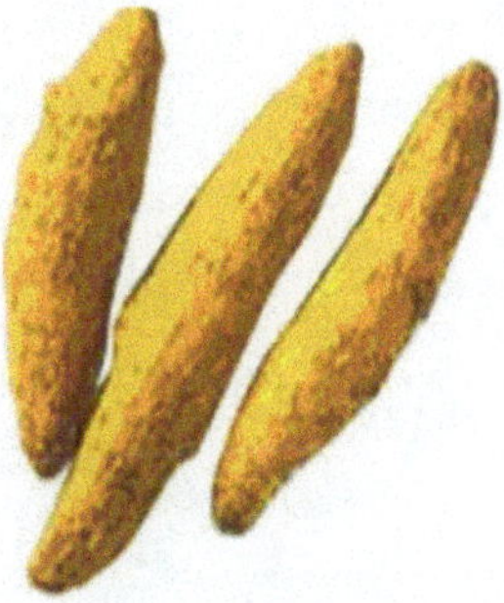

Botanical Name	*Curcuma longa*
Family Name	Zingiberaceae
Name in some International Languages	Spanish-Curcuma, Arabic-Kurcum, Chinese-Yu.Chin
Flavour Characteristics	Musky Flavour, slightly bitter and fragrant
Usage Profile	Foods, medicines and cosmetics
Commercial part	Rhizome or underground stem
Harvesting Season	December to March
Specifications Turmeric Oleoresin	
Description	Extract of dried rhizomes of *Curcuma longa* L. (Family: Zingiberaceae). It is oleoresin obtained by extraction of tubers of Curcuma longa Linn, with volatile solvents and concentration to remove the solvent. The oleoresin chiefly contains volatile oil, resin and yellow colouring matter known as curcuminoids.
Storage	Store in full, tight containers in a cool dry place, protected from sun light.
Appearance	Orange yellow to reddish brown colored semi solid
Odour	Characteristic mild flavour of turmeric.
Dispersibility/solubility	Can be dispersed in dry carriers such as salt, dextrose, etc.
Spice Equivalent	One kg replaces 60 kg of raw Turmeric
Colour Value	14100 to 14500 CU – EOA
Curcumin content	94 to 96.5%
Residual solvent	10 ppm - EOA
Microbiology	Free from microbial contaminants.
Self life	12 months under the specified storage conditions.
Handling	Avoid contact with skin and eyes.

Uses

- The chief component of curcuminoids is curcumin.
- Tumerone, zingiberene are the other constituents of volatile oil.
- It is reported to possess many pharmacological and anti inflammatory actions.

20 Celery Oleoresins

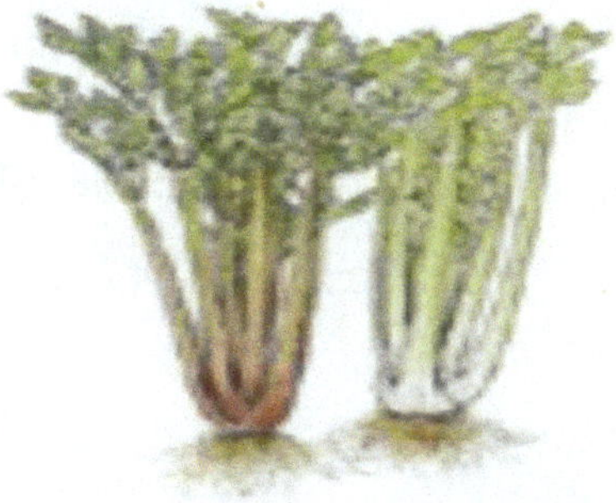

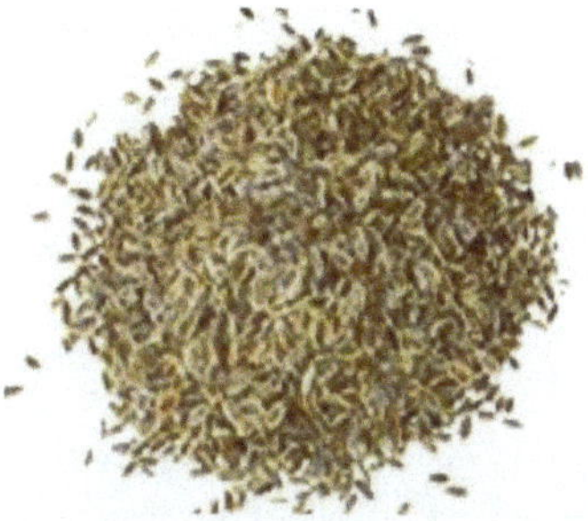

It is olive green free flowing liquid with herbal, slightly lemony and bitter flavour.

Botanical Name	*Apium graveolens*
Family Name	Umbelliferae
Name in some International Languages	Spanish - Aipo, Arabic - Karafs, Chinese - Chin
Flavour Characteristics	Slightly Bitter
Usage Profile	Perfumery, medicines & food
Commercial part	Dried Fruit
Harvesting Season	August to September
Specifications	
Product	Celery Oleoresin
Description	Oleoresin celery is obtained by the solvent extraction of the dried seeds of *Apium graveolens*
Colour & appearance	Greenish yellow in colour & free flowing liquid

Volatile oil content	11%
Residual solvent	<10 ppm
Solubility	Oil dispersible
Yeast & Mould	Nil
Pathogenic microorganisms and their toxins	Absent
Purity	Pure celery oleoresin (no other additives)
Storage	Store preferably in air tight containers and keep in a cool & dry place protected from light.

Uses

- It is the oleoresin derived from the dried rip seeds of the cultivated plants of *Apium graveolens* Linn.
- It contains 1.5-3.0 percent of pale yellow volatile oil; 15-17 percent of fixed oil is resins.
- The volatile oil has a very strong aromatic flavor, which chiefly contains d-limonene and sedanolides responsible for the characteristic flavour.
- Celery Oleoresin is also used as stimulant, carminative, nervine, sedative and even in tonic.
- It is also used to flavour soft drinks and unpleasant medicaments.
- It is used in meat seasoning, flavour soups, gravy, salad dressing confectionary and non-alcoholic beverages.
- Celery salt is a popular flavouring base.

Chapter 9

Plant Amines and Poisonous Plants

The term rare amino acid is misleading in some respects. It refers to all those amino acids that are not incorporated into proteins. We already got to know some of them like ornithine or citrulline that are rather common intermediates of the basic metabolism. Roughly 220 different structures are known, most of which occur in plant cells in a free state though glutamate-, oxalate- or acetyl- derivatives can also sometimes be found.

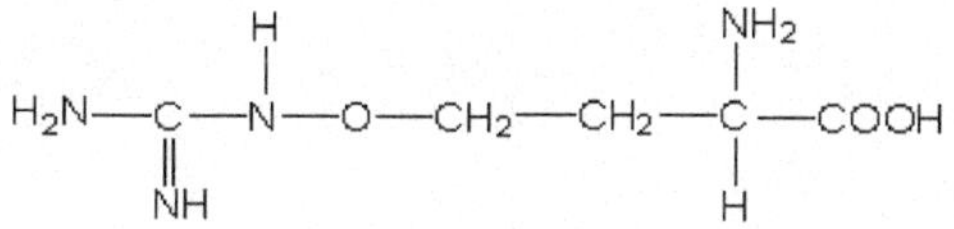

Canavanine

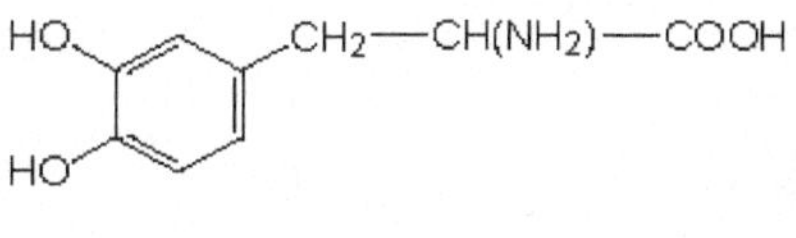

3, 4-dihydroxy phenylalanine

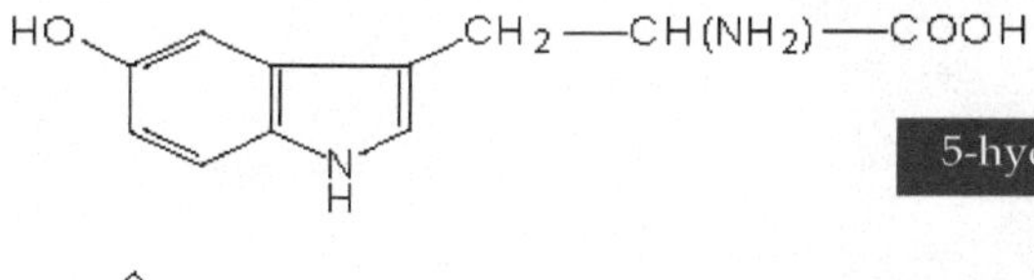

5-hydroxy tryptophane

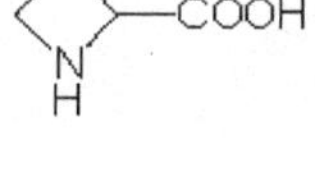

Acetidine-2-carboxylicacide

In some fungi, rare amino acids are polymerized to small, sometimes also cyclic polypeptides like in phalloidine or the amanitins, the toxins of the amanita. Derivatives of nearly all well-known 20 amino acids have been isolated and described. A certain rare amino acid occurs often only in one or a few plant species.

Of the 220 different types of molecules, only the syntheses of two derivatives of arginine, octopine and nopaline are shown here. They became known when it was found out that a plasmid of *Agrobacterium tumefaciens*, the pathogen of crown galls, is the carrier of the genetic information necessary for their syntheses.

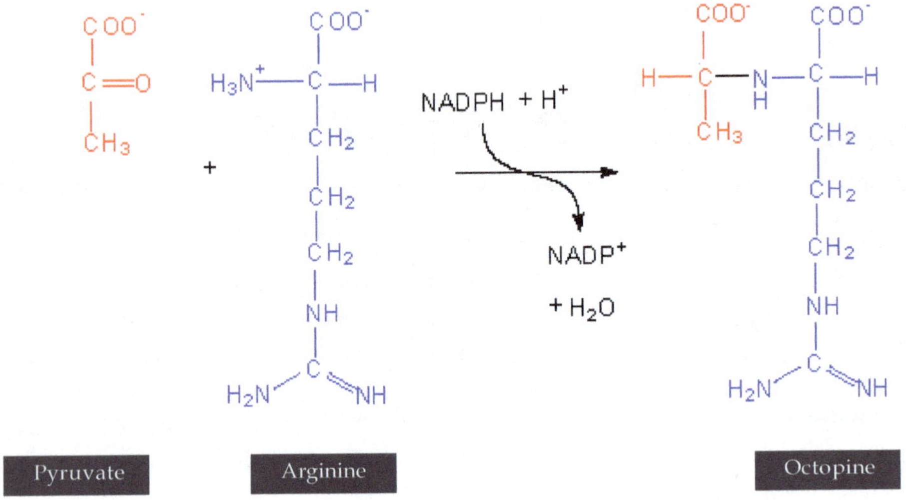

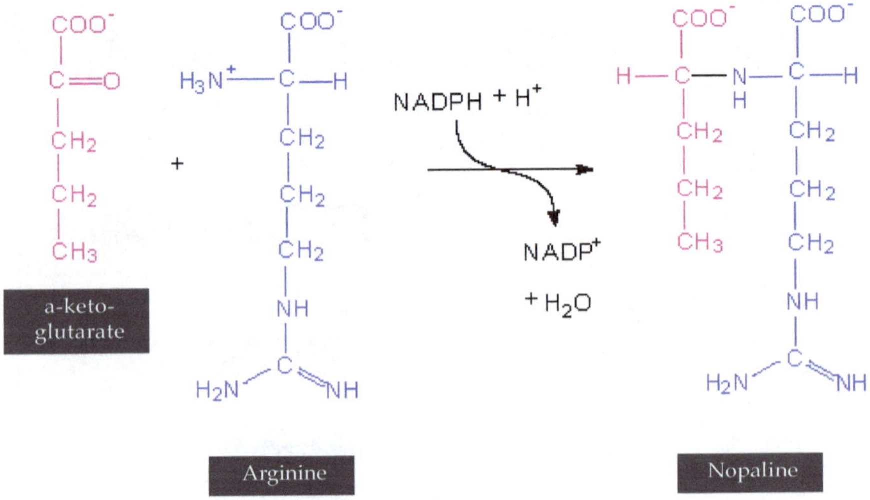

Plant Amines

Plant amines are derivatives of ammonia. Their collective structures are:

Primary amines	NH_2R
Secondary amines	NHRR′
Tertiary amines	NRR′R″
Quaternary amines	$N^+RR'R''R'''(OH^-)$

A wide range of plant amines can be found in the most different plant cells. They are usually generated by the decarboxylation of amino acids or by transamination of aldehydes. The distinction between plant amines and alkaloids is sometimes a little arbitrary. Some, like mescaline, are counted among the alkaloids although in a chemical sense they are amines.

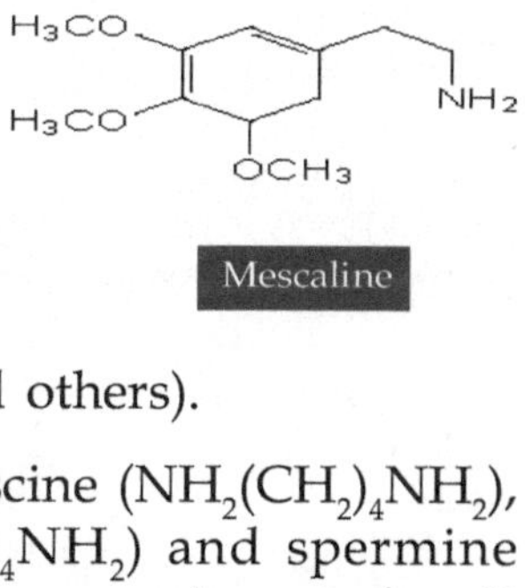

Mescaline

Aliphatic amines are often produced during anthesis, i.e. the opening of a flower or the formation of the fruiting body of certain fungi (like the stinkhorn, for example). They are insect-attractants. A good example of insect attractants is the aliphatic-aromatic amines in Araceae (lords-and-ladies, arum and others).

Among the di- and polyamines are putrescine ($NH_2(CH_2)_4NH_2$), as well as spermidine ($NH_2(CH_2)_3NH(CH_2)_4NH_2$) and spermine ($NH_2(CH_2)_3NH(CH_2)_4NH(CH_2)_3NH_2$). They occur in nearly all eucaryotic cells and interact with the DNA double helix. Among the tryptamines (tryptophane derivatives) are the phytohormone indole-3-acetic acid (IAA) as well as serotonin.

Poisonous Plants

Poisonous plants contain substances that can cause sickness or death if those substances are ingested or come into contact with the body of an animal. These substances are often referred to as "secondary compounds." Primary compounds are chemicals involved in basic metabolism, whereas secondary compounds are chemicals that are generally waste products of metabolism. Secondary plant compounds, the toxic substances, have coevolved in higher plants in response to attack by herbivorous insects for over one hundred million years. Animals are poisoned when the animals' protection mechanisms (detoxification) are inadequate.

Some Plants Poisonous to Humans and Animals.

Plant name and occurrence	**Poisonous plant parts and toxins**	**Comments**
Alfalfa (*Medicago sativa*) - forage and silage	leaves and stems - phytoestrogenic compounds, saponins, bloat-causing proteins	livestock, poultry: bloat, photosensitization (sickness after ingesting plant and subsequent exposure to sunlight), phytoestrogens cause infertility, reduced egg-laying in poultry
Astragalus (*Astragalus lentigenosus*) - rangeland plant	above-ground plant parts - alkaloid: swainsonine	livestock: locoism (erratic behavior), birth deformities, abortion, and (above 2120 m) contributes to congestive heart failure in cattle
Castor bean (*Ricinius communis*) - garden plant	seeds and to a lesser extent the leaves - toxalbumin: ricin	humans, livestock, pets: illness and death; chewing a single seed may sicken a child
Crown-of-thorns (*Euphorbia milii*) - house plant	plant juices or sap - toxic diterpenes including 5-deoxyingenol	humans and pets: irritant in the sap causes irritation of the skin, eyes, mouth
Johnson grass (*Sorghum halepense*) - outdoor weedy grass	leaves and stems - cyanogenic glycoside: dhurrin; nitrate accumulation	livestock: in the animal body dhurrin is converted to cyanide (which may be lethal); can accumulate excessive amounts of nitrates causing death, abortion
Kochia (*Kochia scoparia*) - outdoor and garden plant	leaves, flowers, and seeds - alkaloids, oxalates, and saponins	livestock: photosensitization
Oleander (*Nerium oleander*) - house and garden plant	leaves and stems - glycosides: oleandrin, nerioside	livestock and humans: nausea, vomiting, dizziness, death (e.g. poisoning of humans after eating hot dogs roasted on oleander sticks)
Poison ivy (*Rhus radicans*), Poison sumac (*Rhus vernix*), Western poison oak (*Rhus diversiloba*), - outdoor plants	plant sap - allergin: urushiol containing catechols	humans: allergic reaction causing dermatitis, blisters (many humans develop symptoms after only one exposure); sap contaminates clothing, tools, etc.
Rhubarb (*Rheum raponticum*): - food plant	leaf blade, not the leaf stems - oxalic acid	livestock and humans: leaf stems (petioles) are edible; leaf blades contain oxalic acid crystals causing nausea, vomiting, abdominal pain
Spotted water-hemlock (*Cicuta maculata*) - outdoor plant	all parts, especially roots - alkaloids: cicutoxin, cicutol	animals and humans: most violently toxic plant in North America; symptoms can appear suddenly causing spasms, coma, and death

Secondary compounds include chemicals such as alkaloids, glycosides, oxalates, saponins, tannins, and toxalbumins. These chemicals are toxic in various ways to vertebrates. Some responses are dramatic (violent spasms, death) or subtle (reduced weight gain, birth defects). Other chemicals are only toxic after being altered inside the animal body (for example, cyanogenic glycosides, which produce cyanide) or if the animal is exposed to the sun (photosensitization). Researchers continue to discover new toxins from plants.

In 1986 it was estimated that poisoning of cattle, sheep, and horses grazing western U.S. rangelands cost ranchers $190 million per year. Most cases of human poisoning involve house and garden plants. In 1998 there were 122,578 plant-related calls to poison control centers in the United States, according to information from the American Association of Poison Control Centers. Only 109 of those cases were serious (but included four fatalities).

Some cases of plant poisoning are remarkable. During the nineteenth century tragic loss of human life occurred from a mysterious milk sickness in which cattle ingested white snakeroot and a toxin was passed on to humans through the milk. In 1971 near Garrison, Utah, more than twelve hundred sheep died after ingesting the rangeland plant halogeton. Although these toxic compounds are harmful to most species that ingest them, some insects are not harmed by some of the toxins and actually sequester the poison in their own body as a defense against their own predators.

The apparent lack of primary function in the plant, combined with the observation that many secondary metabolites have specific negative impacts on other organisms such as herbivores and pathogens, leads to the hypothesis that they have evolved because of their protective value. Many secondary metabolites are toxic or repellant to herbivores and microbes and help defend plants producing them. Production increases when a plant is attacked by herbivores or pathogens. Some compounds are released into the air when plants are attacked by insects; these compounds attract parasites and predators that kill the herbivores. Recent research is identifying more and more primary roles for these chemicals in plants as signals, antioxidants, and other functions, so "secondary" may not be an accurate description in the future.

Consuming some secondary metabolites can have severe consequences. Alkaloids can block ion channels, inhibit enzymes, or interfere with neurotransmission, producing hallucinations, loss of coordination, convulsions, vomiting, and death. Some phenolics interfere with digestion, slow growth, block enzyme activity and cell division, or just taste awful.

Most herbivores and plant pathogens possess mechanisms that ameliorate the impacts of plant metabolites, leading to evolutionary associations between particular groups of pests and plants. Some herbivores (for example, the monarch butterfly) can store (sequester) plant toxins and gain protection against their enemies. Secondary metabolites may also inhibit the growth of competitor plants (allelopathy). Pigments (such as terpenoid carotenes, phenolics, and flavonoids) color flowers and, together with terpene and phenolic odors, attract pollinators.

Secondary chemicals are important in plant use by humans. Most pharmaceuticals are based on plant chemical structures, and secondary metabolites are widely used for recreation and stimulation (the alkaloids nicotine and cocaine; the terpene cannabinol). The study of such plant use is called ethnopharmacology. Psychoactive plant chemicals are central to some religions, and flavours of secondary compounds shape our food preferences. The characteristic flavours and aroma of cabbage and relatives are caused by nitrogen-and sulfur-containing chemicals, glucosinolates, which protect these plants from many enemies. The astringency of wine and chocolate derives from tannins. The use of spices and other seasonings developed from their combined uses as preservatives (since they are antibiotic) and flavorings.

Class	Compounds	Sources	Some Effects and Uses
Nitrogen-Containing			
Alkaloids	Nicotine cocaine theobromine	Tobacco coca plant chocolate (cocao)	Interfere with neurotransmission, block enzyme action
Nitrogen-and Sulfur-containing			
Glucosinolates	Sinigrin	Cabbage, relatives	Carcinogenic
Terpenoids			
Monoterpenes	Menthol linalool	Mint and relatives, many plants	Interfere with neurotransmission, block ion transport, anesthetic
Sesquiterpenes	Parthenolid	Parthenium and relatives (*Asteraceae*)	Contact dermatitis
Diterpenes	Gossypol	Cotton	Block phosphorylation; toxic

contd...

Table contd...

Triterpenes, cardiac glycosides	Digitogenin	Digitalis (foxglove)	Stimulate heart muscle, alter ion transport
Tetraterpenoids	Carotene	Many plants	Antioxidant; orange coloring
Terpene polymers	rubber	Hevea (rubber) trees, dandelion	gum up insects; airoplane tires
Sterols	Spinasterol	Spinach	Interfere with animal hormone action
Phenolics			
Phenolic acids	Caffeic, chlorogenic	All plants	Cause oxidative damage, browning in fruits and wine
Coumarins	Umbelliferone	Carrots, parsnip	Cross-link DNA, block cell division
Lignans	Podophyllin urushiol	Mayapple poison ivy	Cathartic, vomiting, allergic dermatitis
Flavonoids	Anthocyanin, catechin	Almost all plants	Flower, leaf color; inhibit enzymes, anti- and pro-oxidants, estrogenic
Tannins	Gallotannin, condensed tannin	Oak, hemlock trees, birdsfoot trefoil, legumes	Bind to proteins, enzymes, block digestion, antioxidants
Lignin	Lignin	All land plants	Structure, toughness, fiber

Chapter 10

Assay of Secondary Metabolites

Isolation and Purification of Secondary Metabolites

Isolation

The act of isolating something; setting something apart from others.

Purification

The process of making pure, free from anything that debases, pollutes, or contaminates, the process of removing impurities.

Crystallization

Crystallization is the (natural or artificial) process of formation of solid crystals from a uniform solution. Crystallization is also a chemical solid-liquid separation technique, in which mass transfer of a solute from the liquid solution to a pure solid crystalline phase occurs. The crystallization process consists, Nucleation Crystal Growth. Nucleation is the step where the solute molecules dispersed in the solvent start together into clusters, on the nanometer scale (elevating solute concentration in a small region), that becomes stable under the current operating conditions. These stable clusters constitute the nuclei.

The crystal growth is the subsequent growth of the nuclei that succeed in achieving the critical cluster size. Many compounds have the ability to crystallize with different crystal structures, a phenomenon called polymorphism. Crystallization may be natural or by artificial methods. For crystallization to occur the solution must be supersaturated. This can be achieved by various methods viz., (1) solution cooling, (2) addition of a second solvent to reduce the solubility of the solute (technique known as anti-solvent or drown-out), (3) chemical reaction and (4) change in pH being the most common methods used in industrial practice. Other methods, such as solvent evaporation, can also be used.

Equipment for Crystallization

1. Tank crystallizers.
2. Scraped surface crystallizers.
3. Double-pipe scraped surface crystallizer.
4. Circulating-liquid evaporator-crystallizer.
5. Circulating-magma vacuum crystallizer.

General Procedure for Extraction and Detection of Alkaloids

Alkaloids are extracted in organic and inorganic solvents depending upon types of alkaloids. The nitrogen generally makes the compound basic and the compound exists in the plant as a salt. Thus, alkaloids are often extracted with water or mild acid and then recovered as crystalline material by treatment with base.

About 5 g dried plant material is kept in 50 ml of 10 % ammonical ethanol for 48 h at room temperature with occasional shaking. The extract then filtered and concentrated under vacuum. The dried/ concentrated extract is acidified with 25 ml of 0.1 N H_2SO_4. The acid extract is centrifuged and the clear supernatant is tested with Mayer's, Wanger's and Dragendorff's reagent.

Solvent Extraction of Alkaloids

Powdered plant material (10 g) wetted with 15 ml NH_4OH (25%, m/m) can be used for solvent extraction performed with 300 mL of ethyl acetate for 72 h. Then after extract is filtered and solvent is evaporated. Dissolve the residue in water, acidify with H_2SO_4. Reextract with petroleum ether & diethyl ether to remove lipophilic, acidic and neutral material. Aqueous phase is made basic by adding NH_4OH. The extract is now washed with distilled water to neutral pH, and finally dried to obtain crude alkaloids. The nitrogen generally makes the compound basic and the compound exists in the plant as a salt. Thus, alkaloids are often extracted with water or mild acid and then recovered as crystalline material by treatment with base.

Alkaloids are also Extracted Using Surfactant

Sample (10 g) suspended in 400 ml of surfactant solution (SDS or Polyethylene glycol dodecyl ether), sonicated in ultrasonic bath (2.5h). Extract is separated by filteration, residual material washed with water. solution acidified with H_2SO_4 & precipitated with 15 ml Mayer reagent. Precipitate dissolved with Na_2CO_3 & extracted with $CHCl_3$.Organic layer washed with water to neutral pH, concentrated to dryness. The extract washed with distilled water to neutral pH, dried to obtain crude alkaloids.

Detection of Alkaloids

Plant extracts are often primarily analyzed by Thin Layer Chromatography (TLC) for qualitative and semi quantitative determination. Colorimetric detection is also possible. Determination of alkaloids by High Performance Liquid Chromatography (HPLC) and capillary Gas Liquid Chromatography (GLC) is more useful because of good resolving power. For small quantities of known alkaloids determination Radioimmunoassay (RIA) or Enzyme Linked Immunosorbant Assay (ELISA) are more appropriate.

Tests for Alkaloids

I. Dragendorff – $NaNO_2$ Reagent

1. Potassium Bismuth Iodide (Dissolve 8 g Bismuth nitrite (Bi $(NO_3)_3$. $5H_2O$) in 20 ml HNO_3)
2. Iodide - 27.2g KI in 50 ml water.

These two solutions are mixed and allowed to stand when KNO_3 crystallizes out. The crystals are allowed to settle and the supernatant is decanted and made up to 100 ml with distilled water.

II. Mayer's Reagent

Mercury chloride $HgCl_2$ (1.36 g) is dissolved in 60 ml distilled water (Solution A) and 5 g of KI in 10 ml water (Solution B). Both the solutions (A & B) are mixed and diluted to 100 ml with distilled water. Since this reagent reacts only with the salts of alkaloids, the alkaloidal solution should be made distinctly acidic with HCl or H_2SO_4 before adding the reagent. Only one or two drops of Mayer's reagent should be added in the beginning because the precipitates of some alkaloids are soluble in excess of the reagent. If no precipitate is obtained with the first two drops of the reagent, more reagents are added. A white precipitate indicates the presence of alkaloids. Mayer's reagent is the most useful reagent since it gives precipitate with hydrochlorides of most alkaloids.

III. Wanger's Reagent

Iodine (1.27 g) and potassium iodide (2 g) after proper mixing are dissolved in 5 ml of distilled water and the solution is made upto 100 ml with distilled water. This reagent gives brown flocculent precipitate with many alkaloids.

IV. Ninhydrin Reagent

Thirty milligram (30 mg) ninhydrin in 10 ml n-butanol + 0.3 ml of glacial acetic acid. After spraying the plate is heated at 110° C for 5-10 min. This test is to detect presence of amino groups which yield violet colour for amino groups.

V. Anisaldehyde – Sulphuric acid Reagent

Prepared by mixing 18 ml ethanol (95%), 1 ml of conc. H_2SO_4, 1 ml anisaldehyde and two drops of glacial acetic acid. The plates, sprayed with this reagent, are heated on a hot plate at 90-100 ° C for 5-10 min.

Estimation of Alkaloids from *Atropa belladonna Spp*

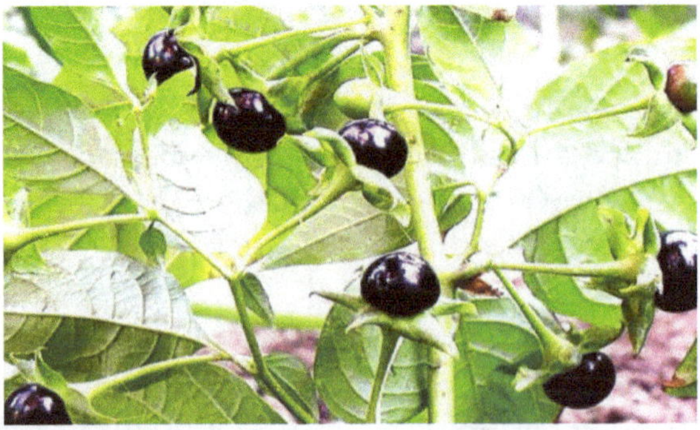

The foliage and flowers, of the three major species of Hyoscymus viz. niger, muticus and albus yield tropane alkaloids which are used in the treatment of asthma, whooping cough and a host of other ailments. Hyoscyamine is indistinguishable from atropine and both are seen together as a spot of low Rf, while scopolamine occupies a higher level. (The colors produced by

Dragendorff's reagent are transient. An over spray of aqueous 5 %-sodium nitrite changes the color of hyoscyamine / atropine to brownish red from orange yellow. Though scopolamine also turns brownish red the color disappears after some time).

Extraction of Atropine

Juice of atropa leaves is treated with potassium carbonate (K_2CO_3) and extracted in chloroform. The chloroform is evaporated and alkaloid atropine is extracted with dilute H_2SO_4 . This is made alkaline by addition of K_2CO_3. The precipitated atropine is purified by washing and crystallization. Tropine and tropic acid can also be converted to atropine with heating in HCl.

A-I. Isolation of Tropane Alkaloid

Finely powdered (100 g) leaves of Atropa (containing chiefly L-hyoscyamine) are extracted exhaustively with 95 % ethanol in a soxhlet extractor. The ethanol is removed by distillation and the syrupy residue is treated with 100 ml 1% HCl. The solution is filtered and the filtrate is shaken with petroleum ether to remove the resinous matter. The acidic solution is made alkaline by the addition of ammonia and the alkaloids are extracted in chloroform. The chloroform solution is shaken with diluted 0.1 N HCl. The HCl solution is neutralized and the alkaloids are again extracted in chloroform. The solvent is removed by distillation and the resulting residue is dissolved in minimum of 0.1N oxalic acid. The oxalates of alkaloids are dissolved in a minimum quantity of acetone and ether is added to the acetone solution slowly till cloudiness appears. On standing, atropine oxalate crystallizes first which is filtered off. The remaining solution is concentrated and more ether is added to it when hyoscyamine oxalate crystals appear. For TLC the solvent system used is : Toluene : Ethyl acetate : Diethylamine (70:20:10) and detection by Dragendorff's reagent.

A-II. Tests for Tropane Alkaloids

1. Vitali-Morin reaction for atropine, hyoscyamine and hyoscine

A little of the solution containing the alkaloid is evaporated to dryness in a porcelain dish on a water bath and the residue is treated with about 0.2 ml of fuming nitric acid and again evaporated to dryness on a water bath. The residue is dissolved in 10 ml of pure acetone (water-free) and a solution 3 % potassium hydroxide in a methanol; added drop wise-a characteristic deep purple colour is produced (This colour is not produced by cocaine).

2. Rathenasinkam reaction for cocaine

To about 0.5 mg of extracted alkaloid in a test tube, 100 mg of potassium nitrate and 10 drops of conc. H_2SO_4 are added and the mixture heated in a boiling waterbath for 10 min. The solution is cooled, diluted with water to about 30 ml and extracted with chloroform. The chloroform is removed and discarded. The aqueous solution is made alkaline with ammonia and again extracted with chloroform. The chloroform is evaporated off and the residue is dissolved in 2 ml of acetone and 1 or 2 drops of 10 % NaOH solution is added-a bluish purple color is formed for positive test.

Estimation of Total Alkaloids from Vinca (*Catharantus roseus*)

Total alkaloid content is estimated by titrimetric method of Masoud *et al.* (1968). Powdered root material (1 g.) is repeatedly extracted with methanol. The extracts are combined and the solvents are removed using a rotary vacuum evaporator. The residue is extracted in 1N HCl and the filtered acid solution is made alkaline with 1 : 3 ammonia to pH 10. The total alkaloid was extracted from this solution with chloroform and the chloroform was dried over sodium sulphate and filtered. After the removal of solvent, the residue is dissolved in glacial acetic acid and titrated against 0.01 N perchloric acid in glacial acetic acid using crystal violet as an indicator. The visual colour is green.

Alkaloids of Adhatoda

A. zelanica is a well-known plant medicine in the Ayurvedic and Unani systems of medicine and is recommended for bronchitis, asthma, fever and jaundice. Leaves and roots are antispasmodic and used as expectorants. Vasicine and vasicinone are known bronchodilators; Vasicine reduces the blood pressure temporarily as slows down the rhythm of heartbeats.

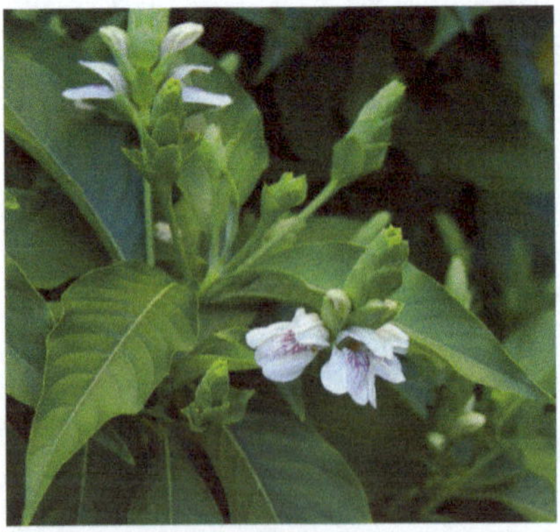

The leaves, bark and roots contain the alkaloids vasicine, vasicinone, pegonine and vasicinol (6-hydroxy peganine). Vasicine, the principal alkaloid ranged between 0.2- 0.4 % in the leaves. However, it was reported upto 0.35 % in the bark. Roots contain vasicine in traces. Leaves contain small amount of a volatile oil.

Extraction of Alkaloids

Twenty gram of powdered leaves are transferred to a soxhlet extractor, kept covered with ethanol and allowed to stand overnight. The extraction is carried out for six h. in the two days in a water bath.Extract is concentrated to dryness and to the residue 20 ml of 5 % aqueous lead acetate solution is added. The flask is shaken well and then stirred with a glass rod so that the entire residue is separated and suspended in the aqueous layer. The solution is filtered to remove the yellow precipitate (lead phosphate). The flask is washed with 20 ml 0.1 N H_2SO_4 and using an acid solution the funnel and the filter paper also are washed down to the filtrate. To the filtrate 10 more ml. of diluted sulphuric acid added and the precipitated lead sulphate is filtered. The precipitate is washed with water until free of alkaloid. The combined washings and the filtrate are extracted thrice with 10 ml portions of chloroform to remove coloring matters and other impurities. The combined chloroform extract is extracted once with 10 ml of 0.1 N H_2SO_4 and this acid extract is added to the original aqueous extract.

The aqueous extract is made distinctly alkaline by the addition of dilute ammonia and is shaken with successive quantities of 40,25,20,15 and 5 ml of chloroform until complete extraction of alkaloids takes place (the aqueous extract is tested with Mayer's reagent). The combined chloroform extracts containing the alkaloids is filtered through a cotton plug (previously soaked in chloroform). The plug is later washed with 5 ml of chloroform and mixed with the original filtrate. The solvent is then removed by keeping in a water bath and the residue is dissolved in 20 ml of 0.1N HCl. The excess of acid is titrated with 0.1 N NaOH using bromothymol blue as the indicator, taking the appearance of a greenish blue colour as the end point. 1 ml of 0.1 N HCl is equivalent to 0.188 g of the alkaloid calculated as vasicine.

Chromatography of Alkaloids

Extracts : 10 % Ammonical ethanol

TLC (silica gel) solvent system : Ethyl acetate : Methanol : Water (100 : 13.5 : 10)

Spray reagent : Dragendorff's reagent

Visicine low Rf : 0.3

Vasicinone Rf : 0.8

Isolation of Vasicine and Vasicinone

Dried leaves (500 g) are refluxed with 2.5lit. of 90 % ethanol for 1 h. The extract is filtered and the alcohol is removed under reduced pressure. The dark green residue obtained is extracted thrice, with hot distilled water and the aqueous extract is filtered. The filtrate is extracted 5 times with chloroform to remove the coloring matters, made alkaline with 5% caustic soda and repeatedly extracted with chloroform till free of alkaloids. The combined chloroform extracts are extracted with 5 % HCl until the chloroform extract is free of alkaloids. The acid solution is made alkaline with ammonia and alkaloids are extracted with chloroform. After repeating the procedure twice the chloroform extract is filtered and concentrated to dryness to a brown powder (approx. 3-4 g). This powder is dissolved in hot ethanol and on cooling crystals begins to appear. The crystals are filtered, dissolved in boiling absolute alcohol and a little ethereal hydrochloric acid appears. These crystals are filtered off and the mother liquor is treated with dry ether till a slight turbidity observed. This is allowed to stand for three days at 15 °C when brown crystals of vasicine hydrochloride appear. Vasicine hydrochloride is dissolved in 95 % alcohol and boiled with charcoal to decolorized and recrystallised to give colorless crystals.

On standing, vasicine, due to auto oxidation in presence of light, gets converted to vasicinone.

Thin Layer Chromatography for alkaloids detection

S. No.	Name of the plant and active components	Extraction solvent	Solvent System	Spray Reagent
1	**Datura** (*Datura metel* L.- Solanaceae) Hyoscyamine, Atropine + Hyoscyamine and Scopolamine	10 % Ammoniacal ethanol	Toluene – ethyl acetate – diethylamine (70:20:10)	Dragendorff – $NaNO_2$ Reagent
2	***Ephedra*** (*Ephedra sinica* Stapf and other sp. Gnetaceae) Ephedrine	$CHCl_3$ – Ether (1:3), 5 ml 10% ammonia solution, 0.5 g sodium carbonate	Toluene-Ethyl acetate-diethylamine (70:20:10)	Ninhydrin Reagent Grey coloured spot against red - violet background

contd....

3	***Rauwolfia*** (*Rauwolfia tetraphylla* L- Apocynaceae) Serpentine, Ajmaline, Reserpine + Rescinnamine, Raubasine	10 % Ammoniacal ethanol	Toluene - ethyl acetate - diethylamine (70:20:10)	Dragendorff Reagent
4	***Liquorice*** (*Glycyrrhiza glabra* L. - Fabaceae) Glycyrrhizin	Extracted in boiling water and concentrated	Ethyl acetate- Formic acid - Acetic acid - Water (100:11:11:27)	Anisaldehyde - Sulphuric acid Reagent

Estimation of Steviocide from stevia *Stevia reboudiani*

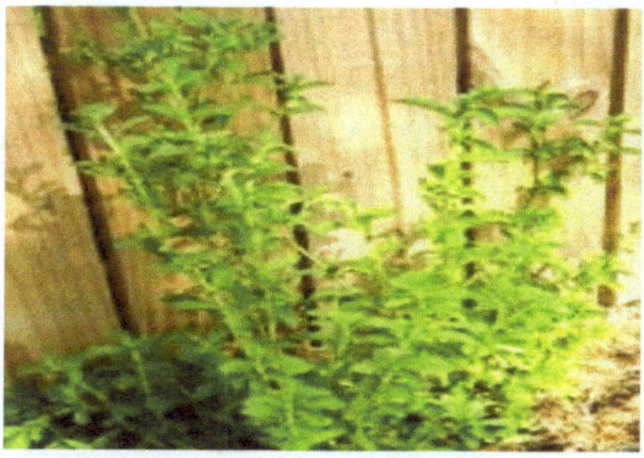

Steviocides are diterpenes glycosides found in *Stevia reboudiani* contain 8-10 %. It is 150-300 times more sweeter than sugar. Stevia is natural sweeter cultivated in Japan, China and North Amrica. It also has antioxidant activity.

Isolation : 2-3 g. fresh weight leaf are ground with methanol and kept at room temperature for more than one day.

- Filter it and the filtrate is evaporated to dryness.
- Water and n-Butenol (BuoH) are added to the residue and the solution is mixed well
- The n-BuoH layer is collected and evaporated to dryness.

Purification

- The residue are dissolved in water and applied to silanized Si gel Colum.(3 g. Si gel/colum)
- The colum is rinsed by water followed by 20 % methanol.
- Stesviode glycosides were eluted with 50 ml of 80 % methyl alcohol (meOH), the fraction are evaporated to dryness. Dissolve in methanol and estimate through HPLC at ambient temperature mobile phase methanol : Deionised water (68:32). How rate 0.9 ml/min. UV detection at 210 nm.

Estimation of Aloin from *Aloe vera*

Chemical Evaluation of *Aloe barbadensis*

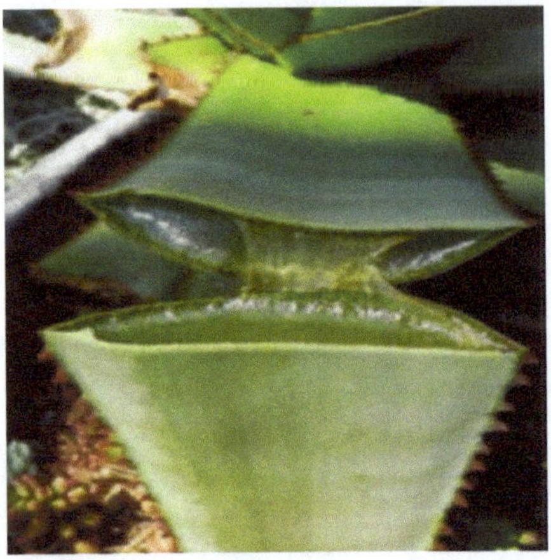

Aloe has been used mainly for therapeutic and cosmetic purposes. Two distinct components can be recognized, the leaf exudates used largely as purgative and the leaf parenchyma, effective against a range of skin lesions. There are many therapeutic actions but the purgative action has received most detailed investigation. Level of barbaloin, a c-glycoside present in the exudates of leaf, is a reliable measure of cathartic response. The second most important use of aloes is in cosmetic, in different blends. The mucilagenous pulp from the leaf parenchyma, which is mainly carbohydrate in nature, is used in skin-disorders.

Above mentioned two important constituents namely barbaloin and aloe-gel can be investigated and chemically evaluated as follows:

I. Aloin Content

The cathartic activity is ascribed due to presence of certain anthroquinones. These are assayed as aloin content, which is mainly barbaloin (10-glucopyranosyl derivative of aloe emodine). Aloin content is assayed in aloe, a commercial dried form of leaf exudates.

1. Leaves of one year old whole plant may be used for chemical assay. It is recommended that plants may be selected at the time of flowering.
2. Transverse incisions are made into leaves. Exudates is allowed to ooze out from the leaves and collected in the beaker.
3. One ml. of leaf exudate is dried and weighed. This is used for calculating percent aloin in dried exudate i.e. Aloe.
4. Another portion of filtered exudates (5-10 ml) was transferred to separating funnel. This is repeatedly extracted with ethyl-acetate (4x25 ml)

5. Total ethyl extract is filtered and evaporated at reduced pressure and low temperature (50 °C).
6. Residue is redissolved in warm water (100 ml) and a little portion (1-2 ml) is taken for chemical assay of aloin.

Recommended Method for the Evaluation of Aloin

The principle constituent of each of the two varieties is barbaloin, a 10- glucopyranosyl derivative of aloe-emodin anthrone [10(1-deoxyglucosyl) aloe-emodin anthrone], small amounts of aloe-emodin is also present. In addition, Curacao aloes contains isobarbaloin and aloinosides A & B.

Principle

Barbaloin reacts with Iron (III) chloride in acidic medium and produced red colour on incubation at 100°C. The colour is eluted in carbon tetrachloride (CCl_4) and then in sodium hydroxide. The colour intensity is measured at 500 nm and 400 nm against blank.

Reagents

1. Carbon tetrachloride (CCl_4)
2. Iron (III) chloride solution, 60 % w/v- Analytical - reagent.
3. Conc. Hydrochloric acid, B.P.
4. Methanol
5. 1N, Sodium hydroxide
6. Distilled water.

Procedure

1. Weigh accurately 0.2 g of powdered curacao aloes or about 0.4 g of powdered aloes and place the sample in a 200 ml conical flask. Moisten with 2 ml of methanol, add 5 ml of water previously warmed to about 60 °C, mix, add a further 75 ml of water at about 60 °C and shake the mixture in a shaker for 30 min. Cool the mixture. Filter through Whatman No.4 filter paper into a 100 ml volumetric flask, wash the conical flask, filter with 20 ml of water, and make up the volume to 100 ml with water.
2. Place 10 ml of this solution in a round - bottomed 100 ml flask containing 1.0 ml of 60 per cent Iron (III) chloride solution and

6.0 ml Hydrochloric acid, Attach a water-cooled, double surface condenser to the flask in a bath of continuously boiling water and heat for 4 h. Cool the solution, transfer it into a separating funnel, rinse out the round-bottomed flask successively with 3-4 ml of water, 3-4 ml of one normal sodium hydroxide and 3-4 ml of water, adding these rinsings to the contents of the separating funnel.

3. Extract the contents of the separating funnel with three 20 ml portions of carbon tetrachloride. Wash the combined carbon tetrachloride layers with two 10 ml portions of water. Reject the washings.

   Extract the carbon tetrachloride layer with one 15 ml portion and with successive 5 ml portions of one normal Sodium Hydroxide (NaOH) until the final Sodium Hydroxide extract is colourless. Combine the alkaline extracts, heat them in a shallow dish on a bath of boiling water for five min., with constant stirring to remove carbon tetrachloride, cool and adjust to 50 ml with 1 N sodium hydroxide. Determine the extinction of the solution in a 1-cm cell at 400 nm. and at the maximum at 500 nm against 1 N sodium hydroxide in similar a cell. The reading should be taken within one h. of beginning the alkaline extraction with one 15 ml portion of 1 N sodium hydroxide and particular care should be taken to carry out these stages of the estimation in subdued light.

4. Calculate the percentage of anhydrous barbaloin present, on the assumption that the E value at 500 nm of the red solution obtained from anhydrous barbaloin is 209. Also calculate the ratio value E 500 nm/E 440 nm. If this ratio is less than 1.9 than the material is of not good quality.

Calibration of Recommended Method with Anhydrous Barbaloin

1. Weigh accurately about 200 mg barbaloin and dry into constant weight at 105 to 110 °C in vacuo, taking due cares to dry the air – re-admitted to the vacuum oven. Calculate the moisture content of the sample of barbaloin. Discard the dried material.

   At the same time weigh accurately about 50 mg of the sample of barbaloin, dissolve it in water and adjust the volume to 500 ml.

2. Follow serial No. (2) onwards and continuing end of section (4) as mentioned in above procedure. Calculate the E value for

anhydrous barbaloin at 500 nm, as examined by this method. Also calculate the ratio value E 500 nm/E 400 nm. If this ratio is less than 1.9, reject the result.

Preparation of Standard Graph

1 mg of Aloin (SIGMA) diluted in methanol and an aliquote is prepared accordingly.

2. Extraction and Purification of Aloe Gel

The second most important use of aloe is in cosmetics. Aloe-gel is the part of mucilaginous pulp and the following method has been standardized for chemical evaluation.

1. Leaves remaining after the removal of its exudate are cut upon and its mucilage is scrapped out with blunt edged knife. This mucilage is stirred vigorously in a blender to make it uniform. This solution is strained through a muslin cloth and filtered. This uniform solution is extracted for cold-extracted gel (CEG) and hot extracted gel (HEG).

Cold-Extracted Gel (CEG)

This solution is acidified with HCl (pH 3.5) and the crude gel is precipitated out from the extract by adding slowly 95 % alcohol while stirring. The gel is obtained by centrifugation.

Hot-Extracted Gel (HEG)

Mass left after passing the blended solution through muslin cloth, is repeatedly treated with hot water until the complete extraction of gel is effected. The crude gel (HEG) is prepared as described above.

Purification

The crude gel obtained by above method, is washed several times with ethanol till free from chloride ions. It is also stirred with absolute acetone and diethyl ether and dried over anhydrous $CaCl_2$ in a vacuum desiccator. The dried gel is also treated with petroleum-ether to remove lipoidal material and greenish tinge of chlorophyll. Dry aloe-gel is white amorphous powder when dried under reduced pressure in a vacuum desiccator.

Isolation, Purification and Crystallization of Aloin

Aloin is isolated from aloe plant (*Aloe barbadanis*) native to Africa.

Source of two herbal preparations:

1. Aloe gel (AG)
2. Aloe latex.

Aloe gel "clear gel" or mucilaginous substance produced by parenchymal cells located in the central region of the leaf. pericyclic tubular cells beneath the outer leaf epidermis produce a bitter yellow substance known as aloe latex, Aloe latex contains a series of glycosides known as anthraquinones, the most prominent being aloin.

Two Classes of Aloin are as Under

1. Nataloins, which yield picric and oxalic acids with nitric acid, and do not give a red coloration with nitric acid.
2. Barbaloins, which yield aloetic acid ($C_7H_2N_3O_5$), chrysammic acid ($C_7H_2N_2O_6$), picric and oxalic acids with nitric acid, being reddened by the acid.

Aloin, has been shown to inactivate various enveloped viruses, such as herpes simplex and also use as laxative.

Isolation and Purification

Aloe Jiuce Extracted from the Leaves of Various Aloe Species

↓

Air Drying or Spray Drying of the Aloe Juice

↓

Extraction in Methanol or higher Alochols

↓

Concentration of the extract

↓

Removal of Sugar, Fats and Colours

↓

Isolation of Cruide Aloin

↓

Purification of Aloin

↓

Crystallization of Aloin

↓

Packing

Crystallization

Crystallizable aloin is the body to which especially all the varieties of aloes owe their bitterness. Its isolation is usually thought to be a matter of some difficulty, but the following simple process.

1. Select a specimen of Barbadoes aloes, the most powerfully odorous that can be procured, bright-looking, and not the most waxy;
2. Break it up and dissolve it in a quantity of boiling distilled water, To which a few drops of sulphuric, sulphurous, or hydrochloric acid have been added.
3. The proportions employed may be those of the Pharmacopoeia for Extractum Aloes, *viz.* one pound to a gallon.
4. Let the liquid stand a night to deposit resin, then pour it off and evaporate quickly till, if 1 lb. of aloes have been used, about 2 lbs. of liquid remain.
5. This left for twenty-four hours will deposit an abundant crop of yellow crystalline matter.
6. The fluid portion poured off and duly concentrated yields a first-rate extract.
7. The yellow crystals must be well drained and pressed, and will yield pure aloin by recrystallization once or twice from water mixed with a small proportion of rectified spirits.

If the selection of the aloes be looked to, the product will amount to about 20 %. of the material employed.

Estimation of Quinones from Aloe

Beside aloin and barbaloin, aloe also contains a group of anthroquinone glycosides and quinones. Isobarbaloin and aloe-emodin (the aglycone of barbaloin) are the minor constituents. The drug also contains a resin composed of resinotannols and aromatic acids like cinnamic and coumaric acids.

Aloes are bitter with a disagreeable taste and are used as cathartics and in the treatment of constipation. It is also used as valuable medicine for the treatment of piles and burnt tissues. The mucilage present in the leaves is cooling and used to poultice inflammations.

Extraction and Separation of quinones by TLC

For extraction of quinones 1g of aloe leaf powder is boiled with 10 ml of methanol for 5 min. The extract is filtered, concentrated to 1 ml and spotted on TLC (Silica gel) plates and developed in ethyl acetate: methanol: Water (100:17:13). Quinones appear as light yellow spots, which on standing exposed to air turns purple in colour. This reaction is enhanced by spraying the plates with 5 % ethanolic potassium hydroxide. Quinones turn bright yellow or reddish pink colour. The plates are then seen in UV (365 nm). Aloin appears as a bright yellow spot having an R_f value of about 0.4, and aloe-emodin is seen as a red spot in the solvent front. A number of blue fluorescing spots in between are of phenolic acids.

Estimation of Tannins

The Tannins are Estimated by the Following Two Methods

1. *Folin-Denis Method* : This is based on the non-stoichiometric oxidation of the molecules containing a phenolic hydroxy1 group.

Principle

Tannin-like compounds reduce phosphotoungstomolybdic acid in alkaline solution to produce a highly colored blue solution, the intensity of which is proportional to the amount of tannin. The intensity is measured in a spectrophotometre at 700 nm.

Reagents

1. *Folin-Denis Reagent*: Dissolve 100 g sodium toungstate and 20 g phosphomolybdic acid in 750 ml distilled water in a suitable flask and add 50 ml phospheric acid. Reflux the mixture for 2 h. and make up to one lit. with water. Protect the reagent from exposure to light.

2. *Sodium Carbonate Solution*: Dissolve 350 g sodium carbonate in one lit. of water at 70-80 °C. Filter through glass wool after allowing it to stand overnight.

3. *Standard Tannic Acid Solution*: Dissolve 100 mg tannic acid in 100 ml of distilled water.

4. *Working Standard Solution*: Dilute 5 ml of the stock solution to 100 ml with distilled water. One ml contains 50 μg tannic acid.

Procedure

1. *Extraction of tannin*: Weigh 0.5 gm of the powdered material and transfer to a 250 ml conical flack. Add 75 ml water. Heat the flask gently and boil for 30 min. Centrifuge at 2,000 rpm for 20 min and collect the supernatant in 100 ml volumetric flask and make up the volume.
2. Transfer 1 ml of the sample extracted to a 100 ml volumetric flask containing 75 ml water.
3. Add 5 ml of Folin-Denis reagent, 10 ml of sodium carbonate solution and dilute to 100 ml with water.
4. Shake well. Read the absorbance at 700 nm after 30 min.
5. If absorbance is greater than 0.7 make a 1 + 4 dilution of sample
6. Prepare a blank with water instead of sample
7. Prepare a standard graph by using 0-100 μg tannin acid.

Calculation

Calculate the tannin content of the sample as tannic acid equivalent from the standard graph.

Estimation of Dihydroxy Phenol

Vanillin Hydrochloride Method : Vanillin method is specific for dihydroxy phenols and is particularly sensitive for meta-substituted, di and tri hydroxybenzene containing molecules.

Principle

The vanillin reagent which react with phenol that has an unsubstituted resorcinol or phloroglucinol nucleus and form a coloured substitution product which is measured at 500 nm.

Reagents

Vanillin hydrochloride reagent : Mix equal volumes of 8 % hydrochloric acid in methanol and 4 % vanillin in methanol. The solution must be mixed just before use and avoid using even if it is slightly colored.

Catechin stock standard solution : Prepare a standard solution containing 1 mg catechin /ml methanol.

Working standard : Dilute the above solution ten times 10 ml to 100 ml (100 μg/ml)

Preparation of extract : Extract 1 g. of ground seed in 50 ml methanol mix occasionally by swirling 20-28 h. centrifuge and collect the supernant.

Procedure

1. Pipette out 1 ml of supernant
2. Quickly add 5 ml of vanillin hydrochloride
3. Read in a spectrophotometer at 500 nm after 20 min.
4. Prepare the blank with vanillin hydrochloride reagent alone
5. Prepare a standard graph with 20-100 μg catechin using the diluted stock solution.

Calculation

From the standard graph calculate amount of catechin i.e. tannin in the sample as per the absorbance and express the result as catechin equivalent.

Purification

Tannins need to be purified from low molecular weight phenolics and pigments that are present in crude plants extracts.

Purification is essential for the preparation of suitable standards. Purification of large quantities of tannins can be done by taking advantage of their absorption by sephadex.

Estimation of Glycoalkaloid from *Solanum dulcamara*

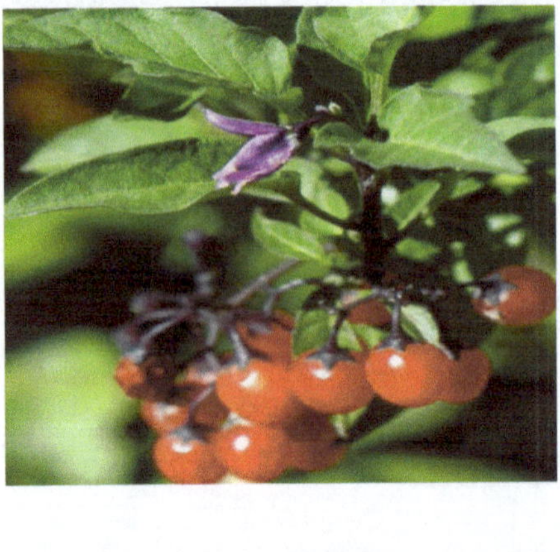

Glycoalkaloids are a family of poisons commonly found in the plant species (nightshade).There are several glycoalkaloids (alkaloids + sugars) that are potentially toxic.

A prototypical glycoalkaloid is called solanine (sugar [solanose] + alkaloid [solanidine] = solanine), which is found in potatoes. The alkaloidal portion of the glycoalkaloid is also generically referred to as an aglycone. The intact glycoalkaloid is poorly absorbed from the gastro intestinal (GI) tract but causes GI irritation. The aglycone is absorbed and is believed to be responsible for observed nervous system signs. Glycoalkaloids are bitter tasting, and produce a burning irritation in the back of the mouth and side of the tongue when eaten.

Potato and brinjal contain two major glyco-alkaloid a-solanin and a chaconin, both of which being triglycosides of solanidine. Bitterness in brinjal and potato is due to the presence of glyco-alkloids, high amount of glycoalkloid produce a bitter taste and off flavor. The variety with low glyco-alkloid content are considered suitable for the processing purpose. It is reported that glyco-alkloid cause human disorder when consumed in high quality including gastro intestinal disturbance nervous depression.

Principle

"Glyco-alkloid from a reddish purple colour when formaldehyde solution is added to the extracted residue in ethanol : sulphuric acid medium, the colour is measured at 562 nm."

Reagent

a. *Chloroform* : acetic acid : methanol solution (50:5:45 v/v) (CAM)

b. Activated charcoal

c. Ethanol : sulphuric acid : half dried rectified spirit to 50 % Solution. To this add conc. sulphuric acid in the ratio of ethanol : sulphuric acid 1: 2 v/v

d. Formaldehyde solution

e. a - solanine standard

Equipment

Tissue homogenizer

Centrifuge

Spectrophotometer

Procedure

1. Take fresh / frozen tissue (1-2 g) and homogenize it in to a tissue homogenizer in present of CAM solvent mixture (apro. 10 volume) containing a pinch of discoloring charcoal. Blend for 10 minute at medium speed.

2. The homogenate is allowed to stand overnight at room temperature.
3. Next morning the solution is filtered and the residue is washed twice with extracting solvent mixture CAM.
4. CAM extract is dried on water bath.
5. Nine ml ethanol-sulphuric acid mixture is slowly added to the residue held in ice bath and 1 ml of formaldehyde is slowly added to the cold solution.
6. The mixture is centrifuged out and the supernant is used for spectrophotometric reading.
7. A reddish purple colour is developed after 90 minute at room temperature.
8. Absorbance is measured at 562 nm against the blank.
9. The blank is prepared by adding 1 ml of formaldehyde solution to 9 ml ice cold ethanol-suphuric acid mixture.
10. A standard curve is prepared using the a -solanine.
11. Read out the glyco-alkloid content from the standard curve.

Calculation

Let a solanine content of the sample aliquot be "X" mg

Glyco-alkloid content (mg/100 gm)=x *100/sample weight in gm.

Estimation of Capsaicine from Chilli

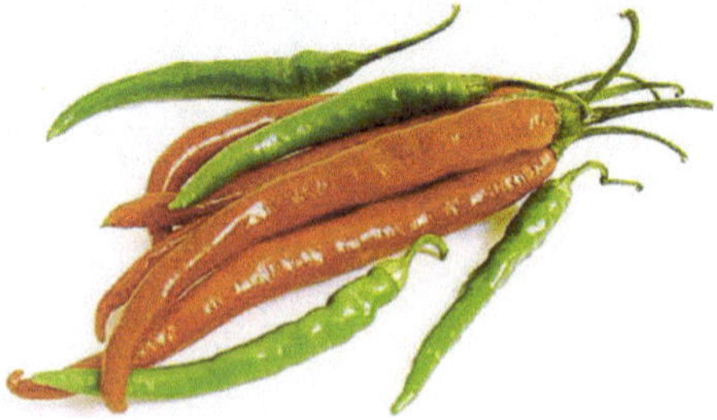

Capsaicin is an active alkaloid present in chili or pepper. There are many varieties available which may be classified as sweet, mild or hot depending upon capsaicin content this material gives pungent taste.

Principle

Capsaicin is extracted alone with other oleo resin, separated paper chromatagraphically and visualized by gibb's reagent the blue colour formed, spot cut out from the paper, extracted in methanol and measured spectrophotomatically at 615 nm.

Reagent

Buffer solution (pH 9.6) : Buffer solution is prepared by dissolving 1 g. of boric acid and 3.7 g. pot. chloride in 750 ml water pH is adjusted using 1 N NaoH solution. The solution is diluted to 1 lit. with water and stored at room temperature.

Chromogenic reagent (gibb's) : Prepare 0.1 % solution of 2-6 dichloroquinone chlorimide in ehtyl acetate and store at room temperature. Reagent is stable atleast for one week.

Developing solvent: Buffer (pH 9.6): methanol (40 : 60 v/v).

Method

Five g. of dry chilly powder is extracted with 100 ml acetone by refluxing for 3 h. the solution is cooled to room temperature and filtered through glass wool. The solution is evaporated using mild heat on water bath. The oily mass is transferred to 10 ml volumetric flask with ethyl acetate and stored under refrigerator.

Prepare Chromatograrphic Separation

Two µl of the above extract is spotted on chromatographic paper and then developed by ascending chromatography with developing solvent. The paper after developing is air dried and quickly passed through Gibb's reagent and again air dried. Next the buffer solution is sprayed when capcaicinoid appear in blue color with varicose intensity depending upon the amount of capcaicinoid Present.The chromatogrphic paper is dried in dark, blue area are cut out and extracted in methanol. The extracted solution is adjusted to 5 ml and optical density is measure at 615 nm against blank using spectrophotometer.

Standard curve of capsaicine is developed exactly the same way by developing the paper chromatograph extracting the colour in methanol and measuring the blue color of incremental doses of capsaicine spotted at 615 nm.

From the standard curve the capsaicine equivalent of the sample is determined.

Calculation

Let the capsaicine equivalent of the sample be X μg.

Then capsaicine content in mg/g = X

Estimation of Gossypol from Cotton

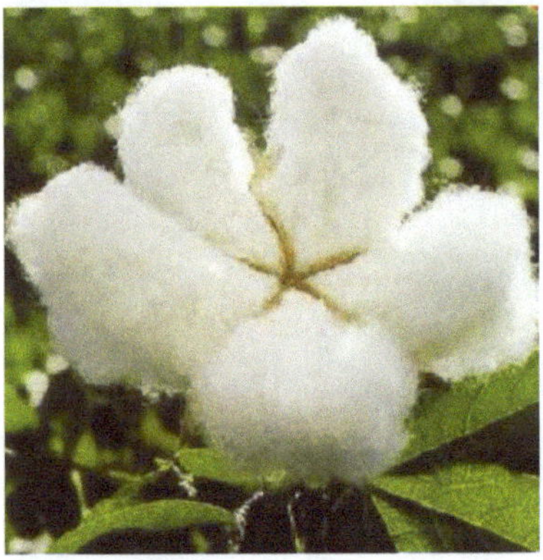

In cultivated cotton, glands in achlorophylllouse plant part contain predominantly the terpenoid aldehydes gossypol in G. *hirsutum* and Gossypol and its methyl and dimethyl derivatives in G *arbadence.* Gland in green tissue contain sesquiterpenoid quinone, para-hemi gossypol as predominance terpene aldehyde in G *hirsutum* and quinone hemi Gossypol 7- methyl ether in G *barbadence.*

"A TLC of separation of extracted crude terpenoid followed by spraying with a visualizing agent quality is estimated by spot size and colour intensity."

Method

1. Take 2 g. of finely chopped fresh tissue in a 50 ml centrifuge tube.
2. Add 30 ml of peroxide free ether and shake on a vortex mixture for 10 minute.
3. Centrifuge out the etheral extract in a 100 ml flask and collect supernatant.
4. Reextracts the tissue with 30 ml of ethyle acetate for 50 minute in a shaker and centrifuge.
5. The extract are combined, reduced to dryness in vaccuo at 30 ^{0}C and taken up in a minimum volume of ethyle acetae for TLC work
6. Prepare silica gel TLC plate and air dry overnight at 40 % to 60 % RH.
7. Plates are developed two dimensionally with ether : hexane : formic acid (15:85:0.5)and cyclohexan : dimethyl ketone (95:5) to estimate the quinone and heliocides.

- Plates are sprayed with a fresh mixture of equal amount of 5 % phlorogucinol in ethanol and conc. HCl. Quinone gives maganta to maroon colour. Heliocides form yellow to orange colour.
- Quantity of compound is estimated from spot size and colour intensity.

Estimation of Medicarpin and Maackiain (Phytoalexins) from Chickpea Leaves

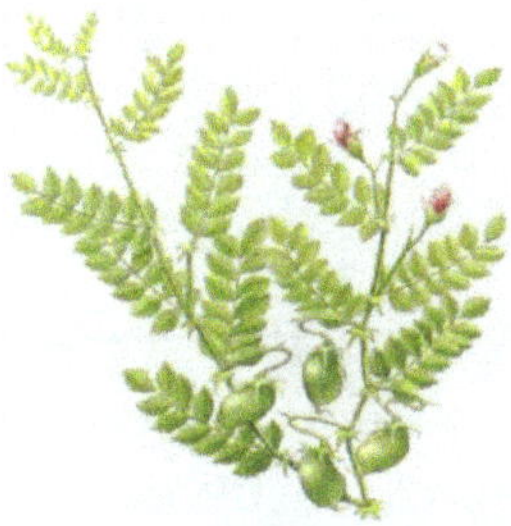

They are phytoalexins synthesised during host pathogen interaction in plant when plant attacked by pathogen.

Preparation of Diazotized p-Nitroaniline

300 mg p-nitroaniline is dissolved in 100 ml 8 % HCl.25 ml of diazotized p-nitroaniline prepared is mixed with 1.5 ml of 5 % sodium nitrate.

Isolation Procedure

- Homogenize 0.5 gm tissue of resistant and susceptible varieties in 8 ml absolute alcohol and then stored at room temperature (22 °C) in the dark over night.
- Collect the alcoholic extract and tissues are socked second time in 8 ml absolute alcohol and kept over night
- Soaking procedure is done three times and three alcohol fraction collected are filtered through whatman filter paper 1.
- Alcohol fractions are evaporated to dryness on water bath at 40°C.
- Residue is dissolved in 200 ml absolute alcohol for thin layer chromatography.
- 10 µl extract is stacked on silica gel plates.
- The plates are developed in two times in n patene: ethyl ether: glacial acetic acid (75:25:1). For detection of phytoalexins diazotized p nitroaniline reagent is used.
- Rf value of separated phytoalexin are noted and compare with standards.

Estimation of Andrographolide from *Kalmegh* (*Andrographis paniculata*)

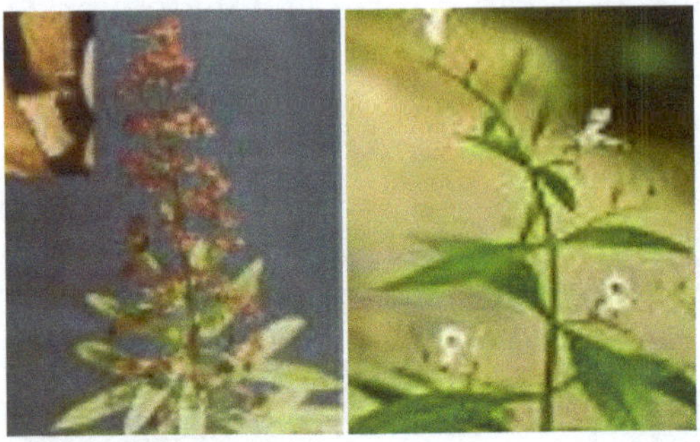

The popular hepato protective Indian herbal drug Kalmegh (*Andrographis paniculata*) can be standardized by high pressure liquid chromatographic determination of its major active constituent, andrographolide. The leaves of the herb are found to contain the highest amount (2.39 % w/w) of andrographolide and the seeds to contain the lowest. The technique is found to be much more sensitive and simple than the known spectrophotometric method. Popularly known as *Kalmegh* is a well known in the Hindu system of medicine and is widely cultivated in India. The extract of the plant is used to relieve griping, irregular stools and loss of appetite, it has the reputation of being febrifuge, tonic and anthelmintic. In view of its importance its dry powder has been included in the Indian Pharmacopoeia. Andrographolide is the main active bitter principle of *Kalmegh.*

1. Chemical Evaluation of Andrographolide from *Andrographis paniculata* by Spectrophotometric Method

One gram of the fine powdered, accurately weighed, is refluxed with 50 ml of benzene on a water bath for 1 h. It is kept at roomtemp 3-4 h. and then filtered under suction. The residue is washed with cold benzene two or three times till no more of the green coloring matter was extracted. The residue is again treated with benzene and filtered to ensure complete removal of the chlorophyll. It is dried to remove the traces of benzene and then mixed thoroughly with 10 g of Kieselguhr. The mixed powder is then extracted in a soxhlet apparatus with pure chloroform for 4 to 5 h. The 5 ml of the extract evaporated to dryness at 50°C in oven and the residue dissolved in spectroscopic grade 10 ml methanol. The tubes subjected to read at 226 nm against methanol as blank. The percent andrographolide calculated using standard graph factor prepared by dissolving pure compounds.

2. Estimation of Andrographolide from *Andrographis paniculata* by HPLC

Extraction

One gm dry powder of Andrographis refluxed with 20 ml of petroleum ether (60-80) for 1 h to remove coloring pigments. Filter it and discard the filtrate. Transfer the residue in a round flat bottomed flask. Add 20 ml of methanol (HPLC Grade) and refluxed it for 1 h, filter it and collect filtrate in 25 ml volumetric flask. Wash the residue with 5 ml methanol. Make final volume of filtrate to 25 ml. Use 10 to 20 μl of the extract for HPLC analysis.

Preparation of Standard solution of Andrographolide

Stock

Weigh 6,25 mg Andrographolide and dissolve in 25 ml Methanol (HPLC Grade).

Working

Pipette out 0.4, 0.8, 1.2, 2.4, 3.2 and 4.8 ml of stock solution in a 10 ml volumetric flask. Adjust the volume to 10 ml with methanol. The concentration of pure Andrographolide is 100 ng/ 10 μl.

HPLC Condition

(i) Column : C_{18} Nucleosil; 10 pi particle (250 X 0.4 mm)

(ii) Mobile phase : Methanol : Water (65 : 35 v/v)

(iii) Flow rate : 0.5 ml / min.

(iv) Detector : 223 n

(v) Retention time : 7.4 ± 0.2 min.

Estimation of Glycirrhizin from *Glycyrrhiza glabra* (Jethimutad)

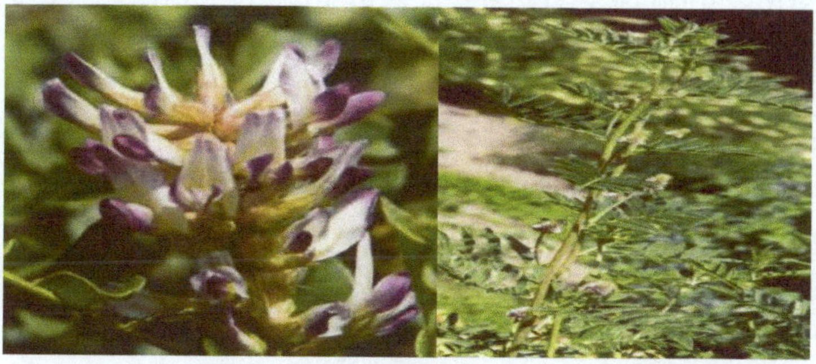

The roots (modified stem) of *Glycyrrhiza glabra* have medicinal importance and is largely imported in to India. During last decade small scale, cultivation was done in Haryana. Licorice is useful in the treatment of ulcers, soar throats, abdominal pains, insomnia, tuberculosis, food poisoning and many other ailments. Glycyrrhizin is about 50 times sweeter than sucrose (cane sugar). A Flavonoid glycoside has been identified: liquiritin. The aglycon liquiritigenin is in part spontaneously formed when the root is dried.

Procedure

Take 1.0 g fine powder in a 150 ml conical flask. Add 50 ml of hot 3% solution of TCA in acetone. Steep for 20 min. while stirring with a glass rod. Allow the mixture to stand for 3 min and transfer the supernatant liquid through whatman No.41 filter paper in to a conical flask. Repeat the extraction two more times with 25 ml of TCA in acetone and steep for 15 min each time. After third extract, transfer the solid to the same filter paper, wash the flask with 25 ml acetone and filter in same flask. To the combined extract, add concentrated ammonia solution drop by drop and stir the content vigorously until the abundant cheesy precipitate is formed (Adjust pH at 8.3 to 8.6 potentiometrically or with the use of moist phenolphthalein paper placed in the neck of the flask which turns pink). Transfer the precipitate together with mother liquor to a filter paper placed in a Buckner funnel and draws the liquid off Wash the flask and filter paper with the residue with 50 ml of acetone four times. Transfer the residue with filter paper to the same flask in which the precipitation made. Dissolve the residue in 50 ml distilled water. Transfer the resultant solution to a 250 ml volumetric flask and make up to volume with distilled water (solution A).

Determination of glycyrrhizic acid may be done by either of the following two methods

1. Take 100 ml of solution A in a 250 ml Erlenmeyer flask add 20 ml of formaldehyde, preliminary neutralized against thymopthalein, stir for two minutes and titrated against standard N/10 NaOH until the yellow colour changes to greenish yellow using same indicator.
2. 1 ml N/10 NaOH = 0.0274 gm of glycyrrhizic acid.

3. Place 10 ml of solution A in 500 ml volumetric flask and make up the volume by adding distilled water (solution B). Determine optical density of solution B at 258 nm in 1 cm cell. Also determine the O.D. of water as blank.

Calculation

Where, D = 0.D of solution

11000 is ml index of absorption.

$$\text{Glycyrrhizic acid (\%)} = \frac{D \times 822 \times 250 \times 600 \times 100}{a \times b \times \underset{(1.0)}{11000} \times \underset{(10)}{1000\ A,}}$$

$$= D \times 93.4$$

a = wt taken in gm, b = Amount of solution, 822 is mol. Wt of glycyrrhizicacid.

Some Reactions of Glycyrrhizin

1. It dissolves in conc. H_2SO_4 with yellow colour, which on slight warming, becomes a violet red and gray powder separates on standing.
2. Add a drop of 0.5 ml HO, CaH_4 CHO to glycyrrhizin, a blood red colour is produced which slowly changes to violet.
3. With para methoxy benzaldehyde give violet colour at once which at first turn to red and finally returns to a persistent violet colour.
4. With cinnamal aldehyde (PH-CH:CH:CHO) glycyrrhizin at once forms intense red colour which turns to intense violet. On warming the colour becomes greenish.Glucose slowly produces a violet colour. Furfural gives at once a beautiful violet colour, which becomes increasingly intense on standing.

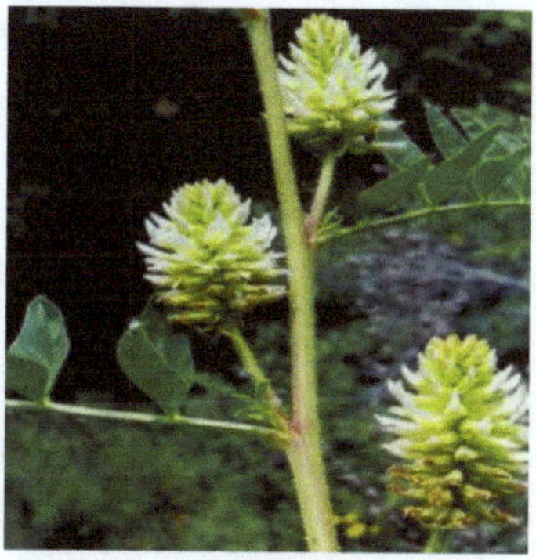

Estimation of Mono-Amonium Glycyrrhizinate &18 B Glycyrrhitinic Acid

Take Glycyrrhiza root powder (100 g). and extract with distilled water on a water bath for several hours, cool and filter. (The water extract is about 20%). Keep the residue for crude fibre determination.

Add to water extract 10 % sulphuric acid to precipitate crude glycyrrhizin (3 to 4 %), filter and keep the filtrate for estimation of deglycyrrhizinised liquorice (D.G.L.).

Wash the precipitate with distilled water to make it acid free (test with barium chloride). Suspend the precipitate in 80 % v/v methanol and add dilute ammonia solution with constant stirring to convert glycyrrhizin into crude ammonium glycyrrhizinate. When precipitate goes completely in solution, filter and distill off methanol. This affords crude ammonium glycyrrhizinate in thick paste form. Crystallize it in equal volume of glacial acetic acid and dry. Dissolve the crystals of crude ammonium glycyrrhizinate in 80 % alcohol. Treat with 2 % activated charcoal. Filter the crystals under vacuum and dry. Weigh as mono- ammonium glycyrrhizinate (2 to 3 %).

Add 10 % sulphuric acid to mono- ammonium glycyrrhizinate and reflux for 8 h. Collect the precipitate on a funnel, wash acid free with distilled water. Dry under vaccum and weigh as 18-B glycyrrhitinic acid (1.5 to 2.0 %).

3. Preparation of Deglycyrrhizinised Liquorice (DGL)

Take filtrate left after precipitation of glycyrrhizine for further estimation of Deglycyrrhizinised Liquorice (DGL) as below.

Add calcium carbonate slowly with constant stirring to the filtrate to make the pH of the solution 6 to 7.5. Settle it for 8 h. Filter the precipitated calcium sulphate. Evaporate the filtrate under vaccum to obtain thick paste. Dry under vacuum at 60° C and weigh. The DGL is about 14 to 18 %.

4. Determination of Crude Fibre Content in *Glycyrrhiza Glabra* roots

Take the residue left after water extract and proceed as follow for determination of crude fibre content. Otherwise, weigh accurately about 2 gm of the powdered sample of the feeding stuff. Treat it with ether on a funnel to make it free from fat.

Transfer the fat free residue to a 400 ml beaker; add 100 ml of 2.5 per cent H_2SO_4 and 100 ml of boiling water make a mark on the beaker with a glass pencil to represent the level of the mixture in it. Bring the contents to boil and continue boiling for exactly 30 minutes. During the boiling, stir with a glass rod to mix the contents and to remove particles from the side of the beaker. Keep the volume of the liquid constant by the addition of hot water from time to time. At the end of 30 min., remove the beaker, filter the contents immediately through a wet piece of linen cloth, and wash the residue with hot till it is free from acid.

Transfer back the entire residue from the cloth to the original beaker, washing the linen with hot water, add 100 ml of 2.5 per cent NaOH solution and then make up the volume up to 200 ml by the addition of boiling water. Boil the contents as before for exactly 30 min., stirring with a glass rod and keeping the volume constant by the addition of hot water. Remove the beaker and immediately filter the contents through the same linen cloth. Transfer the entire residue to the cloth with a jet of hot water. Wash the residue with hot water 3 times, then with dilute 1 % HCl solution and again with hot water till it is free from acid. Finally, wash the residue once with 95 per cent alcohol and once with ether.

Transfer quantitatively the whole residue to a clean dry crucible previously weighed. Dry the residue in the oven at 100° C to constant weight. Cool in a desiccator and weigh. Ignite the residue completely till white or grayish white ash is obtained. Cool in a dessicator and weigh. The difference in the two weights represents the weight of crude fibre. The Glycyrrhiza roots possess about 15 to 20 per cent crude fibre.

Estimation of Withanolides from *Withania somnifera* (Asgand)

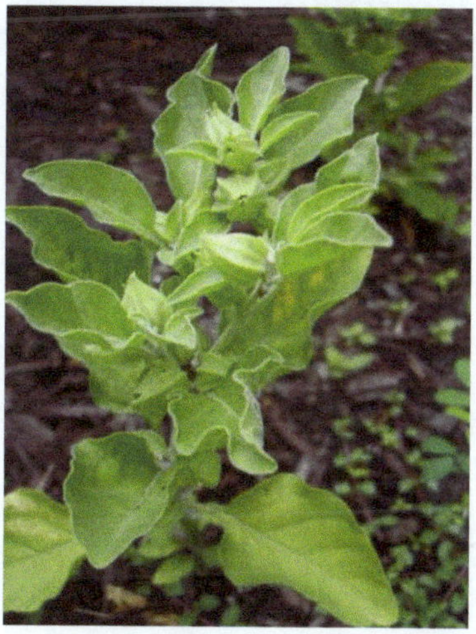

Colorimetric method for estimation of total withanolides (steroidal lactones) from the root of asgand (*Withania somnifera*)

Principle

Withanolides hydrolyzed in presence of concentrated H_2SO_4 and produced δ-lactones, which than reacts with acetic acid and ferric chloride formed a pink colour. The reactions carried out at highly acidic medium.

From Leaf

15 g of dried leaf powder is extracted in soxhlet extractor with the help of ethyl alcohol for eight hours. Extract (30 ml) after distillation and removal of solvent is transferred to a 50 ml centrifuge tube. Mix the content with 10 ml of 0.02 N HCl, keeps for 10 min. It results the precipitation of green sticky mass (Chlorophyll and other impurities). Clear supernatant will be obtained after centrifugation for 5 min. The clear supernatant is collected in 100-ml. vol. flasks. Mix the residue again with 20 ml ethanol with glass rod and centrifuge it. Collect the liquid in the above volumetric flask. It confirms the complete removal of steroid. Make up the volume of flask with ethyl alcohol.

Colorimetric estimation of withanoloides is based on the method used for cholesterol with a few modifications.

Taken (ml)   b = Weight of samples in gm.

Reagents and Chemicals

Ethyl alcohol	:	Absolute alcohol or Rectified spirit dist. over KOH
Iron solution (stock)	:	2.5 g of $FeCl_3.6H_2O$ dissolved in 100ml orthophosphoric acid
Colour solution	:	8.0 ml stock solution of Iron is diluted in 100 ml conc.H_2SO_4 (Prepared in ice bath or use chilled reagent of stock and conc.H_2SO_4)
Cholesterol stock	:	Cholesterol pure 20.0 mg. dissolved in 100 ml. ethyl alcohol.

From Root

Take 1 g of powder of root and add 15 ml ethanol. Shake it on a mechanical shaker for one h. and filter through Whatman filter No. 1.

Collect the filtrate in 50 ml volumetric flask. Wash the matter with another 15 ml ethanol and shake it for 30 minutes on mechanical shaker. Filter it and combine the filtrate. Adjust the final volume to 50 ml with ethanol. Develop the color adding reagents serially in test tubes and read at 540 nm.

Calculation

$$\text{Alkaloid (\%)} = \frac{\text{O.D.} \times \text{GF} \times 50 \times 100}{a \times b \times 1000 \times 1000}$$

OD = Optical density GF = Graph factor a = Aliquot

Thin Layer of Sample Chromatography of Withanoloides

For qualitative determination of various alkaloids a suitable T.L.C. method was developed. A 175 x 60 x 2mm chromatographic glass plates was cleaned by dipping in 10 % sodium carbonate and washed by distilled water. Coated with silica gel G slurry and dried in oven. Plate is spotted with mixture of alkaloids extracted in methanol. Chromatograms are run in the solvent system of n-butanol and HCl (98 : 2) v/v. Time period is 4 h. The plates are taken out and dried. The spots are visualized by spraying Draggendorff reagent. After getting patches of these spots, Rf values are calculated. The identification of alkaloids is done based on respective Rf values.

Profile of alkaloids based on RF values

S. No.	Name of alkaloid	Root	Leaf (Mature & Dry)	Stem (Mature & Dry)	Berry	Seed
		Rf value				
1	3-Tropyl tigloate	0.86	–	–	0.84	–
2	Withanine	0.72	0.71	0.71	0.72	0.71
3	Not identified	0.63	0.63	0.60	0.62	–
4	Not identified	0.55	0.54	0.54	–	–
5	Isopelletierine	0.46	0.43	–	–	–
6	Tropine	0.40	–	–	–	–
7	Anaferine	0.24	–	0.26	–	0.26
8	Pseudotropine	0.18	0.18	–	–	–
9	Anahygrin	0.13	–	–	–	0.11
10	Cuscohygrine	0.07	–	–	–	–
11	Not identified	0.05	–	–	–	–

Estimation of Total Bitter Principle from *Tinospora cordifolia* (Galo)

1. Chemical Evaluation of Total Bitters in *Tinospora Cordifolia* Herb

Tinospora cordifolia is used in a number of formulations in the Indian system of medicine. There are number of chemical constituents reported in it However, therapeutic activity of drug is evaluated in terms of its total bitters content. A study was made to find the chemical nature of total bitters and method was developed for its chemical evaluation.

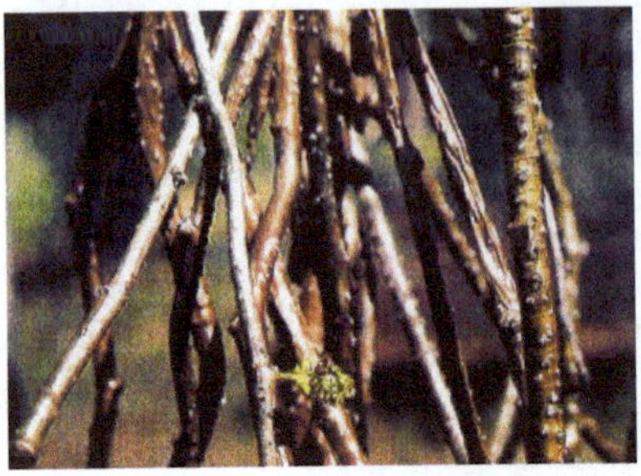

Successive Extraction with Solvents

Samples were subjected to continuous hot extraction with solvents over soxhlet apparatus with petroleum ether (60-80°C), benzene, chloroform, ethyl acetate, ethyl alcohol and water.

Taste of the Extract

Each extract was weighed and tasted after removing solvent. It was found that ethyl acetate and ethyl alcohol extracts were distinctly bitter in taste. Rest of the extracts was found to be tasteless.

Nature of the extract and its treatment over TLC

Chloroform and ethyl alcohol extracts respond to alkaloid test with draggendorff reagent. Ethyl alcohol extract also respond to saponin test.

Thin Layer Chromatography

A suitable solvent system is developed over TLC to test the solvent extracts. Since chlorophyll is interfering in the analysis, attempts were made to remove chlorophyll with minimum of interference. The extracts are treated with different reagents such as alkaline reagent, lead - acetate, activated carbon etc. But these are found to affect the profile of chromatogram. It is also observed that there are two spots over TLC with different Rf responding to Draggendorff reagent.

Column Chromatography

Alcoholic extract of the material is subjected to column chromatography in chloroform with increasing concentration of methanol. Some of the fractions not reported any compounds; however, when the same fraction re-chromatographed the pure compounds are obtained.

1. Analysis for Total Bitters

Dried powdered material is subjected to continuous hot extraction with ethyl alcohol (95%). Solvent is distilled off. Residues are refluxed with benzene and chloroform separately to remove unwanted material. Residues left are redissolved in ethanol, concentrated and diluted with water. This is extracted with ethyl acetate and solvent distilled off. The residue is weighed as total bitters.

2. Water Soluble Extractives

Ten (10g) gram dried powdered drug is macerated with 100 ml of distilled water in a closed flask for 24 h. shaking frequently. Solution was filtered through Whatman Filter paper No. 1 and 25 ml of filtrate is evaporated in a tarred flat bottom shallow dish. Further dried at 100 °C and weighed. The per cent of water extractives is calculated with reference for the air dried drug.

3. Alcohol Soluble Extractive

Successive Steps for Extraction

Dried powdered drug (10g)

↓

Shake frequently in alcohol for 24h.

↓

Filter it, collect the filtrate in 250 ml volumetric flask.

↓

Wash the residue with water several times and combined the filtrate.

↓

25 ml of filtrate was dried in oven at 100°c

↓

Calculate percent Alcohol Extractives by weight differences.

1. Total Alkaloid

A quantitative estimate of alkaloids is carried out by following method of Sairam and Khanna (1971).

Reagents

1. Ethyl alcohol (95%)
2. Ethyl ether
3. Ethanolic (90%) HCl
4. Chloroform
5. Ammonium hydroxide (25 %)

To the fine powdered drug (1g), 0.75 ml of 25 % Ammonium hydroxide, 1.0 ml of 95 % ethyl alcohol and 2.0 ml ethyl ether were added. The material is allowed to shake for 12 h. and dried.

The dried material is extracted with chloroform for 24h. in a soxhlet apparatus. Extract obtained was dried and the residue was redissolved in chloroform. This solution is allowed to evaporate under heat and the residue is mixed with 2.5 ml of 0.1N ethanolic HCl. The extract thus obtained is centrifuged to take supernatant and pellet is discarded. The solution is evaporated and the total alkaloids are weighed after drying it 100°C.

Estimation of Guggal sterones from *Commiphora wightii* (Guggal)

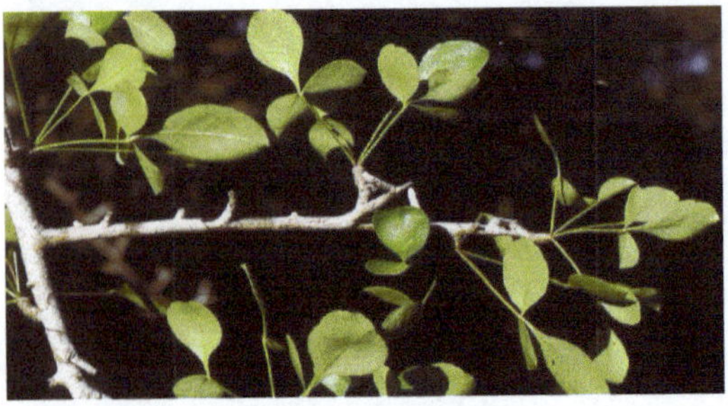

Gum of Guggal is an, consisting of ethyl acetate soluble-resin, ethyl acetate insoluble-gum and a small amount of essential oil. The ethyl acetate soluble fraction consists of sterones and other ingredients. These sterones (Z & E guggal sterones and others) are pharmacologically active and represent the quality of the gum, which can be analysed on U.V. Spectrophotometer.

Separation Scheme

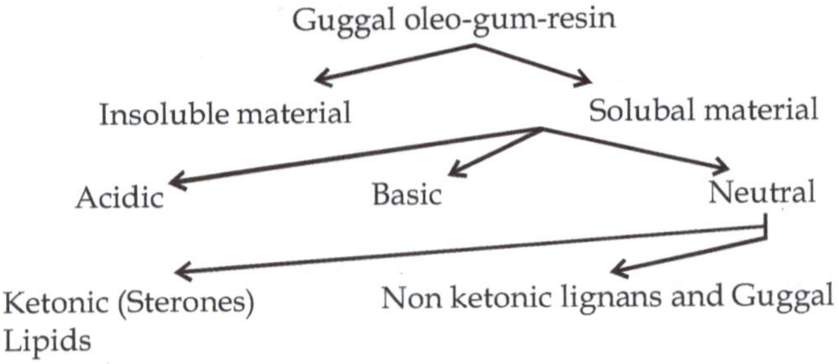

The Method to Determine Total Ketonic Fraction as Z and E Guggal Sterones

One gm of guggal gum and 25 ml of ethyl acetate are mixed thoroughly in a mortar and filtered through Whatman filter No. 40. The residue is again washed with ethyl acetate and filtered. The residue is again washed with ethyl acetate and filtered. The process is repeated several times until the entire soluble portion comes into the solution or until the ethyl acetate fraction is colorless. Total ethyl acetate extract thus obtained is then distilled under vacuum and weighed to obtain resin fraction, i.e. Ethyl acetate soluble material. One to two mg of resin weighed accurately is taken in a 25 ml volumetric flask, dissolved in double distilled ethanol and volume is made up to 25 ml. Optical density is read at 241 nm in a U.V. spectrophotometer and percentage of total ketonic fraction as Z and E guggal sterones was calculated taking the value E=25000 as for standard (100 per cent pure compounds)using the equation.

C = Molar concentration

l = Cell path in cm

A = Absorption

Mole wt. 312 gms EtoH max = 241 nm Z & E Guggal sterones (E = 25000), M.P. - 193°C

Thin layer chromatography of resin (Ethyl acetate soluble fraction)

Ethyl acetate solution is spotted on activated silica gel coated plates and developed with the solvent system of 25 per cent ethyl acetate in benzene. Developed plates after drying in air are sprayed with DNP (Dinitro Phenyl Hydrazine) reagent in hood. After some time when spots appeared, the plates are subsequently sprayed with concentrated H_2SO_4 and heated for charring in oven at about 120°C. The Rf values of separated components are calculated E and Z guggal sterones showed R_f values about 0.4 depending upon the thickness of coating material.

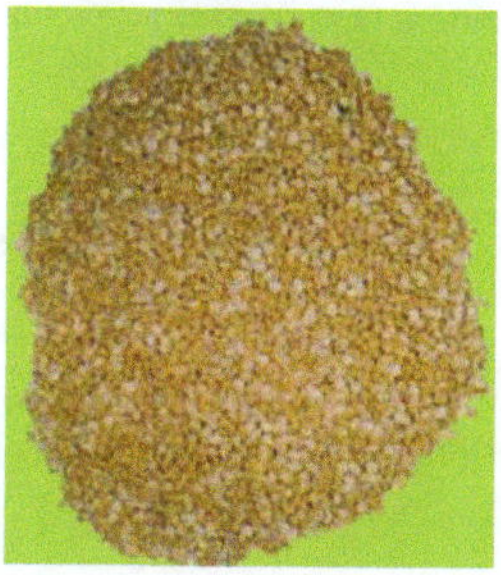

Estimation of Mucilages from *Plantago ovata* (Isabgol)

The Isabgol husk is used for its mucilage content. Mucin or mucilage are generally acid mucopolysacharides. They are usually attached to proteins to form proteoglycans in which the polysaccharides makeup most of the weight. Normally mucin consist of recurring disaccharide units each of which contains a derivative of an aminohexose, usually D-glucosamine or D-galactosamine. The polysaccharides isolated from mucin are slippery viscous and lubricating proteoglycan of mucous. These are jelly like ground substance or intercellular cement. There is scanty information available regarding the composition and quality of mucilage of Isabgol germplasm, it is necessary to test the Isabgol mucilage for its quantity and quality parameters.

Following the method suggested by Karawya *et al.* (1971), the mucilage material was fractionated into two parts : one soluble in cold water called Cold Extractable Mucilage (CEM) and the second fraction soluble in hot water called Hot Extractable Mucilage (HEM) materials.

a) Cold Extractable Mucilage (CEM)

One gram of the entire seed is mixed with 100 ml of distilled water, slightly acidified with 0.5 % hydrochloric acid, stirred for 12 h. at about 25°C and left to stand at the same temperature for another 12 h. The solution is passed through a two layer of -muslin cloth. The process was repeated thrice and the mucilage is precipitated from the combined aqueous extract by adding four volumes of 95 % ethanol slowly while stirring. The precipitate obtained by centrifugation is washed several times with ethanol until free from chloride ions. The mucilage (CEM) is then vigorously stirred in absolute acetone, filtered through Whatman filter No. 1 and then dried in vacuum desiccators over anhydrous calcium chlorides.

b) Hot Extractable Mucilage (HEM)

The matter, after the exhaustive extraction with cold water, is washed with water until free from chloride; then repeatedly treated with boiling water until complete extraction of mucilage is effected (tested by giving no cloudiness or precipitate on the addition of 4 volumes of 95% ethanol to one volume of the extract). The mucilage (HEM) was precipitated by 95 % ethanol and purified as described under CEM.

c) Hydrolysis of Mucilage

Hundred milligram (100mg) purified mucilage (CEM and HEM) was accurately weighed separately and refluxed with 20 ml of 4 % H_2

SO_4 for 20 h., on boiling water bath. The solution is filtered after cooling. The filtrate is made free of sulphate by precipitating the anion with barium carbonate powder. The filtrate from barium sulphate is allowed to pass over a column of cation exchange resin "Amberlite I.R. 120 H" (2.5 x 15 cm), to remove most of cations. The elute is concentrated on boiling water bath to a syrupy consistency, diluted with 10% isopropanol in water to make 4 ml volume and used for paper chromatography of hydrolysed sugars as per the method suggested by Karawya *et al.* (1971).

d) Chromatographic Resolution and Identification of Sugars

One dimensional double development ascending paper chromatography is employed to separate the hydrolysed sugars in the two fractions of the mucilage's. The separated sugars are identified by comparing the Rf values with that of the standard sugar mixture chromatographed from the same paper.

Thirty microlitre (30 µl) solution of mixed sugars from the hydrolyzed mucilage of each sample is spotted on a chromatographic grade whatman filter paper (42 cm x 50 cm) on the base line drawn 2 cm above the edge on the length of the sheet. A total of 10 samples are spotted at an interval of 4 cm, keeping the pure sugar mixture was reference standard at the center. For this purpose a standard sugar mixture was prepared as follow:

An equivalent of 10 mg of chromatographically pure homogenous sugars (BDH biochemical) was weighed and dissolved in 10% isopropanol, made up the volume to 10 ml to get a working solution of concentration 1 µg/ml. The following sugar solutions were made and mixed in equal proportion to make the standard sugar mixtures.

1. D - glucose
2. D - galactose
3. D - xylose
4. L - rhamnose
5. L - arabinose
6. D - galacturonic acid

The paper is saturated in the solvent system ethyl acetate: pyridine: water (2:1:2) in a glass chamber for 12 h. and then developed from the same solvent system (Jermyn and Isherwood, 1949 and Karawya *et al.*, 1971). The solvent was allowed to raise up to 26 cm. The paper is taken out, dried and again run for the same distance (Jeanes *et al.*, 1951). After the second development the paper was dried, sprayed with aniline-pthalate (Aph) reagent (Meites, 1963 and Karawya *et al.*, 1971) prepared in the following way : 1.66 gm pthalic acid and 0.91 ml aniline were taken in 100 ml volumetric flask. They are dissolved in n-butanol with mild heating. Ultimately volume is made up by n-butanol. Next, the paper is heated at 105°C for 10 minutes. The reagent gives yellow color with glucose, rhamnose, galactose and galacturonic acid (6-carbon sugar) and brown red colour with xylose and arabinose (5-carbon sugar) (Karawya *et al.*, 1971).

The R_f value of each well-defined separated spot was calculated and individual sugars in mucilage samples were identified in comparison with standard sugars.

e) Quantitation of Resolved Sugars

After the sugars are chromatographed on the paper, the colour is developed with aniline-pthalate reagent. The individual coloured spots are cut out of the paper and extracted for 15-30 min. with 3 ml of 80 % ethanol v/v (Vernon and Aronoff, 1952). The colour is read in a spectrophotometer at 480 nm for pentoses and 490 nm for hexoses. The results are deduced from the corresponding standard curves. The absorbance versus concentration in (mg) is plotted for each sugar for standard curves.

Quality Evaluation of Isabgol Seeds

The pharmacopoeia standards prescribe swelling factor which is a measure of swelling capacity of seeds in cold water. The method may be useful for determining wide differences between different species but is not suitable for detecting smaller differences in agricultural research. Further, the top layer consisting of dispersed seeds does not permit accurate reading. Actual separation of husk through mechanical means was suggested by D. Greenberg in 1948. (Journal Amer. Assoc. 37: 139-145). Such separation normally allows some husk particles to pass along with the seed particles; purification is cumbersome or will require special grinder. Another method followed for mucilage estimation is extraction with hot water and precipitating it with alcohol. However, even after prolonged hot water extraction, Isabgol seeds are found to be sticky. All these three methods are standardized/modified suitably for the estimation of husk content in Isabgol seeds. The procedures are given below. Further work requires to be done for statistical treatment and recommendation of the procedure. Certain observations made on the quality aspects of Isabgol seeds are also presented.

(i) Swelling Factor of Seeds

One-gram seeds are placed in a 25 ml graduate stoppered cylinder and distilled water is added up to 20 ml, agitated immediately for through wetting and allowed to stand for about 20 min. Then it is agitated again for uniform distribution of swollen seeds and was allowed to stand for 6 hr. Thereafter the volume of the swollen seeds is recorded (*Indian Pharmacopoeia* 1955; Patel et.al., 1978)

The Indian Pharmacopoeia prescribes, "1g agitated gently and occasionally during 24 h. and allowed to stand for 1 h ." However, it is observed that Isabgol seeds form a gel after ½ h. and then it is difficult to shake. Further keeping the swollen seeds after 6 h. is not desirable because the swollen seeds separate partly and move to the top of the water column. Hence the modifications suggested above make the method easy, quick and accurate. Tap water should not be used as the dissolved salts decrease the swelling factor. The values are 12 and 9.5 cc/g for distilled water and tap water respectively.

(ii) Mechanical Separation

Seeds of 15 g were churned for 30 sec. in third speed in a Braun Warring blender. The dehusked seeds and husk were separated by sieving through 40 mesh sieve followed by manual winnowing. The method required relatively higher amount of seed sample and was laborious. Besides, some broken seed particles pass along with the husk particles.

Chemical Method (I)

In this indirect method, the seeds are treated with hot 0.1N HCl to dissolve the husk and then the dehusked seeds are weighed and from this weight the husk content is worked out after applying necessary correction factor for the weight loss due to soluble portion of the dehusked seed.

Ten ml. of 0.1N HCl was heated to boiling in a 100 ml beaker for 2 minutes. The beaker was removed from the flames and then the seed sample of 1 g was quantitatively transferred to 0.1 N HCl without being deposited on the sides of the beaker to the possible extent. The heating was continued at boiling temperature for 2 minutes. The process of dissolution of husk from the seed was watched and when all the seeds turn into pale yellow colour (wheat colour) from the original colour of reddish brown and are visibly free from husk, the beaker was taken off from the flames and the seeds are allowed to settle.

The hot supernatant acidic solution is decanted off through previously weighed porcelain gooch crucible (The pore size should not be big enough to allow the dehusked seed to escape). The seeds are washed twice with hot water by decanting the water. The crucible was dried at 110° C for 3 h. and the weight of dried dehusked seeds is recorded.

Mechanically separated dehusked seeds of 1g were subjected to the same procedure and a weight lose of 0.2g is noted. The weight of dehusked seed obtained from the sample may be multiplied by 1.2 and the value obtained may be subtracted from 1g to get husk content of 1g seeds.

(iii) Chemical Methods (II)

The 0.1 N HCl extract obtained above may be treated with alcohol (1:3) to participate the mucilage and the precipitate may be dried and weighed. The dissolution of seed portion other than husk does not interfere in this method.

Ten ml of 0.1 N HCl was heated to boiling and 1g seeds was added. When the husk was removed, the solution was filtered through gooch crucible and seeds were washed twice by adding 5 ml of hot water through pipette each time. The filtrate taken in a 100 ml of beaker was treated with 60 ml alcohol, stirred and allowed to stand for 5 hr. The clear supernatant liquid was decanted off and the beaker with the precipitate was kept in warm water at 50°C in a thermo state water bath. (Drying this way was quicker and more effective than drying over calcium chloride).

The commercial husk weighing 0.2, 0.3, 0.4 and 0.5g was subjected to the above method. A linear relationship was obtained between the weight of husk and the corresponding weight of the precipitate. From this it is derived that 1g husk was equivalent to 0.75g of the precipitate.

Gum Determination in Clusterbean Seed

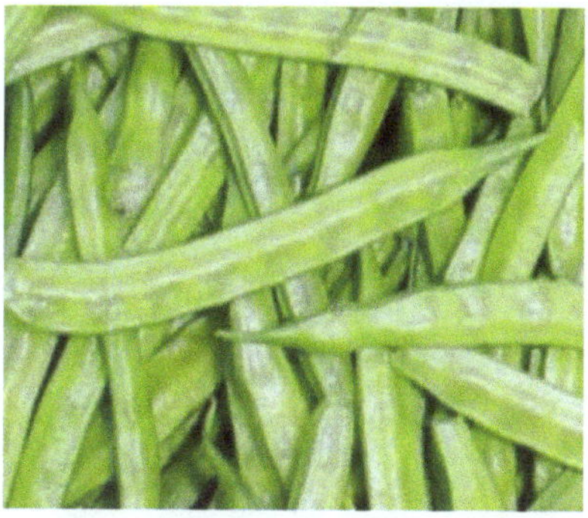

Take 0.1 gram of cluster bean seed in a conical flask and 40 ml D.W. mix the content thoroughly and than autoclave at 15 psi pressure for 4 h. as per method of Mital et.al.(1971). Later on cool the content and filter thoroughly a filter through a filter paper. Take 0.1 ml filtrate in a test tube and 1.9 ml of D.W. Follow the other steps as describe above for the standard curve.

Reagents

1. Concentration sulphuric acid (H_2SO_4)
2. 5 % Phenol (C_6H_5OH) : Dissolve 5 gram phenol in D.W. and make a
3. 100 ml volume.
4. Stock solution of Guar Gum: Weigh 200 mg D-mannose and 100 mg of D-galactose and dissolve in D.W. and make final volume of 1 liter. This solution contains 300 ppm Guar Gum.
5. Working solution: Dilute 10 ml of stock solution to 100 ml in volumetric flask.
6. This will give 30 microgram per ml. i.e. 30 ppm.

Procedure for Standard Curve

From the working solution pipette out varying quantities viz. 0.0, 0.4, 0.6, 0.8, 1.2, 1.6 and 2.0 ml in duplicate to the tube and add 2.0, 1.6, 1.2, 0.8, 0.4 and 0.0 ml D.W. respectively. Thus, a series of 0, 12,24,36,48 and 60 microgram per 2 ml are prepared. Then add 1 ml of 5 % phenol in each of the test tubes. And then add 5 ml of con.sulphuric acid rapidly in such a way that the stream of acid being directed the liquid surface rather than against the side of the test tube in order to obtain good mixing. Allow the test tube to stand for 10 min. and then place them for 15-20 min. ia a water bath at 25.0 to 30.0°C. Read the developed color on spectronic -20 at 485 nm wavelength. Draw standard curve (as drawn in figure given below) for the amount of gum against the optical density.

The amount of gum can be calculated from the standard curve. This value is used for calculating yield per hectare.

$$\%\,GUM = \frac{Sample\ O.D \times G.F}{R \times G.R.} \times \frac{40}{0.1} \times \frac{2}{0.1} \times \frac{100}{1\,000000}$$

Estimation of L-Dihydroxy phenyl alanine (DOPA) / Methyl DOPA from *Mucuna prurita* (Kaucha)

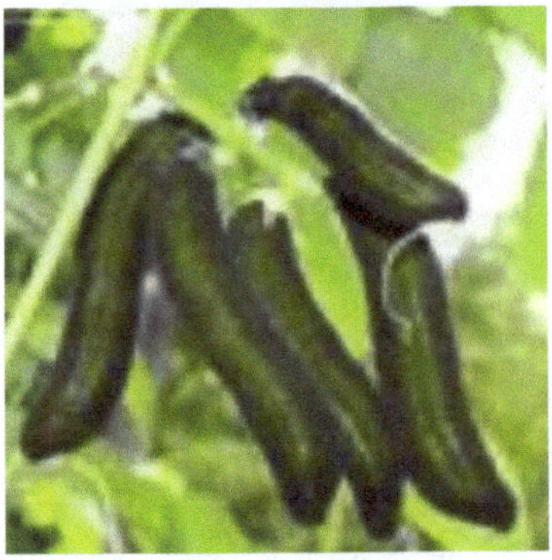

L-DOPA is found in several plant species belonging to different genera. However, the best source of natural L-DOPA is a few Mucuna species. L-DOPA is used in the treatment of Parkinson's disease while methyl DOPA is used in hypertension

Estimation of L-DOPA/Methyl DOPA

Reagents

1. Sodium nitrate (10% W/v.)
2. Sulphuric acid (10% W/v.)
3. Sodium hydroxide (20% W/v.)
4. Hydrochloric acid (1M)
5. Standard solution of methyl DOPA prepared in 1 M HCl to obtain final conc.of 200/ml.

Assay

A quantity of powdered sample equivalent to 0.2 g of methyl dopa was dissolved in10 ml of 1 N HCl and filtered. Wash the filter paper with 10 ml 1 N HCl. From the combined filtrate, an aliquot of 10 ml was further diluted to 100 ml with 1 N hydrochloric acid.

Five ml of sample and standard solutions as well as 5.0 ml of 1N hydrochloric acid is taken in three separate 50 ml volumetric flasks. To each one of them 5.0 ml of sodium nitrite solution is added and shaken for 2 minutes. After addition of 5 ml of sulphuric acid solution the resultant solutions were again kept for 2 minutes and then 6.0 ml of sodium hydroxide solution was poured to each one of them. The volumes are made up to the mark with water. The absorbance of the standard and the samples are measured at 490 nm using the solution containing 1M hydrochloric acid as blank.

Estimation of Gymnemic acid content from *Gymnema sylvestre* (Madhunashini)

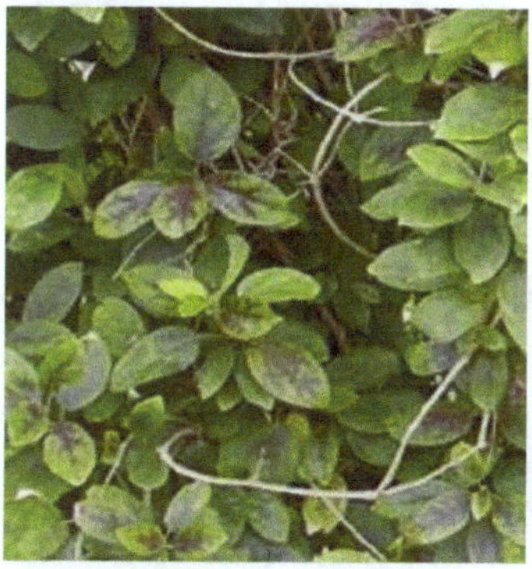

Twenty-gram (20 g) sample is soaked in water for 5 hours. The aqueous extract is filtered and dilute HCl was added to make it acidic. A dark brownish mass was obtained. This was extracted with chloroform to remove the inactive substances. The chloroform fraction is evaporated under reduced pressure and the weights of the crude gymnemic acids are recorded. The yield of crude acid obtained with this method are 1.5 % to 1.75 %.

Gymnemagenins

Treatment of the chloroform extract: The residue (15 g) from the chloroform extract is sparingly soluble in water but readily dissolved in dilute ammonium hydroxide solution. The alkaline solution is acidified with diluted HCl until a dark viscous material was obtained. Refluxing with 6 % ethanolic sulphuric acid for 3 h. hydrolysed it. The alcohol is evaporated off keeping the acid strength more or less constant by frequent addition of water. The crude sapogenine is filtered and the residue is washed repeatedly with distilled water until free from acid and dried at 60 ° C. The yield of crude sapogin from 15 g crude residue is 12.4 g.

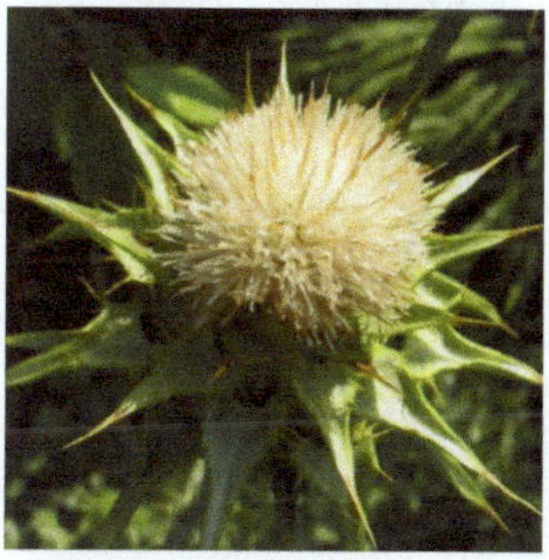

Estimation of Flavanolignans from *Silybum marianum* (Silybium)

The seeds of *Silybium marianum* Gaertn (Milk thistle- Asteraceae) are the only drug showing genuine antihepatotoxic properties. It is antagonistic to to a α-amanitine poisoning and thus exhibit a protective effect on liver.

The seeds contain three flavanolignans, silybin, silidianin and silychristin collectively known as silymarin.

Isolation of Flavanolignans

Powdered seeds (10 gm) are extracted successively with petroleum ether (40 - 60°), benzene and ethanol in a soxhlet. The petroleum extract is concentrated and shaken with methanol. The insoluble precipitate/ residue (R) is separated by filtration and the methanol solution is concentrated and loaded on silica gel column and eluted with petroleum ether. The eluted on concentration gives thick oil, which on keeping in a refrigerator yields crystals of myristic acid. The methanol insoluble residue contains other fatty acids *viz.* stearic, palmitic and oleic acids. The benzene fraction on concentration, chromatography on silica gel column and elution with benzene yields β-sitosterol.

The flavanolignanss get extracted in ethanol only and this extract is concentrated, loaded on columns of silica get and eluted with benzene:ethyl acetate (1:1). The first fractions yield a mixture (M_I) and the later fractions contain silybin which can be crystallized from methanol. The column is then eluted with ethyl acetate to get another mixture M_2.

The mixture M_I is concentrated and rechromatographed in silica gel column. On elution of the column with benzene:ethyl acetate (3:1) the first fractions yield dehydrosilybin (crystallized from methanol) and the later fractions silybin.

The mixture M_2 on column chromatography (silica gel) with benzene: ethyl acetate (1:1) yields taxifolin (flavanol) in first two fractions, silybin in later fractions and silychristin in final fractions. The UV absorption spectra of these compounds are:

Dehydrosilybin	λ max	287 nm. (major) peak	360 nm. (minor peak)
Silybin	MeOH	265 nm. (major)	350 nm. (minor)
Silychristin	MeOH		289 nm.

Analytical method to determine betain hydrochlorides in *Silybum marianum*

Betain hydrochlorides donate methyl groups in the synthesis of choline in the liver in the antihepatotoxic principle of the drug.

Method of Analysis

Air dried; finely ground seeds (500 g) are extracted with petroleum ether (40-60°). The defatted seeds are then extracted with 70 % ethanol by cold percolation. The extract is divided into two parts. In the first part, the solvent free extract is acidified with dilute hydrochloric acid (0.1N). The acidic solution is found to contain considerable amount of water-soluble quaternary bases which are readily precipitated by addition of ammonium solution. The ammonia solutions are dissolved in acetone and decomposed with freshly prepared silver sulphate solution. The residue obtained on evaporation to dryness is dissolved in ethanol. This is chromatographed through activated alumina. Elution is with chloroform, mixture of chloroform and ethanol (1:1) and finally with pure ethanol. Pure ethanol fraction gave white crystalline powder (40 mg) m.p. 229-31° with decomposition $(a)^D$ 20-30°. The total yield of betain hydrichloride was 0.008 %.

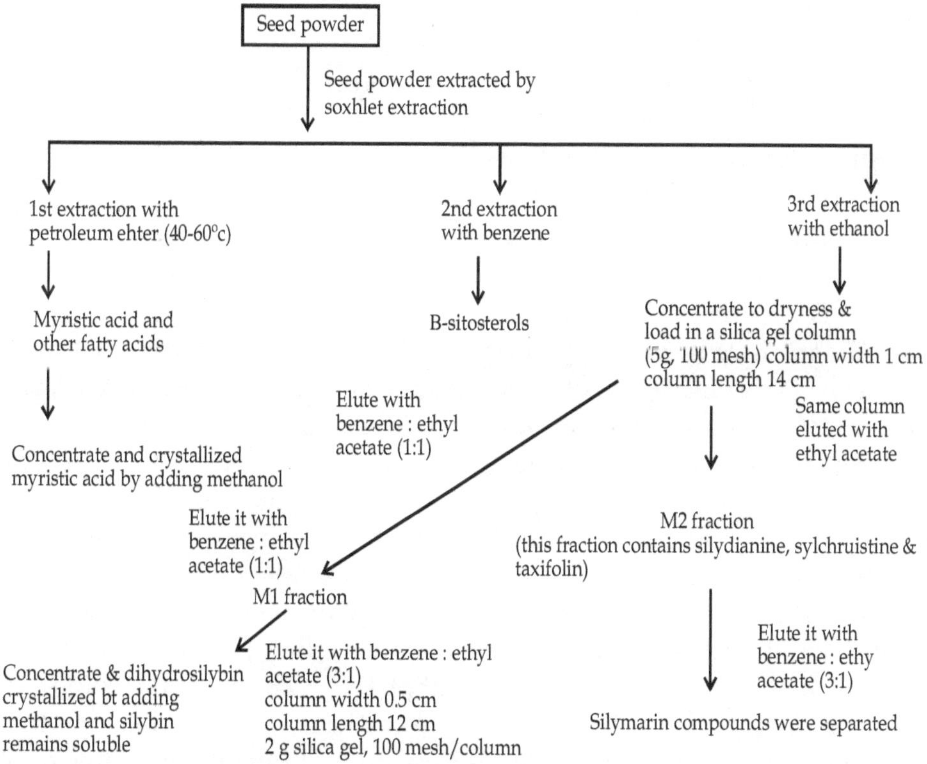

Fig. 10.1. Schematic diagram for isolation of Silymarin compounds

Estimation of Sennoside and Quinones from Senna (*Cassia angustifolia*)

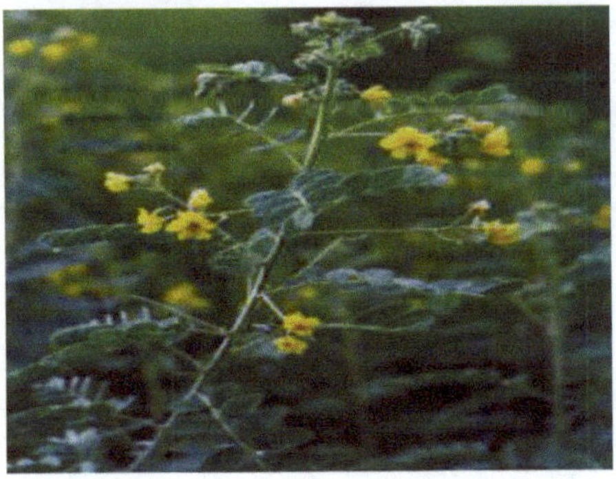

Ten gram (10 gm) plant material is warmed with 50 % methanol. The extract is filtered, concentrated and spotted on TLC plates. The chromatogram developed in n-Propanol: Ethyl acetate : Water (40 : 40 : 30). For visualizing the plates are first sprayed with conc. Nitric acid and heated for 15 min. at 120° C. The plates are cooled and sprayed with 10 % ethanolic KOH. The quinines of Senna appear as red-brown spots of 7-9 compounds. The major spots at R_f. about 0.4 (lowest spot) are of Sennoside B & A. Sennoside C is seen as a diffuse spot at R_f. 0.7 and Sennoside D at R_f. 0.55. Rhein is seen near the solvent front at R_f. 0.8. All these spots fluoresce lemon yellow when viewed on UV-365 nm. Senna fruits show five red-brown spot corresponding to Sennoside A, B, C, D and rhein.

Estimation of Sennoside Content

Extract 500 mg. of powdered leaves or pods with 30 ml water by warming on a boiling water bath for 15 minutes. Cool the solution to room temperature and make the volume to 50 ml with water. Then shake the solution and filter. Transfer about 20 ml of the filtrate to a separating funnel. Add a drop of conc. HCl and extract it twice with 20 ml of chloroform. Discard the chloroform layers and transfer 10 ml of the aliquot to a 100 ml vol. flask. Adjust the pH of the solution at 7 to 8 with a 5 % W/V solution of Na_2CO_3 (about 0.5 ml). Add 20 ml of 16 % $FeCl_3$ solution to the flask and digest it on a water bath for about 20 min. by which time ppt gets dissolved. Allow to cool, then transfer the mixture to a separating funnel and extract thrice with 25 ml of solvent ether. Combine the ether extract and make up the vol. to 100 ml with solvent ether. Evaporate 10 ml of this and dissolved the residue in 10 ml of 1N KOH. Filter the coloured solution if necessary, through a sintered glass filter. Measure the extinction of the solution at 500 nm (or green filter) using water as a blank.

Modified Procedure given in British Pharmacopoeia is as Under

The modified BPC; 1973 method gave value of only sennosides and not of total anthroquinone. The method has been modified with a view to develop a simple and cheaper method that gives consistent results, is less time consuming and estimate total anthroquinone laxative Principles of Senna calculated as Sennoside-B.

Methods for Extraction and Estimation

Two hundred fifty milligrams (250 mg) of the dried powdered senna leaves are taken in a flask, 2- ml of water is added and heated over a boiling water bath with occasional shaking to digest the material (about 15 min). The flask was shaken thoroughly and the material was allowed to settle. The contents are again heated over boiling water bath. The solution is decanted and taken in a 50 ml volumetric flask. This procedure is followed twice for complete extraction and volume of the pooled extract was made exactly to 50 ml. 20 ml of this solution is taken in a conical flask and made alkaline with a drop of 5% sodium bicarbonate solution in water. 20 ml of 6.3 % freshly prepared solution of ferric chloride in water, mixed and heated over a water bath for about 20 min (up to appearance of precipitate). Heating was continued and 2- ml of HCl was added and the contents are shaken thoroughly to dissolve the precipitate and allowed to cool. The liquid is then transferred to a separating funnel and extracted with two 20 ml portion of solvent ether, after using each portion to rinse the flask first. The ethereal extracts are then combined and the final volume is made to 50 ml. 10 ml of this solution is taken in a separating funnel and the color was extracted with 10 ml of 1 N NaOH. The extinction is measured immediately at 500 nm using water as blank.

1 mg of 1-8 Dihydroxy anthroquinone = 1.797 mg of Sennoside B

From the standard curve 1 OD = 0.045 mg Sennoside B/ml.

0.25 g. → 50 ml → 20.0 ml → 50 ml → 10 ml

$$\text{Sennoside (\%)} = \frac{\text{Sample O.D.} \times 0.045 \times 50 \times 50 \times 100}{10 \times 20 \times 0.25 \times 1000}$$

$$= \text{O.D.} \times 0.225$$

Sennoside Content

Another Procedure of Sennoside Content

- 250 mg powder of dry leaves was weighted and 50 ml distilled water is added.
- The material was reflexed for 15 min. at 90° C temp. in water bath, it was allowed to cool at room temperature and centrifuge at 5000 RPM for 10 min. The extract was collected
- An aliquot of 20 ml extract is taken in 25 ml volumetric flask and acidify with one ml conc. HCl (pH 6.5) and then one ml of 6.3 % $FeCl_3$ was added. The solution is heated in water bath for 2 min. and cools down at room temperature. The solution is neutralized using 0.5 % Na_2CO_3 and final volume was adjusted 25 ml with distilled water.
- For colour development and aliquot one ml was pipetted in test tube and 4.0 ml freshly prepared 5% KOH is added. The tubes are heated in boiling water bath for 2 minutes and cooled down in ice bath and centrifuge at 5000 RPM for 10 min. The supernatant is read against blank at 500 nm
- The percentage of sennoside B was calculated using standard graph factor of 1-8 dihydroxy anthraquinone.

Standard

- 10 mg 1-8 dihydroxy anthraquinone
- Dissolved in 100 ml absolute alcohol.

Estimation of Sapogenine from safed Musli (*Chlorophytum borivilianum*)

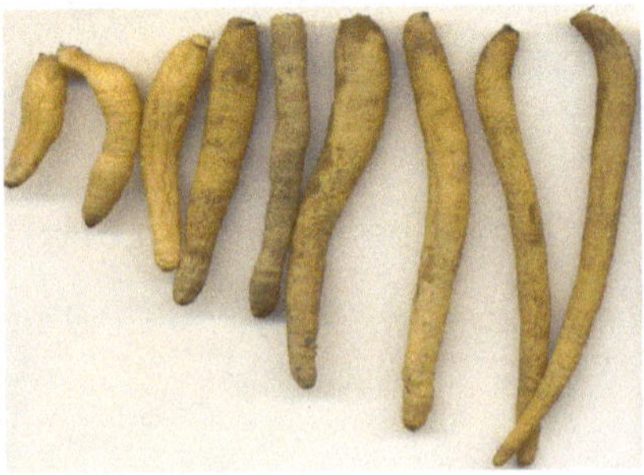

The economic part of *safed musli* is roots, which is extensively used in ayurvedic medicines. It grows on steep sloppy hills in the forests and is a source of income for the local tribal.

1. Colorimetric Method for Estimation of Total Sapogenin

Reagents

1. *Solvent mixture* : Chloroform : Methanol (4 :1)

2. Modified L.B. Reagent
3. *Conc.* H_2SO_4 : Acetic anhydride (3:1)

   [The mixture is prepaid fresh while keeping the flask in the ice bath]
4. *Preparation of Standard* : Twenty-milligram (20 mg) pure cholesterol is dissolved in 100 ml chloroform.

Extraction of Sapogenine

Weigh 0.5 gm of dry root powder and mix it well in 10 ml of solvent mixture. Keep it overnight and filter through glass wool. Wash the crude residue 3 times with 5 ml of solvent mixture each. Collect the filtrate in a beaker and evaporate the liquid up to 3-4 ml. Transfer the content in a measuring cylinder, wash the beaker with solvent chloroform. Collect the washings in the same measuring cylinder and make the volume exactly 10 ml with the help of solvent chloroform. Aliquotes of 0.2 to 0.5 ml of this solution are taken for colour development. The reagents are added serially as given in following table:

S. No.	Standard (ml)	Solvent Chloroform (ml)	Conc. of Standard (µg.)	L.B. Reagent (ml)		O.D. at 530 nm.
1	0.1	0.9	20	4.0	Keep all the tubes in boiling water bath for five (5) minutes. Cool it and read at 530 nm.	
2	0.2	0.8	40	4.0		
3	0.3	0.7	60	4.0		
4	0.4	0.6	80	4.0		
5	0.5	0.5	100	4.0		
Sample	0.5	0.5	----	4.0		
Blank	----	1.0	----	4.0		

2. Separation of Saponin by Thin Layer Chromatography

Saponins are glycosides of triterpenoids or steroids and very hygroscopic in nature. Saponins are readily soluble in water and foam when shaken. They are in soluble in non-polar solvents. The foam-forming activity of saponins is detected by method of O'Del et al. (1959), which involves shaking of 5.0 ml of 0.01 – 1.0 % saponins in M/15 K_2HPO_4 for one minute in a 25 ml graduated cylinder and measuring the amount of foam after another minutes.

Thin Layer Chromatography of Saponins

Saponins are water soluble and hence they may be extracted in water and hydrolysed with 2N HCl. The precipitated aglycones are taken up in ether and hydrolysed further.

Hundred gram (100 g.) of plant material or 20 g. of dry powder is boiled with 500 ml of water. The extract is filtered and about 82 ml of Con. HCl added (to make the solution 2N for HCl) and the mixture is refluxed for 3 h. The mixture is cooled and extracted with solvent ether. The concentrated ether fraction is spotted on TLC plates (silica gel) and developed using solvent systems (1) Chloroform : Ethyl acetate (1:1) or (2) hexane : acetone (4:1). The developed plates are dried and sprayed with 50 % H_2SO_4 or Liberman-Burchard reagent (2 ml Con. H_2SO_4 + 40 ml acetic anhydride + 100 ml chloroform) On heating the plates for 5 minutes saponins develop purple/ violet colors. Water can be used as a non-destructive spray to smoothly moisten the silica gel. It leaves the sapogenins as white spots on a wet translucent background. The common sapogenins and their relative positions in thin layer hromatograms are presented in following Figure.

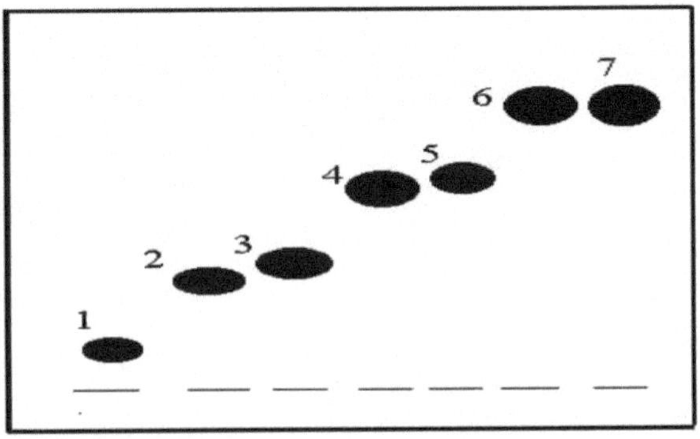

TLC (silica gel) of sapogenins

1. Gitoxigene
2. Hecogenin
3. Glycyrrhetinic acid
4. Yamogenin
5. Diosgenin
6. Smilogenin
7. Sarapogenin

3. Extraction and Purification of Mucilage from *safed musli*

Five hundred milligram (500 mg) of dry powder of Safed musli is soaked in 15 ml cold distilled water containing 0.5 % HCl for 1 h. The material is kept for overnight at room temperature and centrifuged it. Collect the extractions in 50 ml vol. flask. The residue is washed two times in 15 ml cold distilled water and the supernatants pooled. Adjust the vol. with water to 50 ml. Pipette 5.0 ml of aliquot in pre-weighed glass centrifuge tube and add 4.0 ml of ethanol to precipitate mucilage. The mucilage then separated by centrifuging it at 5000 rpm and supernatant was discarded. The mucilage is then washed three times with 5.o ml ethanol to remove chlorides. Dry the mucilage in oven at 65° C for overnight. Cool the tubes and weigh it. Calculate the percent Cold Extracted Mucilage (CEM) by weight differences.

The percentage of Cold Extracted Mucilage ranged between 20-35 % on dry weight basis.

Volatile Oils from Different Aromatic Species

I. Steam Distillation

Weigh 100-200g. of fresh material of aromatic plants such as Ocimum spp., Roisa grass, Palmarosa, Citronella, Jammu-lemon grass, Marjorum and Davana or any aromatic flowers e.g. Rose, Jasmine etc. and transferred in a distillation unit. Add approximately 1 L of water. The contents of flask are heated to boiling. The boiling is controlled so that the rate of distillation is not more than 2-3 ml per minute. The distillation is continued for 3 – 4 h. The volatile oil which distils over condenses along with the water vapor and remain as a layer above the water in the receiver. When the distillation is over the contents of the receiver is shaken with 50 ml ether. The ether layer is collected and the aqueous fraction is re-extracted with 20 ml of ether. The ether fractions combined, the solvent is allowed to evaporate in a desiccator and the oil remaining weighed, calculated to percentage.

II. Solvent Extraction

Organic solvents such as petroleum ether, toluene, chloroform etc. are used to extract the oil. 10 g. of the plant material is extracted with 100 ml solvent, at room temperature with occasional shaking, for 1 h. The extract is filtered through ordinary Whatman filter paper and the residue is put back into the beaker and re-extracted with 50 ml more of solvent for 30 min. After filtration, the filter paper and the residue are thoroughly washed with solvent and the washings added to the oil extract. The extract is distilled under reduced pressure and the oil in the flask is quantitatively transferred to a preweighed beaker by washing the flask 2-3 times with ether and adding the washings to the beaker. The ether is allowed to evaporate at room temperature to a constant weight. The increase in weight due to oil is calculated to percentage.

III. TLC of Volatile Oils

5 g of dry powdered aromatic materials/spice is kept covered with 50 ml solvent ether in a conical flask for 30 min. with frequent shaking. The clear supernatant is decanted into a 100 ml beaker and the extract is kept below a ceiling fan to concentrate. When the extract is reduced to 5 ml, it is spotted on TLC (silica gel) plates. The plates are developed in benzene or benzene: chloroform (1:1). [In benzene, the monoterpenes have higher Rf values and therefore this solvent is preferred over the second system in winter. In benzene: chloroform the monoterpenes has lower Rf values and therefore it is recommended for summer]. The chromatograms are dried and sprayed with vanillin-sulphuric acid (spraying the plates first with a solution of 5 % ethanolic sulphuric acid, followed by an overspray of 1 % ethanolic-vanillin). The plates are then warmed over a hot plate for 3-5 min. (or by keeping in an oven at 110 °C for 5 min.) when the monoterpenes appear as colored spots.

Extraction of "Biocrude" from Plants

'Biocrude' refers to the total lipids isolated and which can be converted to gasoline or other petroleum products. A general method for the evaluation and identification of the hydrocarbon and rubber producing crops, prescribed by Buchanan *et al.*, (1978), is as follows:

Dry plant material (500 g) ground to fine powder, is extracted with acetone for 24 h. The extract is concentrated, dissolved in 90% aqueous methanol (MeOH : H_2O, 9:1) or 87% ethanol (EtOH- H_2O, 7:1) and this solution is shaken with hexane. The hexane fraction contains the oils and the methanol fraction contains polyphenols and complex lipids. The oil fraction (hexane solubles) is concentrated and transferred to a preweighed beaker, the solvent evaporated and the increase in weight is calculated. This is the biocrude. The biocrude is fractionated after saponification. The biocrude is saponified and the saponified extract is taken in 50% aqueous ethanol and shaken with hexane. The unsaponifiable matter (phytosterols, terpenes, wax components) may be quantified (by weighing the dry matter after the removal of solvent). The saponified fraction (ethanol fraction) is acidified to pH 6 and the precipitated lipids are extracted in hexane. The hexane fraction contains the fatty acids, carboxly acids and some organic acids while the aqueous ethanol fraction contains glycerol.

The plant material left after acetone extraction is extracted further with benzene - hexane (2 : 3) or cyclohexane. Isoprene polymers, waxes and other terpenoids are extracted in this solvent/mixture. This fraction also is quantified and added to the biocrude to get the total biocrude from the plant.

In, a modified method of Calvin and Coworkers (1981) recommend extraction of dry plant material directly with heptane to isolate the biocrude.

The plant material left after extractions with acetone and benzene - hexane (heptane) is the oil and hydrocarbon - free residue. This residue contains cellulose, lignin, proteins, polysaccharides and inorganic components. Each one of these plant products may be quantified using appropriate methods. The scheme of extraction is presented in Fig 10.2

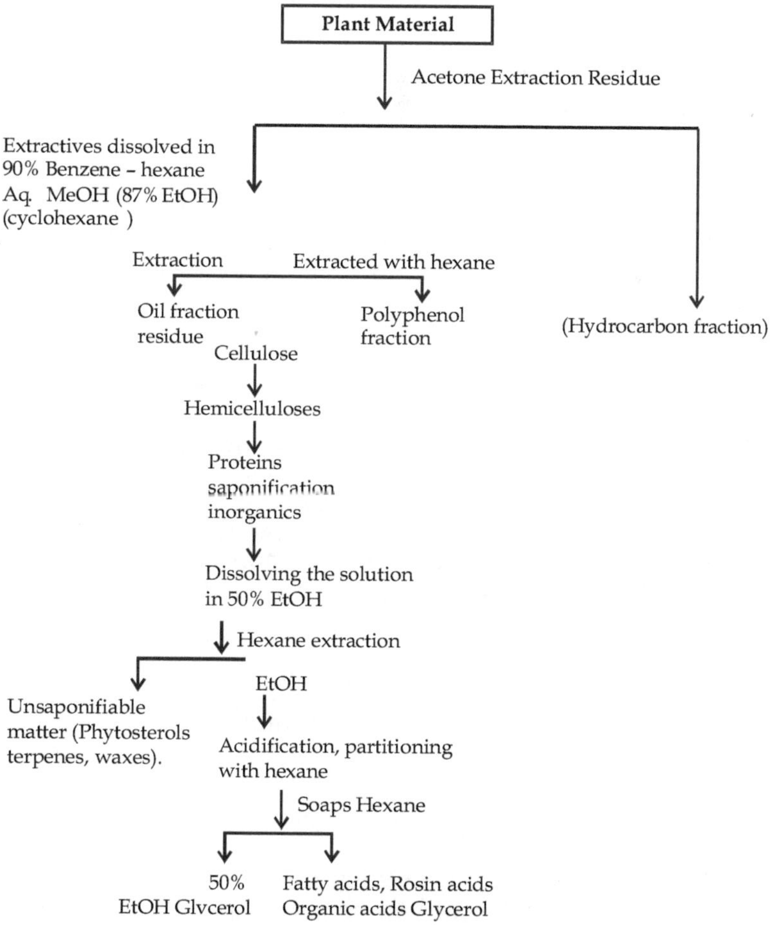

Fig. 10.2 : Scheme of extraction to isolate biocrude from plants

Solvent Extraction

When the water-insoluble compounds are to be extracted oil or an organic solvent is used. This is done in a soxhlet extractor. The organic solvent (Acetone, benzene etc.) dissolves wax. Chlorophyll oil etc alongwith the desired compound. Therefore, normally the extract is coloured. Solvents like methanol and alcohol dissolves many water-soluble compound also.

Steps for extraction

Sovent extration (by soxhlet)

↓

Plant material (1g : 100 ml)

↓

Solvent extration (100 ml solvent, at room temperature)

↓

Extract

↓

Distilled under reduced pressure

↓

Oil

Advantage

Extract the volatile oils from plant material.

Disadvantages

1. The preparation of volatile oils, contain many other organic compounds such as waxes, fats and pigments.
2. The removal of solvent needs other techniques, like distillation and therefore, need additional equipment.
3. Solvents used are to be chemically pure and therefore incur higher expenditure.

Water Extraction (Aqueous Medium)

This is the most common method of extraction. The water-soluble compounds will be extracted by this method. In cold extraction, the plant material is kept in water for 24 hrs. In hot extraction the material is boiled in water for 2-6 hrs. These extracts contain a large number of other compounds besides the active principles. These compounds include carbohydrates (Sugar & Starch) amino acids, proteins, phosphatides, amines, minerals and vitamins, which are the building blocks of the body. Therefore, in a formulation of aqueous extract a number of raw materials are available which help the body to repair itself. That is why the herbal preparations are slow to act, but leads to improvement of the body as a whole.

This is the most common method of extraction. All water-soluble compounds will be extracted by this method.

Steps for extraction

Steam distillation

↓

Plant material (10g)

↓

Water 250 ml (in distillaion Appartatus)

↓

Glycerine (few ml.)

↓

Heated to boiling (boiling controlled distributes ethanol more than 2-3 ml/min.)

↓

3-4 hrs. Distillate

↓

Volatile oil
(Condenses in water, remains in water level)

Advantages

1. Oils obtained in pure form
2. The equipment needed is relatively inexpensive.

Disadvantage

The temperature of steam distillation is 100° C at which some of the unstable compounds of oil get decompose.

Precautionary Steps During Quantitative and Qualitative Analysis of Secondary Metabolites

1. Cleaning of glassware's : All glasswares are cleaned in running tap water followed by dipping in 5% chromic acid solution for 3-4 h. Chromic acid solution prepared by dissolving 5 g of potassium dichromate in 100 ml concentrated H_2SO_4. This solution further diluted in 10 lit. water. After chromic acid treatment, glasswares rinsed with tap water and washed with 5 % soap solution and finally with tap water until free from soap. All the glasswares rinsed with distilled water and dried in oven at 100° C for 6 h.

2. Chemicals and Solvents – For evaluation of drug plants, AR grade chemicals or solvents are used.

3. Weighing of the Chemicals and Samples - These should be accurate.

4. Temperature - It should be maintained constant as per the procedure.

5. Processing of Plants -

   - Collected plants washed with water and remove excess water by pressing in cloths or ordinary filter paper so that all the dust particles removed.
   - Crude drug then dried under the shade
   - Powdered the drug in a blender and pass through 60 or 80 mesh sieve
   - Powdered drug analysed as early as possible to avoid deterioration.

Chapter 11

Biotechnological Approaches and Application of Plant Secondary Metabolites

Role of Biotechnological Approaches

In our fore-going chapters, we have studied variety of plant products such as alkaloids, glycosides, volatile or essential oils, gums and mucilage and oleoresins with varied role to play to the plants as well as to human.Knowledge of plants and knowledge of healing have been closely linked. It is well established that industries have many direct and indirect effects on human population. Increased stress is most evident at the same time health awareness goes parallel in the recent times. Most of the natural plant products are compounds biosynthetically derived from primary metabolites such as amino acids, carbohydrate metabolic intermediates and fatty acids. These secondary metabolites are the major sources of pharmaceuticals, food additives, fragrance and pesticides.

Application of biotechnology know how helps to synthesize the novel molecules and also could be beneficial to enhance the production of secondary metabolites. Classical definition of biotechnology states that it is "The use of living organisms or their products to enhance our lives and our environment." The word Pharming is commonly use to describe genetically engineered plants or livestock to produce medically useful products –predominantly protein drugs. Plants or animals are genetically engineered to contain genes capable of producing a biologic or drug compound. Therapeutic proteins are designed to treat illness includes serum proteins, cytokines, growth regulators, anti coagulants, antbiotics, lysosomal enzymes and plant secondary metabolites.

Apart from micoorganisms plants are preferred due to :

- Their flexibility and could produce a wide variety of proteins.
- They can synthesize a wide variety of metabolites (proteins) that are free of mammalian toxins and pathogens.
- They produce large amounts of biomass at low cost and require limited facilities.
- Crops are therefore well suited for the production of safe low-cost therapeutic proteins.
- Stability
- Safety
- Production cost
- Storage cost
- Ethical reasons

Why plants for secondary metabolites ?

Expressions System	Yeast	Bacteria	Transgenic Plants
Cost of maintaining	inexpensive	inexpensive	inexpensive
Type of storage	-2.0°C	-2.0°C	RT*
Gene size (protein) restriction	Unknown	Unknown	Not limited
Protein yield	High	Medium	High
Therapeutic risk	yes	yes	Unknown

Phenolics & Polyphenols, Terpenoids & essential oils, alkaloids, lecitins, etc.are the major groups of antimicrobial compounds from plants responsible for antimicrobial activity. Tobacco has been engineered to manufacture numerous products including antibiotics, novel polymers, a dental treatment, and anti-cancer drugs.Research is going on at The Tobacco and Health Research Institute (THRI)It is in late-stage of clinical trials and are expected to reach the market in the very near future. It is estimated that one-third of the world's population is infected with *Tuberculosis bacillus*. There is an urgent need to search for and develop new, effective and affordable anti-TB drugs. In this scenario, the plant kingdom with enormous chemical diversity may be looked as an important source of new anti-TB agents. Ø17,500 higher plant species occurring in India, out of that only 365 species have been evaluated so far for antimycobacterial activity. 70 % of 365 plant species from a wide range of families that have shown antimycobacterial activity. Most of the plant species have shown strong positive ethno pharmacological correlation with the traditional knowledge however, none of these product are currently commercially available. Three plant products: noni juice, spider plant root, and garlic are known for their abilities to inhibit bacterial growth. Noni juice is currently a $2 billion dollar industry, but many of its medicinal claims haven't been scientifically tested.

The garlic extract and spider plant extract at the test concentrations were unable to significantly inhibit the growth of *E. coli*. However, this study did demonstrate that noni juice at a concentration of at least 12 % completely inhibits the growth of *E. coli* on nutrient agar plates. clinical trials using noni might prove interesting. Preparations of aqueous and ethanolic extracts of 38 medicinal plant species commonly used in Thailand to cure gastrointestinal infections were tested for their antibacterial activity against different strains of *Escherichia coli*, including 6 strains of *Escherichia coli* O157:H7, *Escherichia coli* O26:H11, *Escherichia coli* O111:NM, Escherichia coli O22; 5 strains of *Escherichia coli* isolated from bovine; and *Escherichia coli* ATCC 25922.Among the medicinal plants tested 21.05 % exhibited antimicrobial activity against *Escherichia coli* O157:H7. These plant species may provide alternative but bioactive medicines for the treatment of *Escherichia coli* O157:H7 infection.

MeOH and EtOH resin extracts from *Larrea tridentata* (Chapparal) and *Flourensia cernua* D.C. (Asteraceae) against some fungi and bacteria that affect crops, foods and humans. The antimicrobial activity was evaluated using fresh cultures of bacteria prepared by inoculating 5 mL of brain-heart infusion with a loop ful of the stock cultures. The tubes were incubated at 30°C for 18-20h.; in the case of fungi they were activated by growth in PDA for 7 to 10 days at 25°C. It is also tested in albino rabbits for an in vivo assessment of skin irritation by plant extracts. The results showed that *L. tridentata* and *F. cernua* extracts had antimicrobial activities against 8 fungi, 8 bacteria and yeast species tested.

Biotechnological Advances in Secondary Metabolites is Useful to

- Increase secondary product synthesis by modifying the pathways for the secondary products.
- Cloning a specific gene(s) into plant or non-plant species which are not conventionally producing the secondary metabolites.
- Under standing the pathways for secondary metabolites and altering the directed metabolism in plant.

  e.g. Shikimate $----\alpha$ phenyl propanoid alkaloid
- Evolution of genetically engineered plants to produce less toxic bye-products. e.g. bromoxynol resistant cotton.
- Genetic engineering to produce new type of secondary metabolites generally not produced by the plant
- Over production of primary metabolites in micro-organisms which are required for the synthesis of secondary metabolite synthesis. e.g. Over production of Shikimic acid or aromatic amino acid such as tryptophan for alkaloid synthesis.
- Production of low nicotine or chlorogenic acid type of tobacco or erucic acid of mustard.
- Elimination of toxic secondary metabolites from plant for improving the crop quality.
- Production of hybrid secondary metabolite such as semi-synthetic derivatives of morphine and codeine in *E.coli* to be used in

pharmaceutical industry, which are more potent than original products.

- To develop new, structurally unique antibiotics with increased activity.
- Genetic manipulation to enhance yields & thus increase the cost of production.
- The biosynthetic pathways are complex i.e. 10-30 enzymatic steps. Moreover there is little or no information about genes or proteins.

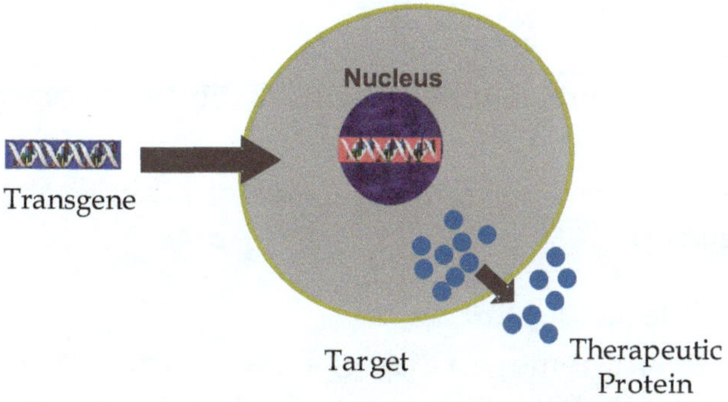

Advantages of Biotechnological Approaches

- It is difficult to increase the area under plantation for a particular species and the growth of plants takes its own time.
- To meet the ever increasing demand the natural resources are not sufficient.
- The world political scenario may also affect the supply of a particular raw material.
- To overcome these hurdles, the industry requires alternative methods of assured supply of uniform material throughout the year.
- Harvesting of plants from natural forest resources is not only difficult but also makes them endangered species.
- When plant material is not available throughout the year in a quantity sufficient for industrial production and chemical synthesis is not possible, particularly for large complex molecules, biotechnological methods offer an excellent alternative.

But before implementing this approach, cost of the product and its demand should justify production by such means.

Steps Involved for Gene Transfer

- A segment of DNA containing a gene sequence which has been isolated from one organism & is introduced into a new organism
- It must include promoter, gene to be expressed & termination sequences.
- Transgenic plants are plants that possess gene or genes that have been transferred from a different species.

Produced by

- Cross-pollination based hybridization between different plant species
- Laboratory manipulations to insert additional genes (Genetic Engineering)

Stage 1: Selecting gene

- Locate and remove DNA of interest using restriction enzymes that recognize specific target DNA sequences
- Place into a plasmid for amplification in a bacterium

Stage 2: Insertion gene into tissue

- Involves tissue culture techniques
- Often use sterile young leaf segments as targets

Stage 3: Get DNA into the target plant

- Chemical method
- Electroporation
- Gene gun method
- Agrobacterium mediated
- Transformation
- Micro injection
- Macro injection

Stage 4: Regenerate transgenic plants

- Transformation is not 100% efficient – not every targeted plant cell will be transgenic.

- Transformed explants taken through a dedifferentiating callus stage.

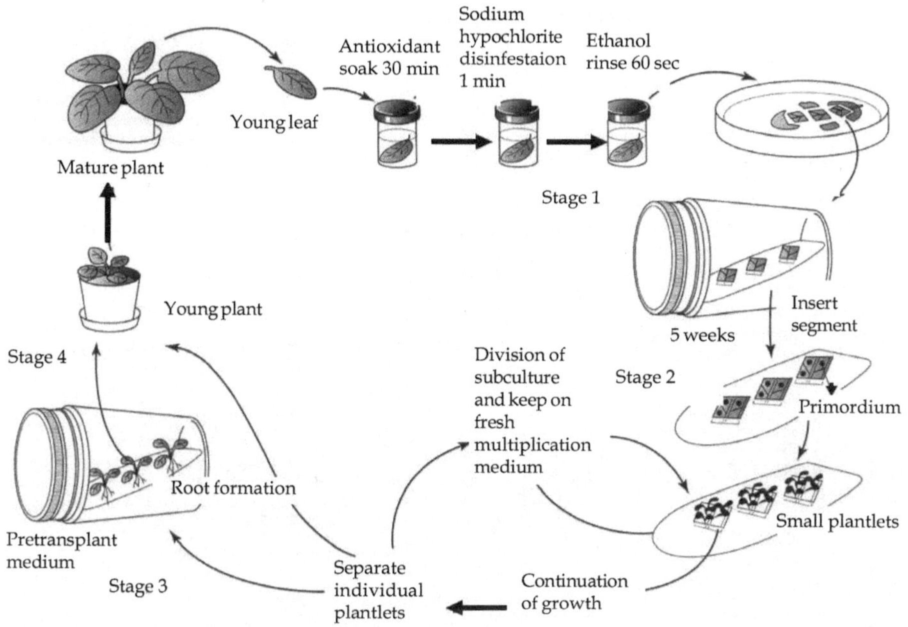

In vitro grown plant cells and tissues have been used extensively for the production of secondary metabolites (Fig.11.1). Depending on the objectives, a system such as callus, cell suspension or root/shoot culture is used. Once the *in vitro* culture system is established it is used to achieve objectives through different approaches *viz.*, micropropagation, genetic manipulation or cultivation in a Bioreactor (Fig. 11.2). The following applications of biotechnology are being pursued in the subject of secondary metabolites.

1. Development of seed material for domestication and micropropagation.
2. Continuous improvement of plants for secondary metabolites through somaclonal and genetic variation.
3. Understanding metabolic pathways.
4. Alternative methods using Bioreactors (biomass); immobilization, organ culture (shoot/hairy root).
5. New compounds in tissue culture.

Common name	Scientific name	Compound	Class	Activity[d]
Alfalifa	*Medicago sativa*	?		Gram-positive organisms
Allspice	*Pimenta dioica*	Eugenol	Essential oil	General
Aloe	*Aloe barbadensis* *Aloe vera*	Latex	Complex mixture	Corynebacterium, Salmonell, *Streptococcus, S. aureus*
Apple	*Malus sylvestris*	Phloretin	Flavonoid derivative	General
Ashwagandha	*Withania somniferum*	Withafarin A	Lactone	Bacterial, fungi
Aveloz	*Euphorbia tirucalli*	?		S. aureus
Bael tree	*Aegle marmelos*	Essential oil	Terpenoid	Fungi
Balsam pear	*Momordica charantia*	?		General
Barberry	*Berberis vulgaris*	Berberine	Alkaloid	Bacteria, protozoa
Basil	*Ocimum basilicum*	Essential oils	Terpenoids	Salmonella, bacteria
Bay	*Laurus nobilis*	Essential oils	Terpenoids	Bacteria, fungi
Betel pepper	*Piper betel*	Catechols, eugenol	Essential oils	General
Black papper	*Piper nigrum*	Piperine	Alkaloid	Fungi, Lactobacillus, Micrococcus, E. coli, E. faecalis
Blueberry	*Vaccinium spp.*	Fructose	Monosaccharide	*E. coli*
Brazilian pepper tree	*Schinus terebinthifolius*	Terebinthone	Terpenoids	General
Buchu	*Barosma setulina*	Essential oil	Terpenoid	General
Burdock	*Arctium lappa*		Plyacetylene, tannins, terpenoids	Bacteria, fungi, viruses
Buttercup	*Rantunculus bulbosus*	Protoanemonin	Lactone	General
Caraway	*Carum carvi*		Coumarins	Bacteria, fungi, viruses
Cascara sagrada	*Rhamnus purshiana*	Tannins	Polyphenols Anthraquinone	Viruses, bacterial, fungi
Cashew	*Anancardium pulsatilla*	Salicylic acids	Polyphenols	P. acnes Bacteria, fungi
Castor bean	*Ricinus communis*	?		General

Contd...

Table Contd...

Ceylon cinnamon	*Clinnamommum verum*	Essential oils, others	Terpenoids, tannis	General
Chamomile	*Matricaria chamomilla*	Anthemic acid	Phenolic acid	*M. tuberculosis, S. typhi* murium, S. aureus helminths
		-	Coumarins	Viruses
Chapparal	*Larrea tridentata*	Nordihydroguai aretic acid	Lignan	Skin bacteria
Chilli peppers, paprika	*Capsicum annum*	Capsaicin	Terpenoid	Bacteria
Clove	*Syzygium aromaticum*	Eugenol	Terpenoid	General
Coca	*Erythroxylum coca*	Cocaine	Alkaloid	Gram-negative and positive cocci
Cockle	*Agrostemma githago*	?		General
Coltsfoot	*Tussilago farfata*	?		General
Coriander, cilantro	*Corandrum sativum*	?		Bacteria, fungi
Cranberry	*Vaccinitum spp.*	Fructose Other	Monosaccharide	Bacteria
Dandelion	*Taraxacum officinale*	?		C. albicans, S. cerevisiae
Dill	*Anethum graveolens*	Essential oil	Terpenoid	Bacteria
Echinacea	*Echinaceae angustifolia*	?		General
Eucalyptus	*Eucalyptus globulus*	Tannin	Polypehnol	Bacteria, viruses
		-	Terpenoid	
Fava bean	*Vicia faba*	Fabatin	Thionin	Bacteria
Gamboge	*Garcinia hanburyi*		Resin	Bacteria
Garlic	*Allium sativum*	Allicin ajoene	Sulfoxide Sulfaed terpenoids	General
Ginseng	*Panax notoginseng*		Saponins	*E. coli*, Sporothrix schenckii, Staphytococcus, Trichophyton
Glory lily	*Gloriosa superba*	Colchicine	Alkaloid	General
Goldenseal	*Hydrastis canadensis*	Berberine, hydrastine	Alkaloids	Bacteria, Giardia duodenate, trypanosomes Plasmodia

Contd...

Table Contd...

Gotu kola	*Centella asiatica*	Asiatocoside	Terpernoid	M. leprae
Graperfruit peel	*Citrus paradisa*		Terpernoid	Fungi
Green Tea	*Camellia sinensis*	Catechin	Flavonoid	General
				Shigella Vibrio S. mutans Viruses
Harmel, rue	*Peganum harmala*	?		Bacteria, fungi
Hemp	*Cannabis sativa*	β-Resercylic acid	Organic acid	Bacteria and viruses
Henna	*Lawsonia inermis*	Gallic acid	Phenolic	S. aureus
Hops	*Humulus lupulus*	Lupulone, humulone	Phenolic acids (Hemi) terpenoids	General
Horseradish	*Armoracia rusticana*		Terpenoids	General
Hyssop	*Hyssopus officinalis*		Terpenoids	Viruses
(japanese) herb	*Rabdosia trichocarpa*	Trichorabadal A	Terpene	Helicobacter pylori
Lantana	*Lantana camara*	?		General
-	*Lowsonia*	Lawsone	Quinone	M. tuberculosis
Lavender-cotton	*Santolina chamaecyparissus*	?		Gram-positive bacteria, Candida
Legume (West Africa)	*Millettia thonningii*	Alpinumisoflavone	Flavone	Schistosoma
Lemon balm	*Melissa officinalis*	Tannins	Polyphenols	Viruses
Lemon verbena	*Aloysia triphylla*	Essential oil	Terpenoid	Ascaris
			?	E. coli, M. tuberculosis, S. aureus
Licorice	*Glycyrhiza glabra*	Glabrol	Phenolic alcohol	S. aureus, M. tuberculosis
Lucky nut, yellw	*Thevetia peruviana*	?		Plasmodium
Mace, nutmeg	*Myristica fragrans*	?		General
Marigold	*Calendula officinalis*	?		Bacteria
Mesquite	*Prosopis juliflora*	?		General
Mountain tobacco	*Arnica montana*	Helanins	Lactones	General
Oak	*Quercus rubra*	Tannins	Polyphenols	
		Quercetin (available commercially)	Flavonoid	

Contd...

Table Contd...

Olive oil	*Olea europaea*	Hexanal	Aldehyde	General
Onion	*Allium cepa*	Allicin	Sulfoxide	Bacterial, Candida
Orange peel	*Citrus sinensis*	?	Terpenoid	Fungi
Oregon grape	*Mahonia aquifolia*	Berberine	Alkaloid	Plasmodium Trypansomes, general
Pao d'arco	*Tabebuia*	Sesquiterpenes	Terpernoids	Fungi
Papaya	*Carica papaya*	Latex	Mix of terpenoids, organic acids alkaloids	General
Pasque-flower	*Anemone pulsatilla*	Anemonins	Lactone	Bacteria
Peppemint	*Mentha piperita*	Menthol	Terpenoid	General
Periwindle	*Vinca minor*	Reserpine	Alkaloid	General
Peyote	*Laphophora williamssi*	Mescalline	Alkaloid	General
Poinsettia	*Euphorbia pulcherrima*	?		General
Poppy	*Papaver somniferum*	Opium	Alkaloids and others	General
Potato	*Solanum tuberosum*	?		Bacteria, fungi
Prostrate knotweed	*Polygonum aviculare*	?		General
Purple prairie clover	*Petalostemum*	Petalostemumol	Flavonol	Bacteria, fungi
Quinine	*Cinchona sp.*	Quinine	Alkaloid	Plasmodium spp.
Rauvolfia, chandra	*Rauvolfia serpentina*	Reserpine	Alkaloid	General
Rosemary	*Rosmarinus officinalis*	Essetential oil	Terpenoid	General
Sainfoin	*Onobrychis viciifolia*	Tannins	Plyphenols	Ruminal bacteria
Sassafras	*Sassafrasa albidum*	?		Helminths
Savory	*Satureja montana*	Carvacrol	Terpenoid	General
Senna	*Cassia angustifolia*	Rhein	Anthraquinone	S. aures
Smooth hydrangea, seven barks	*Hydrangea arborescens*	?		General
Snakeplant	*Rivea corymbosa*	?		General
St. John's wort	*Hypercum perforatum*	Hypericin others	Anthraquinone	General

Contd...

Table Contd...

Sweet flag, calamus	*Acorus calamus*	?		Enteric bacteria
Tansy	*Tanacetum vulgare*	Essential oils	Terpenoid	Helminths, bacteria
Tarragon	*Artemsia dracunculus*	Caffeic acids, tannins	Terpenoid Polyphenols	Viruses, helminths
Thyme	*Thymus vulgaris*	Cafferic acid Thymol Tannins	Terpenoid Phenolic alcohol Polyphenols Flavones	Viruses, bacteria, fungi -
Tree bard	*Pdocarpus nagi*	Totarol	Flavonol	P. acnes, other gram-positive bacteria
		Nagilactone	Lactone	Fungi
Tua-Tua	*Jatropha gossyphiifolia*	?		General
Turmeric	*Curcuma tonga*	Curcumin Turmeric oil	Terpenoids	Bacteria, protozoa
Valerian	*Valeriana officinalis*	Essential oil	Terpenoid	General
Willow	*Salix alba*	Salicin Tannins Essential oil	Phenolic glucoside Polyphenol Terpenoid	
Wintergreen	*Gaultheria procumbens*	Tannins	Polyphenol	General
Woodruff	*Galium odoratum*	-	Coumarin	General Viruses
Yarrow	*Achillea millefolium*	?		Viruses, helminths
Yellow dock	*Rumex crispus*	?		E. coli, Samonella, Staphylococcus

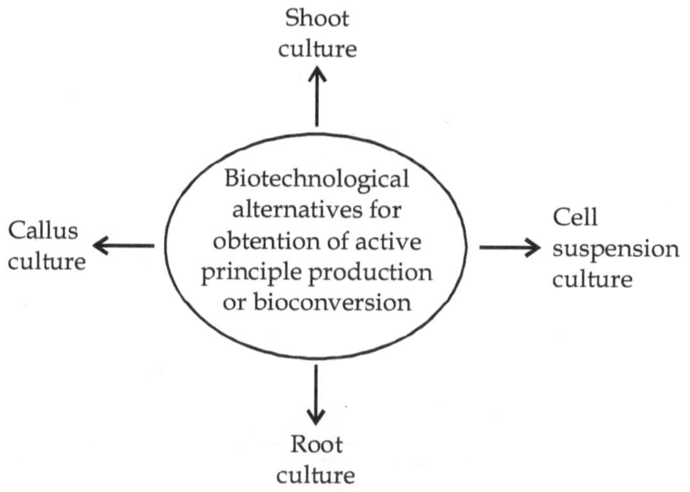

Fig. 11.1 : Different ways to obtain a product *in vitro*

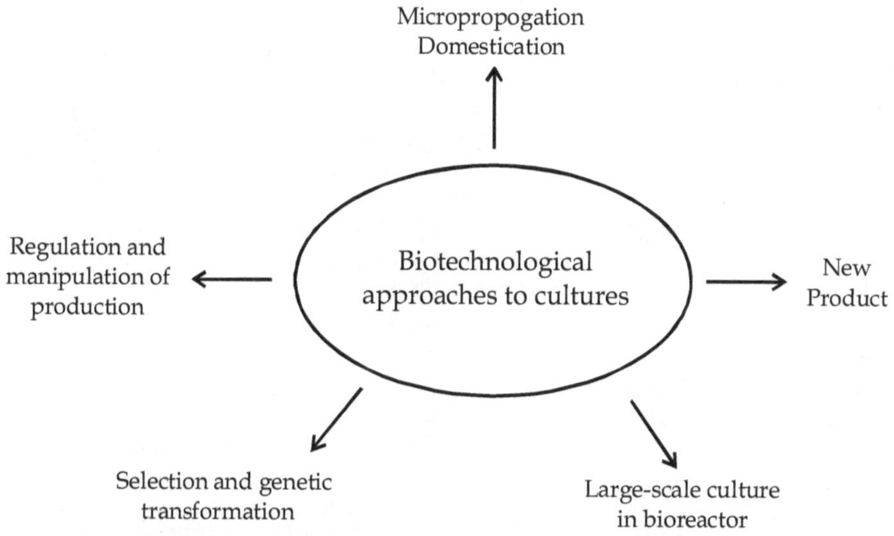

Fig. 11.2 : Different approaches for the production of secondary metabolites

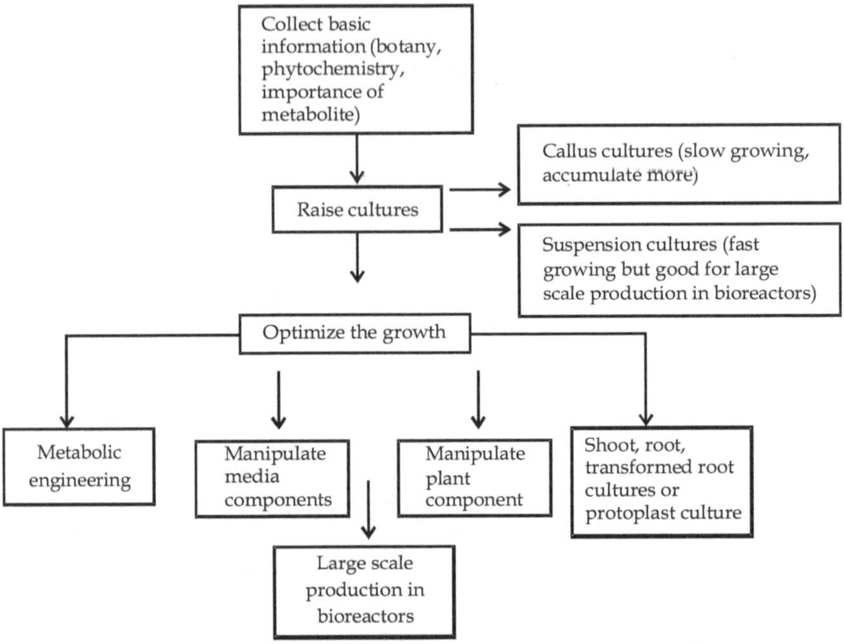

Fig. 11.3 : Application of tissue culture in secondary metabolites productions.

Table: A list of selected antibiotics produced commercially

Antibiotic	Produced by	Activity	Chemical Nature
Amphotericin B	*Streptomyces nodosus*	Antifungal	Polyene
Bacitracin	*Bacillus subtilis*	Gram +ve bacteria	Peptide
Cephalosporin C	*Cephalosporium acremonium*	Gram +ve & -ve	Peptide
Cycloheximide	*S. griseus*	Antifungal	--
Gentamicin	*Micromonospora purpurea*	Gram +ve bacteria	Aminoglycoside
Gramicidin	*Bacillus brevis*	Gram +ve bacteria	Peptide
Kanamycin	*S. kanamycetius*	Gram +ve & -ve bacteria & mycobacteria	Aminoglycoside
Pimaricin	*S. natalensis*	Anti tumor	Polyene
Penicillin G	*P. chrysogenum*	Gram +ve bacteria	Peptide
Polymixin B	*Bacillus polymyxa*	Antifungal	peptide
Streptomycin	*S. griseus*	Gram +ve & -ve bacteria & mycobacteria	Aminoglycoside
Tetracycline	*Streptomyces* spp.	Gram +ve & -ve bacteria	Tetracycline

Development of Seed Material for Domestication

Plants are collected from their wild habitats for medicinal uses. This supply is unable to meet the demand if a plant finds multipurpose uses or applications. Under such conditions, uniform and large supplies can be assured only by systematic cultivation on a large scale. This requires planting materials such as seeds, tubers or other vegetative parts. There are several examples of insufficient availability of planting material necessitating, raising it through biotechnological method as the only way to get a sufficient amount. This approach has been used for the domestication of such plants as *Digitalis* species, *Dioscorea* species, *Chlorophytum* species, *Commiphora wightii* and many others.

Micropropagation

Micropropagation is the most widely used application of plant tissue culture and micropropagation protocols for a large number of medicinal plants have been reported. Micropropagation is routinely used wherever a particular selected or unselected genotype has to multiply at an enormous rate to meet the demand of cultivators to replace the existing stock of material (perhaps having inferior characters such as low productivity, disease susceptibility, poor responsiveness) or for introduction to a new state/country for cultivation, e.g., *Atropa belladonna, Rauwolfia serpentina, Dioscorea floribunda, Mentha* species etc.

Improvement-Somaclonal Variation and Genetic Engineering

Decline of potential for the production of active principle or essential oil content is a common feature with cultivation of medicinal plants and a continuous selection is required to maintain the high yield of active constituents for commercially viable programmes. Therefore, selection through conventional breeding as well as in cell culture is explored for obtaining high-yielding cultivars. Once selected, this material is multiplied by the micropropagation technique to provide seedling material to the farmers, e.g. *Mentha, Citronella* and *Cymbopogon* species. Though genetic engineering offers great promise for improving the existing genotype, the work is still in its infancy in relation to medicinal plants because more vigorous efforts are put into cereals and pulses. Genetic manipulation has been employed to obtain hairy root cultures of a large number of solanaceous plants and manipulation of biosynthetic pathways to obtain a desired product, e.g., change in flower colour by blocking the chalcone synthase gene responsible for flower colour.

Understanding Metabolic Pathways

Plant tissue culture has been extensively used to understand the nutrition of the plant cell and the secondary metabolites it can produce. All the earlier work regarding the production of the active principle concentrated on the possibility of producing a compound by the cell culture of a plant species. Subsequent efforts were devoted to learning about the factors, governing the production of secondary metabolites (optimization). Later, selection of cell lines for high yield of secondary metabolites and enzymes involved in the biosynthesis were investigated using radioactive precursors wherever considered necessary. Growth of the cell in a totally controlled environment of physical and chemical factors provides an excellent system for studying changes in the production of secondary metabolites, which are always present in small quantities. This basic information has provided significant clues for genes and their functioning, leading to genetic manipulation for biosynthetic pathways so as to obtain desired products by either blocking a pathway or enhancing the metabolic reaction.

Metabolic Engineering

The goal of metabolic engineering is to improve cellular activity by manipulating enzymatic, transport and regulatory functions of a cell. This is accomplished through the use of recombinant DNA technology.

This approach may lead to an increase of some enzymes involved in metabolism and consequently results in the accumulation of the target products.

Methods Involved

There are two different categories of transformation methods based on the type of genes to transfer, which are as follows.

1. Utilizes the foreign genes that encode enzyme activities not normally present in a plant. This may cause the modification or diversion of plant metabolic pathways. Two direct repeats of a bacterial lysine decarboxylase gene expressed in the hairy roots of *N. tabacum* markedly increased cadaverine and anabasine (Fecker *et al.*, 1993). The production of anthraquinone and alizarin in hairy roots of *Rubia peregrina* L. was enhanced by the introduction of isochorismate synthase (Lodhi *et al.*, 1996). The hairy roots of *A. belladonna* transformed with the rabbit *P450 2E1* gene displayed increased levels of the metabolites (Banerjee

et al. 2002). *Catharanthus roseus* hairy roots harboring hamster 3-hydroxy-3-methylglutaryl coenzyme A (CoA) reductase (HMGR) cDNA without the membrane-binding domain were found to produce more ajmalicine and cantharanthine or serpentine and campesterol than the control (Ayora-Talavera *et al.* 2002).

2. Over expression of enzymes that are already located in a plant. The tobacco putrescine *N*-methyltransfersase (PMT) was transformed into *Datura metel* L. and *Hyoscyamus muticus* L. (Moyano *et al.* 2003). The enzyme catalyzed the first committed step in the tropane alkaloid pathway and stimulated the growth of transgenic roots and the accumulation of tropane alkaloid.

   Oxygen deficiency is a usual problem in hairy root culture caused by poor mixing and mass transfer conditions. To improve the low oxygen conditions that affect growth during fermentation, two enzymes, namely dehydrogenase and pyruvate decarboxylase, were transferred into the hairy roots of *Arabidopsis thaliana* L. The transformant root lines maintained a similar growth rate under conditions of low oxygen to the rate achieved with full aeration (Shiao *et al.* 2002).

New Compounds/Derivatives Production

Plant cell cultures have produced (a) new compounds previously not known in the intact plant, (b) new derivatives of a known compound and (c) new derivatives by biotransformation of molecules incorporated in the medium. Such results provide unlimited opportunity to screen the cultures for new compounds. It is presumed that production of new compound/derivatives might be due to altered gene function in the cultured cells compared to the *in vivo* grown mother plant. Production of new alkaloids in cultures of *Catharanthus roseus, Ochrosia elliptica, Papaver somniferum* and *Ruta graveolens* are frequently cited examples.

Research on Metabolic Engineering of Terpenoids

- Petunia was transformed with the **(S)**-limonene synthase gene from *Clarkia breweri* resulting in the production of linalool, which repels aphids
- Same gene was introduced into tomato, under the control of a fruit-specific promoter, resulting in the accumulation of linalool in tomato fruits

- Transgenic tomatoes have also been described expressing phytoene synthase and total carotenoid content was increased up to four fold in transgenic tomatoes than normal varieties.

Scaling up Technology Through Bioreactors

Plant cell cultures grown in a Bioreactor enable biomass production of a desired medicinal plant or its active principle through transformation. Such a system has been used for a long time for the production of antibiotics using fungi. The basic technology was derived from microbial systems and has been continuously improved for the growth of plant cells and organ cultures on a large scale. Bioreactors up to 20,000 litres have been designed and tested for the growth of plant cell cultures. Such a culture system produces a huge biomass in a short duration (10 to 20 days) but there are still several challenges to resolve before wider applications. However, several pharmaceuticals are produced or are on the verge of being produced at the commercial level using large Bioreactors, e.g., shikonin from *Lithospermum erythrorhizon,* taxol from *Taxus brevifolia* and berberine from *Coptis japonica*.

The demand for natural products will increase in the coming two decades. This demand will exert tremendous pressure on already scant natural resources. Therefore, biotechnological alternative methods hold great promise for meeting the demand and the challenge. The demand for natural products is also increasing day by day because of increased health and antipollution awareness as exemplified by the use of natural dyes instead of synthetic dyes for coloruing clothes, biofertilizers and biopesticides. Health care products for improving skin colour and texture, antiageing and vitalizing drugs, medicines for hyperlipidemia and hypercholesterolemia are already in great demand.

Bioreactors

Scope of bioengineering ranges from simple wine-bottle microbiology to industrialization of not only beer, wine, cheese, and milk production , but also the production of biotechnology's newer products-antibiotics, enzymes, steroidal hormones, vitamins, sugars, and organic acids Concept of bioreactors-Fermentation technology emerged when Louis Pasteur defined fermentation as a biological activity of microscopic plant called Yeast and his work laid foundation for Bioreactors, because once the process was identified and understood, it can be controlled. Bioreactor is a system in which a biological conversion is effected, organisms are cultivated in a controlled manner and materials are converted or transformed via specific reactions. Bioreactors are specifically designed to influence metabolic pathways. The term "Bioreactor" is often synonymously used with "Fermenter". Fermenter is a system that provides an anaerobic process for producing alcohol from sugar. The majority of fundamental bioreactor engineering and design issues are similar, maintaining the desired biological activity and eliminating or minimizing undesired activities often presents a great challenge. The goal of an effective bioreactor is to control, contain and positively influence the biological reaction.To accomplish this, two areas must be taken in to considerations. One is the suitable reactor parameters for the desired biological , chemical and physical (macro kinetic) system

- Macro kinetic system includes organism growth and metabolite production and the other areas of major importance in bioreactor design involves the bioreactor parameters , including:
- Controlled temperature
- Optimum pH
- Sufficient substrate (usually a carbon source)
- Water availability
- Salts for nutrition
- Vitamins
- Oxygen (for aerobic purpose)
- Gas evolution
- Product and byproduct removal
- In addition to these, the bioreactor must be designed to promote
- Optimal formation of morphology of the organism
- To reduce contamination by unwanted organisms or mutation of the organism

Various Types of Bioreaction Systems

These systems are batch, continuous, surface/tray, submerged, air-lift loop and trickle bed setups.

Batch Bioreactors - Methodology

- Sterilization
- Inoculation of medium with specific organism

- Agitation
- Aeration and gas-removal
- Maintenance of optimum pH
- Harvest of product

Secondary Metabolism of Hairy Root Cultures in Bioreactors

Hairy roots are the result of genetic transformation-*Agrobacterium rhizogenes.* Hairy root cultures have the same or greater biosynthetic capacity for secondary metabolite production.Wide range of secondary metabolites are synthesized in roots and their synthesis is linked to the differentiation of the root. Hairy root cultures have been shown to accumulate secondary metabolites, which were normally accumulated in the aerial parts of the intact plants. Genetic stability is the another characteristic of hairy root cultures. Based on continuous phase, reactors used to culture hairy roots can be roughly divided in to three types (1) Liquid-phase (2) Gas-phase and (3) Hybrid reactors.

Hairy Root Culture

Hairy root culture - culture of fast-growing roots by:

- Inoculation with *Agrobacterium rhizogenes* (esp. useful where differentiated cells are required for secondary metabolite production)
- Transfer of T-DNA causing hairy roots, then elimination of Agrobacterium by antibiotic
- Transformed hairy roots are first subcultured to solid, then liquid medium.
- Sec. metabolite is released in the Medium and then harvested.

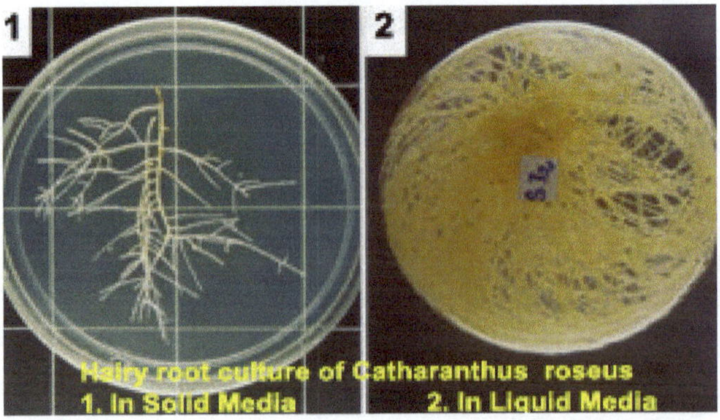

Advantages of Hairy Root Culture

Agrobacterium rhizogenes causes hairy root disease in plants. Hairy root-infected *A. rhizogenes* is characterized by a high growth rate and genetic stability. Hairy root cultures have been proven to be an efficient means of producing secondary metabolites that are normally biosynthesized in roots of differentiated plants. Furthermore, a transgenic root system offers tremendous potential for introducing additional genes along with the Ri plasmid, especially with modified genes, into medicinal plant cells with *A. rhizogenes* vector systems. The cultures have turned out to be a valuable tool with which we study the biochemical properties and the gene expression profile of metabolic pathways. Normally, root cultures need an exogenous phytohormone supply and grow very slowly, resulting in the poor or negligible synthesis of secondary metabolites. The hairy root system is stable and highly productive under hormone-free culture conditions. The fast growth, low doubling time, ease of maintenance, and ability to synthesize a range of chemical compounds of hairy root cultures offer additional advantages as continuous sources for the production of valuable secondary metabolites. Hairy roots are also valuable source of phytochemicals that are useful as pharmaceuticals, cosmetics, and food additives. These roots can also synthesize more than a single metabolite and, therefore, prove economical for commercial production purposes.

Many medicinal plants have been transformed successfully by *A. rhizogenes* and the hairy roots induced show a relatively high productivity of secondary metabolites, which are potentially important pharmaceutical products. Moreover, the cultures can be used to elucidate the intermediates and key enzymes involved in the biosynthesis of secondary metabolites. However, sometimes the efficiency of secondary metabolic production is not so desirable. Metabolic engineering offers new perspectives for improving the production of secondary metabolites by the over expression of single genes.

Liquid-Phase Bioreactors

- Stirred tank, Bubble column, Air lift, Liquid-impelled loop and Submerged convective flow reactors belong to this category
- In this reactors roots are submerged in medium
- Steel cage or mesh are used to isolate the roots from the impeller

- Mechanical agitation is replaced by using sparger technology
- Oxygen is growth limiting factor due to mass transport limitation
- Introduce gas at multiple points in to bubble column reactor that was divided into three segments by wire mesh, with each segment containing a sparger. It is proposed the use of a microsporous polypropylene membrane tubing that is inserted in to gas-driven reactor along with sparger to provide additional oxygen to the root bed. Convective flow reactor developed consist of a stirred tank, a peristaltic pump, and a tubular culture chamber. The medium is oxygenated in the stirred tank and a positive displacement pump recirculates the liquid between the stirred tank and the tubular reactor.

Convective reactor cannot be applied on large- scale system due to the pressure required to circulate the culture medium at a high velocity to overcome the flow resistance of the root bed.

Gas-phase Reactors

- Trickle bed, liquid-dispersed and nutrient mist reactors belong to this category
- Roots are exposed to air or other gas mixtures
- Nutrients are delivered to the roots as droplets
- The roots must be immobilized, since the continuous phase is gas
- Disadvantage of gas-phase reactors is that there is no way to uniformly distribute the roots in growth chamber without manual loading. It is proposed that a solution to overcome this problem. The reactor is initially run as a bubble column in order to suspend, distribute and attach the roots to the packing rings in the reactors. After few weeks, when root clumps are dense, the reactor is switched to trickle bed operation, thus exposing roots to the gas environment. The roots are mechanically chopped in a blender and then pumped as a slurry in to the reactor.

Hybrid Reactors

- Root inoculation step is completed mechanically and required and no manual labor is required. In a seed vessel placed on the top of reactor, the roots are grown as an inoculum. A helical screw with a blade located in the bottom of the seed vessel was used to cut and transfer the roots to the reactor. The main reactor contains assemblies of wire chains and bars to immobilize the roots.

Secondary Metabolite Production

- *Strain selection* : Selection of good hairy lines is a prerequisite, and plants producing high levels of secondary metabolites usually generate high-producing cell lines
- Relation ship to growth phase
- Production of secondary metabolite can occur at any growth stage and production is therefore growth-related
- For effective production of secondary metabolites on large scale, it is important to understand when in a growth phase a specific product is formed
- If a product is mainly formed during exponential growth, one should use a fed-batch culture strategy to keep the culture at active growth stage
- Medium composition
- Nutrients in the culture medium can be easily manipulated and have a great impact on secondary metabolite production
- *Example* : Ammonium ion altered the secretion pattern of products from hairy root cultures of *Lithospermum erythrorhizon.* In ammonium-free MS medium L. *erythrorhizon* normally accumulates shikonin on the surface of roots and in border cells. When ammonium ion is present, hydroxyechinifurn and a potent antifungal agent rhizonone were secreted in to medium
- Exogenous addition of phytohormones effects secondary metabolite production
- The total content of alkaloids is increased in *Hyoscyamus albus* when roots were grown in indole-3-acetic acid (IAA) and kinetin in dark
- Gases
  - CO_2, O_2, C_2H_4 also effect secondary metabolite production
  - Many studies emphasized on the role of oxygen in growth and secondary metabolism

- More artemisinin is produced in *Artemisia annua* hairy root grown in nutrient mist reactors in contrast to bubble column reactors where oxygen is limitation

❑ *Elicitors*

- Elicitors can be used to induce secondary metabolite production
- Pitta –Alvarez *et al.*(2000) tested the effects of different biotic (salicylic acid, yeast extract) and abiotic ($CaCl_2$, $AgNO_3$, $CdCl_2$) elicitors on accumulation and release of scopolamine and hyoscyamine in *Brugmansia candida* hairy root cultures
- Elicitors are always added after growth is completed

❑ Light plays important role in both growth and secondary metabolite production. Sauerwein *et al.* (1992) found that alkaloid content of both normal and hairy roots of *Hyoscyamus albus* was greater in roots grown in light compared to roots grown in the dark. Other factors influencing secondary metabolite production are temperature, subculture cycle, shear and medium pH. Sub culture cycle has shown to effect growth and production of indole alkaloids in *Catheranthus* hairy roots. Culture temperature has shown to influence hyoscyamine production in *Datura stramonium* hairy roots. Changes in medium pH can change the permeability of cell membranes, resulting in release of products in to the culture medium. Reactor operation will also effect the secondary metabolite production. Continuous cultures instead of batch cultures stimulated product release and an increase in the rate of production of both hyoscyamine and nicotine in Datura.

Bioreactors are integral to the development of many new high-value products. The proper selection and design of the bioreactor will determine the optimal commercial bioprocess and the corresponding capital investment. The synthesis of secondary metabolites is triggered and regulated by nutrient availability and environmental factors. Metabolic engineering of key regulatory enzymes may enable to control nutrient flux to desired compound or allow us to selectively control a desired pathway. This type of genetic engineering, together with proper reactor design, is essential to the success of large-scale production of secondary metabolites.

Comparative Growth and Secondary Metabolie Production in Bioreactors

Reactor type	Working volume (liter)	Root Culture	Culture period (d)	Inocuhum	Final density (g DW 1-1)	Biomass producti vity (g DW1-1 d-1)	Secondary metabolite productivity[a]
Isolated impeller - batch	12	*Datura stramocium*	35	n.a.	8.4	0.24	Hyoscyamine, 66.5 mgl^{-1}
Isolated impeller-continous	12	*Datura stramocium*	33	n.a.	20.4	0.62	Hyoscyamine, 211.2 mgl^{-1}
Isolated impeller-batch	25	*Atropa belladonna*	30	60g FW l-1	60.2	1.81	Atropine, 325.1 mgl^{-1}
Sagmented bubble column	2.5	*Atropa belladonna*	43	0.06g DW l-1	9.9	0.23	Atropine, 14 mg l-1
Bubble column	2	*Hyoscyarmus muticus*	30	0.16g DW l-1	14.3	0.47	n.a.
Bubble column	1.5	*Arternisia annua*	38	0.34g DW l-1	15.3	0.39	Artemisirin, 0.025 mg l-1
Bubble column-convective flow	2	*Hyoscyarmus muticus*	11+19 = 30	0.16 g DW l-1	25.3	0.83	n.a.
Radial flow	0.39	*Beta vulgaris*	11.7	77g FW l-1	51	3.73	n.a.
Sumerged-droplet phase	500	*Datura stramonium*	21+40 = 60	n.a.	8	0.13	n.a.
Bubble colum-trickle bed	14	*Hyoscyannus muticus*	15+10 = 25	0.16g DW l-1	20	0.79	n.a.
Bubble column-nutrient mist	1.5	*Artenisia annua*	21+17 = 38	0.33 g DW l-1	14.4	0.37	Artemisinin, 0.031 mg l-1
Modified inner loop nutrient mist	2.3	*Artemisia annua*	25	0.2 g DW l-1b	13.6b	0.53	n.a.
Erlenmeyer flask	1	*Artemisia annua*	10	10g FW l-1	13.4	1.24	Artermisinin, 0.088 mg l-1

Advantages of Bioreactors

- The advanced bioreactor culture system is the key step towards commercial production of secondary metabolites by plant biotechnology.
- Bioreactors with computer control systems theoretically offer various advantages over conventional culture procedures due to the possibilities of automation, labour savings and reduction of production costs.
- Therefore, a series of experiments are conducted to establish efficient adventitious roots and somatic embryos growth and secondary metabolite production using the bioreactor technology for natural products.
- Most bioactive compounds/secondary metabolites are obtained directly from plant tissue whose availability may be limited.
- The use of cell culture for producing these natural products has long been considered as an attractive solution to the problem of extracting the metabolites/bioactive compounds from the whole plant, since the cells can be cultured in large quantities under controlled conditions and harvesting of the desired product could be less problematic

Enhancement of Alkaloid Production through Biotechnological Means

1) Producition under stress

Plants adapt themselves to changed environment by modifying their physical & chemical composition. Stress can be generated by altering any of environmental, water hormonal factors. Biotic & abiotic stresses can be induced.

Osmotic stress: Addition of osmoticums. Sucrose increases production of alkaloids, anthocyanins, terpenoids.

Biotic stresses: are by infection, plant will generate defence related compounds to combat infection which are secondary metabolites. Most fungal metabolites are used which have shown success in production of catharanthine, morphine, saguinarine.

2) Alkaloids from cultured plant cells

Refined culture systems have improved biochemical yields considerably, many cell cultures produce 2g/l or more of biochemical.

Biochemical produced in high concentration by plant suspension

Compound	Plant species	Yield (g/L)
Ajmaline	*Rauwolfia serpentine*	2
Berberine	*Coptis japonica*	7
Raucaffricine	*Rauwolfia serpentine*	1.6
Taxol	*Taxus sps.*	

The biochemicals obtained from plant cell cultures are comparable in quality & activity to those derived from intact plants in their chemical, biochemical & biological property. In many instances, plant cells cultured in vitro accumulate a much higher level of the biochemical than the concerned intact plants.

Accumulation of higher levels of biochemicals in cultured plant cells than in concerned intact plants.

Biochemical	Plant species	Biochemical content (% dry weight)	
		Whole plant	Cultured plant
Berberine	Coptis japonica	4.0	13.4
	Thalictrum minor	0.01	10.0
Diosgenin	Dioscorea deltoidea	24	7.8
Serpentine	Catharanthus roseus	0.3	2.0

Alkaloid Production by Transformed Root Cultures of *Cinchona Ledgeriana* Transformed Root Cultures of *Cinchona ledgeriana* generated by Infecting Shoots Cultured in vitro with *Agrobacterium rhizogenes.* These root cultures grow on media containing Gamborg B5 Salts at Half or Full Strength with 3 % (W/v) sucrose as the carbon source. They Show a 6- to 8-fold increase in fresh weight in 28 Days. Transformation was confirmed by Southern Blotting Using [32P]-labelled Fragments from both the T L- and T R-DNA of the Ri Plasmid. The cultures were shown to synthesise a range of Quinoline alkaloids, of which Quinine, Cinchonidine, and Quinidine were the major components. The level of these alkaloids changes with the age of the cultures, reaching a Maximum at about 50 µg/g Fresh Weight after 45 Days. This compounds are having medicinal value.

Improvement of Biochemical Production Includes 2 Steps

Increasing the Cell Biomass Yield Per Unit Volume of the Culture

The production stratergy should consist of 2 distinct phase

(i) Growth phase for cell biomass accumulation and

(ii) Production phase for biosynthesis & accumulation of the biochemicals

In some cases culture growth & biochemical production occur together e.g. berberine production in *Thalictrum minor*.Enhancing the biochemical content of the cell biomass

Improving Biochemical Content of Cells

(i) Devising suitable culture medium & conditions- such as Temperature, light, innoculum size. In case of *C. japonica*, a 10-fold increase in copper concenteration of medium enhanced berberine content of cells by 20-30% without reducing biomass accumulation.In case of *C. roseus*, light influences ajmalicine/ serpentine ratio (less than 15hr photoperiod favors serpentine accumulation) & site of product accumulation.

(ii) Selection of high producing cell clones- Reduces cost of production. Highly productive cell clones have been successfully selected in case of *C. japonica*; it has facilitated commercial production of berberine from cell culture.

(iii) *Use of elicitors* : Some molecules stimulate the production of secondary metabolites these are called elicitors. Biotic (pectin, pectic acid, cellulse, chitin, chitosan or glucans), Abiotic (UV light, salts of heavy metals, chemicals that disrupt membrane integrity).

Biochemicals induced by elicitors are releazed in the medium.

(iv) *Use of two- phase culture system* : Culture medium constitutes the 1st phase, adsorbant compound makes up the 2nd phase. Adsorbants remove even traces of secondary metabolites, protect biochemicals from degradation.

(v) *Use of organ culture* : Growth of organized tissues like shoots, roots is another approach to enhance the production of active principle in the higher amount than unorganized cultures. e.g. production of vincristine by shoot cultures of periwinkle.

Production by Micropropagation & Hairy Root Cultures

Method for rapid clonal propagation by using tissue culture is known as micropropogation. It is only process of plant biotechnology which is being utilized by industries in India for commercial production of mainly ornamental plants & fruit trees. Many of the root synthesized compounds including tropane alkaloids, atropine, steroidal precursors such as solasidine,& catharanthus alkaloids are of sufficient high values (1000US$/kg) to justify the exploitation of hairy root culture for their commercial production.

Production in Bioreactors

Bioreactor is a large vessel in which a substance of low value is utilized by living cells or enzymes to generate a product of higher value. Various strategies have been applied to optimize active principle production in bioreactor. They are as below,

Establishment of cell suspension cultures of plant with high content of desired drug.

- Selection of highly productive clone
- Optimization of cultural conditions
- Culture of plant cells on large scale in bioreactor.

3) By Altering the Metabolism of Plant

Using antisense/cosuppression technologies or over expression, medicinal plants can be tailored to produce pharmaceutically important alkaloids by eliminating interfering metabolic steps or by introducing desired metabolic steps.

(A) To accumulate more of the end product alkaloid, a side pathway that also uses the same precursor may have to be blocked.

(B) To accumulate an alkaloid not normally produced in a particular plant species, a transgene (from another plant or a microorganism) may be introduced.

(C) If the end product alkaloid would be more useful as a particular derivative, a gene that encodes that particular enzyme may be introduced.

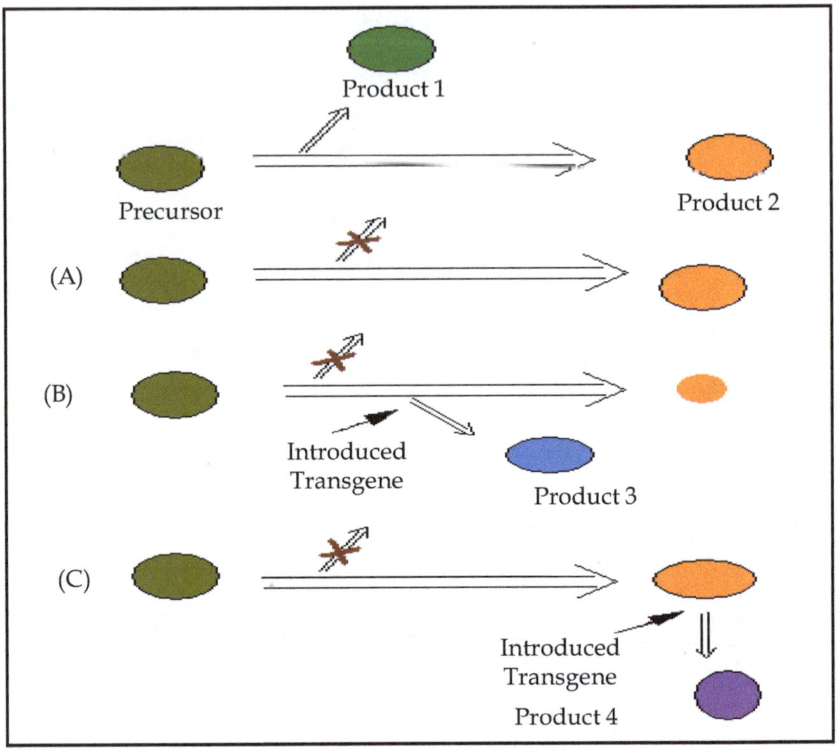

Metabolic engineering of medicinal plants may be pharmaceutical biotechnology of the future

A cDNA encoding hyoscyamine 6β-hydroxylase from *H.niger* has been introduced into *Atropa belladona* by using *Agrobacterium tumerificans & A. rhizogenes* mediated transformation. The resulting transgenic plants & hairy roots each contained greater concentrations of scopolamine than the wild types. These transgenic Atropa plants provided the 1st e.g. of how medicinal plants could be successfully altered by using molecular genetic techniques to produce increased quantities of a medicinally important alkaloid. One alternative approach to the use of metabolically engineered plants is to use microbes to produce alkaloids. Short biosynthetic pathways can be expressed in either yeast or bacteria & used as a source of alkaloid. Plant alkaloid genes can be functionally expressed in microorganisms to produce either single biotransformation steps or short biosynthetic pathways. For e.g. a known plant biosynthetic pathway contains an enzyme encoded by gene 3 which catalyzes a transformation step that is difficult to achieve by chemical synthesis. After heterologous expression of gene 3 in a microorganism the protein product can be used in a biomimetic synthesis of alkaloid D. (that is, the microorganism is supplied with compound C and produces alkaloid D).

Likewise, a short pathway consisting of enzymes encoded by genes G1, G2, G3, and *G4*, could be expressed in a microorganism to produce alkaloid E directly from precursor A.

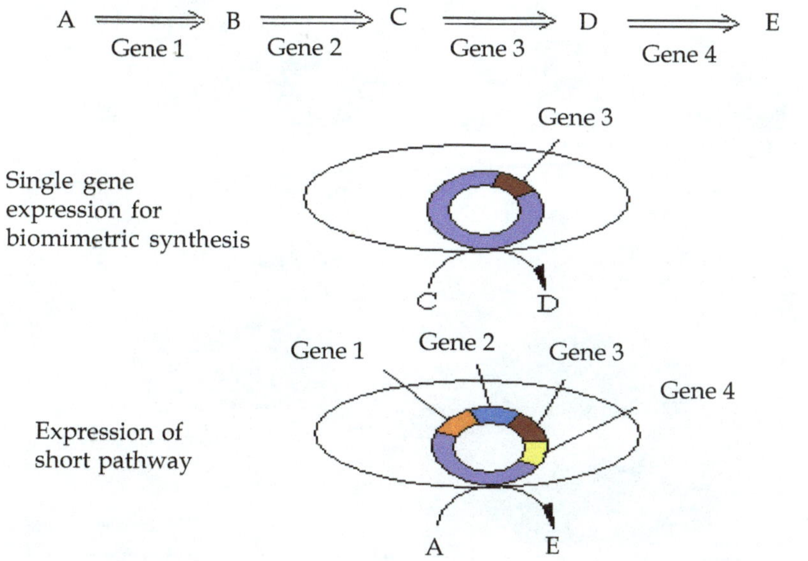

Metabolic Engineering of Caffeine

In coffee plant caffeine is synthesized from xanthosine through three successive methylation and ribose removal steps. All the genes coding for the corresponding enzymes have been isolated. Using these genes caffeine production has been engineered in 2 ways. The first is to decrease the caffeine content in coffee plants to cope with occasional health problems caused by caffeine uptake, and the other is to produce caffeine as an insect repellant in crop plants originally not synthesizing caffeine. The first approach was performed using an RNAi for *MXMT*, yielding a 70% suppression of the caffeine level in leaves of transgenic coffee plants. The other approach was carried out by simultaneous introduction of three genes, *XMT*, *MXMT* and *DXMT*, into tobacco plants, which produced up to 5mg caffeine per g fresh weight of leaves. This amount of caffeine was enough to repel tobacco cutworms (*Spodoptera litura*), suggesting the method to be practically efficient for construction of herbivore tolerant crops.

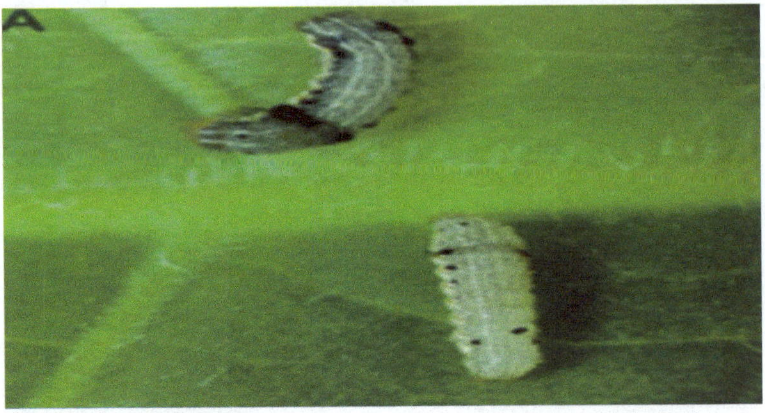

(A) Tobacco cutworm

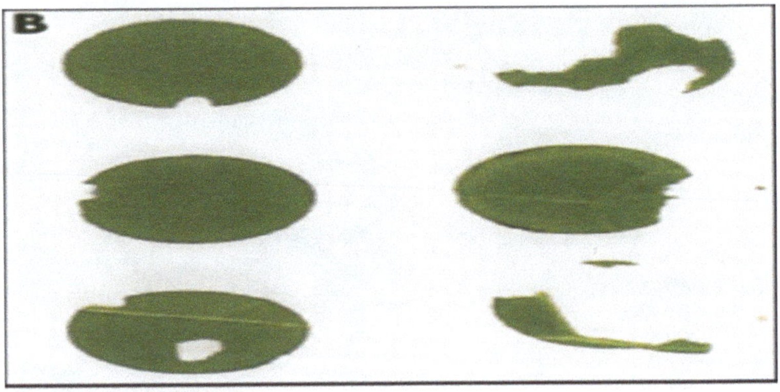

B. Leaf disc choice test

Larvae were allowed to feed on six leaf discs, three from caffeine producing, and three from control plants. After feeding for 3 h in the dark, each disc was collected and photographed. The tested transgenic plant contained caffeine at average 5 µg/g fresh weight. Disc samples are from caffeine containing (left) and control leaves (right).

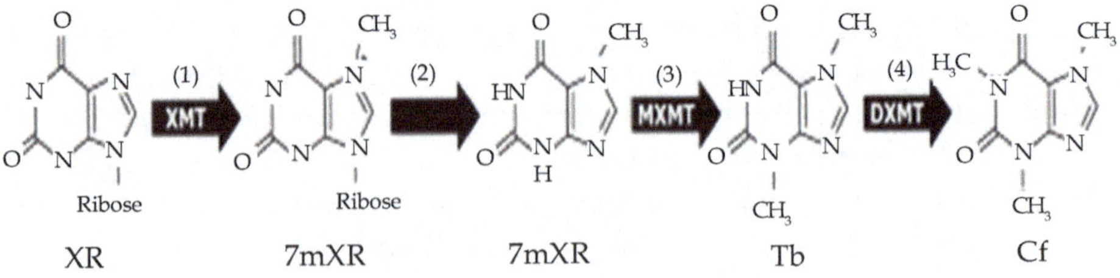

Caffeine Biosynthetic Pathway in Coffee Plants

The first (1), third (3) and fourth (4) steps feature methyl group transfer, and the second(2) step involves ribose(Rib) removal, XR, xanthosine; 7mXR, 7-methylxanthosine; 7mX, 7-methylxanthine; Tb, theobromine; Cf, caffeine; XMT, xanthosine methyltransferase, MXMT, 7-methylxanthine methyl transferase, DXMT, 3,7-dimethylxanthine methyl transferase.

Strategy to Produce Novel Flavonoids in Tomato

In cultivated tomato fruits flavonoids are only found in the peel. The main flavonoids accumulating are naringenin-chalcone and the flavonol rutin (quercetin-3-rutinoside). In fruit flesh, the pathway is hardly active and structural genes required for the production of flavonoids are expressed at very low levels, relative to fruit peel.

In order to introduce new flavonoid biosynthetic branches, three binary gene constructs were made. To target the pathway towards the production of stilbenes, we introduced a gene construct expressing the grape stilbene synthase *(STS)* cDNA under control of the constitutive cauliflower mosaic virus double 35S promoter (CaMV d35S).

Schematic Overview of the Flavonoid Pathway

In wild type tomato fruit peel the flavonoid pathway is active leading to the accumulation of 6-hydroxychalcones and flavonols (solid black arrows). Over expression of flavonoid pathway genes (black) led to a stimulated flux through the pathway (bold black arrow) and the introduction of new branches of this pathway (bold grey arrows).The dotted arrow represents the pathway leading to anthocyanins, which normally is not active in tomato fruit. Abbreviations: CHS, chalcone synthase; STS, stilbene synthase; CHR, chalcone reductase; CHI, chalcone isomerase; F3H, flavanone 3 hydroxylase; FNS, flavone synthase; FLS, flavonol synthase; DFR, dihydroflavonol reductase; ANS, anthocyanidin synthase.

This enzyme acts independent of CHS (Schröder and Schröder, 1990) and therefore it was expected that expression of the corresponding gene alone would result in the accumulation of stilbenes in both peel and flesh. However, to produce deoxychalcones independently of the endogenous tomato *CHS* geneexpression levels during the tomato fruit ripening, we reasoned that both chalcone synthase *(CHS)* and chalcone reductase *(CHR)* genes were required. Therefore, a double gene construct was made, consisting of the petunia *CHS1* cDNA and the alfalfa *CHR* cDNA, both expressed under control of the d35S promoter.

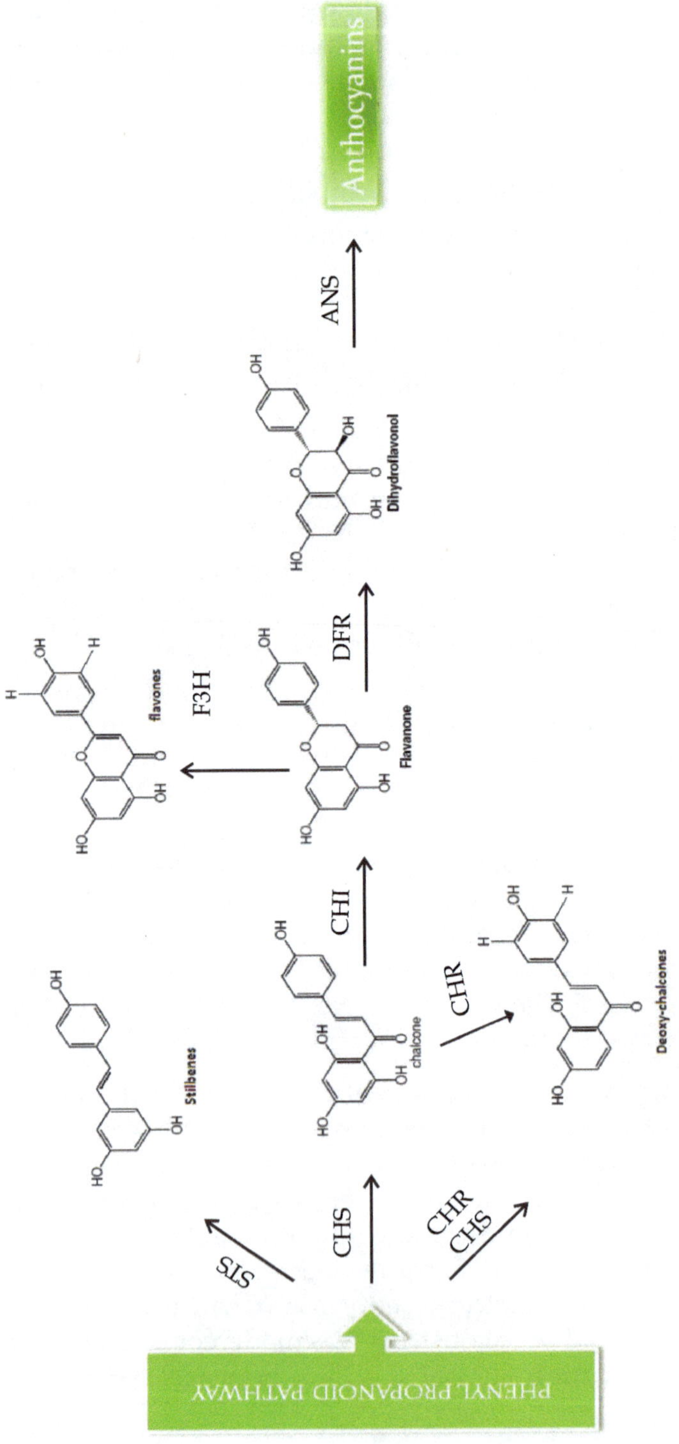
PHENYL PROPANOID PATHWAY
STS
CHS
CHR
CHS
Stilbenes
chalcone
CHR
Deoxy-chalcones
CHI
Flavanone
F3H
flavones
DFR
Dihydroflavonol
ANS
Anthocyanins

The third construct aimed at producing flavones, which are produced from flavanones through the action of flavone synthase (FNS).We reasoned that at least two genes are required to target the pathway in tomato peel towards flavones: a gene encoding chalcone isomerase (CHI) to relief the block in the pathway in the fruit peel at *CHI* and an *FNS* gene to convert the CHI product 2S-naringenin into flavones. So, the third construct used consisted of the petunia *CHI* gene in combination with the *Gerbera FNS-II* gene, both expressed under control of the d35S promoter.

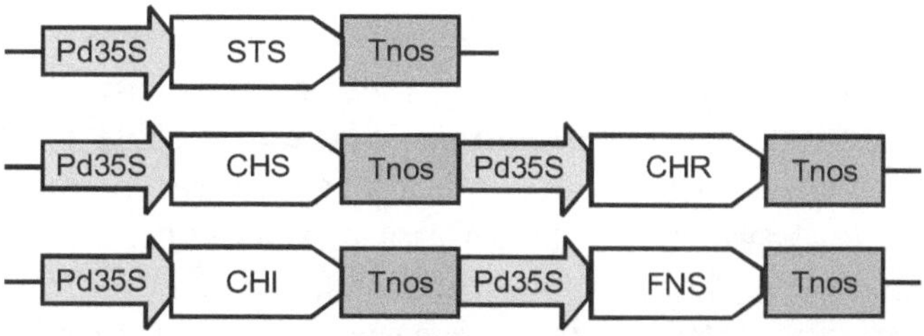

Schematic Overview of Gene Constructs

In all gene constructs, transgene expression was under control of the CaMV double 35S promoter (Pd35S) and terminated by the *Agrobacterium tumefaciens* nos terminator (Tnos). Abbreviations of transgenes: *STS* (Stilbene synthase), *CHS* (Chalcone synthase), *CHR* (Chalcone reductase), *CHI* (Chalcone iso-merase), *FNS* (Flavone synthase); RB, right border; LB left border.

These three gene constructs were expressed in tomato cv. Moneymaker through *Agrobacterium tumefaciens*-mediated transformation. In total 10 *STS*, 16 *CHS/CHR* and 17 *CHI/FNS* primary transformants were obtained carrying one to three copies of these transgenes. Plants were grown to maturity and fruits were harvested when visually ripe.

From each plant at least 3 fruits were harvested, and peel tissue was screened for flavonoid composition by HPLC. This initial screening revealed that several transgenic lines accumulated the expected compounds in the peel of their fruits: stilbenes in *STS*, deoxychalcones in *CHS/CHR* and flavones in *CHI/FNS* transgenic plants.Transgenic plants producing highest levels of stilbenes (3 plants), deoxychalcones (6 plants), and flavones (5 plants) were selected for detailed molecular and biochemical analyses. Of each selected transgenic plant and of a wild-type plant three cuttings were made and all plants were simultaneously grown to maturity. Ripe fruits from individual plants were pooled and peel tissue was analysed for the composition and levels of flavonoids by HPLC.

Applications of Secondary Metabolites

In our fore-going chapters, we have studied variety of plant products such as alkaloids, glycosides, volatile or essential oils, gums and mucilage and oleoresins with varied role to play to the plants as well as to human.

Knowledge of plants and knowledge of healing have been closely linked. It is well established that industries has many direct and indirect effects on human population. Increased stress is most evident at the same time health awareness goes parallel in the recent times. Most of the natural plant products are compounds biosynthetically derived from primary metabolites such as amino acids, carbohydrate metabolic intermediates and fatty acids. These secondary metabolites are the major sources of pharmaceuticals, food additives, fragrance and pesticides. Most of the spices and some medicinal plants are rich sources of oleoresins. Spice oleoresins are derived through non-aqueous volatile solvent extraction of powdered and dried spices. These spices are mixed with a suitable solvent and subsequently removed at the end of the process through evaporation. Spice oil, being volatile in nature, is distilled from the grounded spice and thereafter the wet spice, is dried and extracted with a solvent to produce oleoresins. The extraction method will also vary depending on the properties of the spice being extracted.

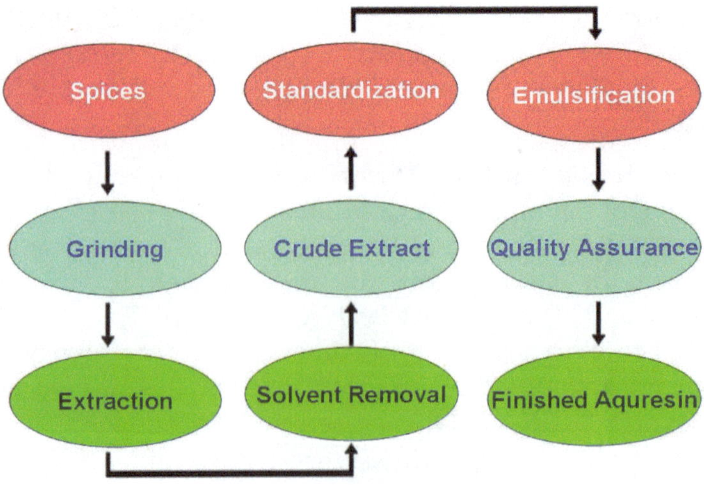

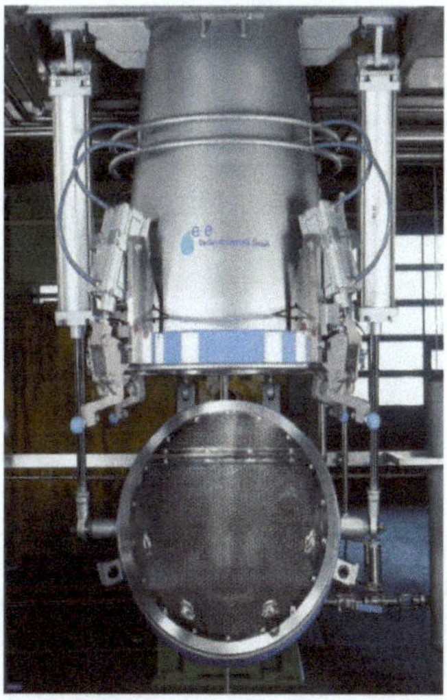

Plant derived natural products and their industrial uses

Industry	Plant Product	Plant spp.	Industrial Use
Pharmaceutical	Codeine	*Papaver* spp	Anti-tussive
	Diosgenin	*Dioscorea* spp	Anti-fertility
	Quinine	*Cinchona* spp.	Anti-malarial
	Digoxin	*Digitalis* spp.	Cardiac tonic
	Ajmalcine	*Catharanthus* spp.	Anti-hypertensive
Agrochemicals	Pyrethrin	*Chrysanthemum* spp	Insecticide
	Azadirachtin	Neem tree	Insecticide
	Quinine	*Cinchona* spp	Bittering agent
Food and Drink	Thaumatin	*Thaumatococcus* spp	Artificial sweetener
	Mucilage	Many plant spp	Ice-cream stabiliser
	Pepper alkaloid	*Piperene* Spp	Condiment
Cosmetics	Jasmine	*Jasminium* spp	Perfumery
	Alloe vera	*Aloe* spp.	Facial cosmetics
	Atropine	*Atropa* spp.	Dilation of pupil
Medicinal	Morphine	*Sertwener* Spp.	Pain killer
	Cocaine	Cocca	Local anaesthesia
	Strychine	Strychnos plants	Anti-helmentics
	Raserpine	Raserpinous spp	Anti-hypertensive
	Caffeine	Coffee plants	Sedative in surgery
	Eucalyptus oil	Eucalyptus tree	Medicinal property

The concept of extraction is simple. Take an organic material, mix it with a solvent which dissolves the required components, and then remove the solvent.

The flow chart below outlines these basic steps

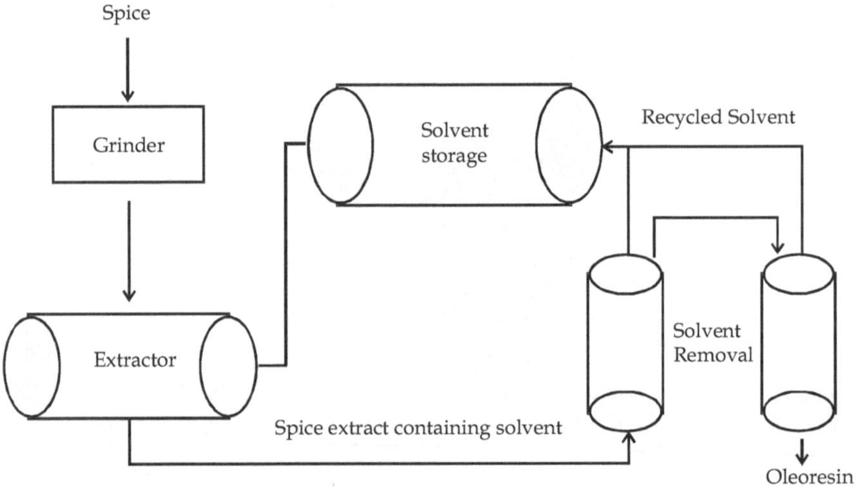

Within this basic framework, there are many variables. For example, the choice of solvent will determine which components will be dissolved. For many spices hexane provides a suitable profile, while types of alcohol are used for some (some gingers and vanilla), and even liquid carbon dioxide has specific applications.

Industrial Uses of Essential Oils

They have a wide and varied use in perfumery, cosmetics and additive in food industry. In the course of a single day, from morning to night, we use or consume a great variety of volatile oils either in spices and condiments or in perfumes or in toilet soap or as scent or in food.

Here is the list of some industries, wherein, the essential oils are used.

Animal Feed Industry	Cat food, cattle feed, dog foods etc.
Baking Goods Industry	Biscuit, cake, icings, minced meat, puddings, sandwich, pies
Canning Industry	Meat, fish, sauces, soups
Chewing Gum Industry	Variety of chewing gums and chocolates

Condiments	Chilli sauces, salad dressing, pickled fish, table sauce, vinegar etc.
Confectionary	Chocolates, jellies, soft centre candies
Food Industry	Cheese, puddings, dehydrated soups, rennet desserts.
Household	Deodorant, furniture polish, laundry Soap, room spray
Insecticide Industry	Attractants, insect repellents. Disinfectant sprays
Paint Industry	Bituminous paint, enamels, paint and varnish removers, synthetic coatings, varnish
Pharmaceutical Industry	Cough drops, antacids, elixir, hospital sprays, laxatives, ointments, tonic, vitamin flavour preparation
Perfume and Toilet Industry	Baby soap, Face cream, cologne, lip-stick, lotion, shaving cream, eye shadow, mask etc.
Pickle Industry	Sweet and sour pickle preparation
Wine Industry	Rum, whisky, wine etc
Rubber Industry	Toys, waterproofing, glove, surgical supplies.
Soap Industry	All kind of ordinary and luxury soaps.
Soft Drink	Cola drinks, syrups and soft drink powder
Tobacco Industry	Chewing and smoking tobacco
Ice-Cream Industry	Used in the preparation of ice-cream

The list of industries, where the essential and volatile oils are used, is endless suggesting its industrial demand and the potential in driving the economy of the country. *Please note that the list is not complete.*

Important Spices, Medicinal Plants and their Uses

1. Mace (*Myristica spp*)(*Jayfal*)

Myristica spp (Jayfal) contains 93 % terpenes and 77% aromatics. The volatile oils comprise of camphene, di-pentene, eugenol, myristicin, safrole, geraniol, β -penene etc.

Uses : It acts as stimulant and carminative (act on the flatulence or gas problem), used in the preparation of medicinal soap. It is also useful in preparation of dental paste, flavouring chewing gums. It is used in perfumery, dentifrices and tobacco industry.

2. Turmeric *(Curcuma longa)*

Curcuma longa (Turmeric) has essential oil content is 5–8 % containing di-phellandrene, d-sabinene, cineol, borneol, zingiberebe, sesqui-terpene. Colour is due to curcuminoids (0.2 to 2.0 %) and β – carotene.

Uses : It is used in the cooking, curry powder, cosmetics, natural dye for colouring wool, silk and cotton. It acts as anti-septic having anti-microbial activity. Curcumin has anti-oxidant property, inhibit cancer, anti-inflammatory and lowers blood cholesterol.

3. Cardamom (*Ellettaria* spp*)*

They contain volatile oil such as cineol, α –terpneol, terpinene, d-limonene, sesqui-terpene and α and β - pinene, linalool acetate etc. The chief constituent is borneol.

Uses : It is used as flavouring agent, beverages, liquor, sweet preparation and culinary (it is the product which is used in kitchen and cookery). It is also used in the treatment of inflammation of eyelids, carminative. Roots and fruits are known as laxative, diuretic and stimulant.

4. Clove (*Myristica spp.) (Laving)*

It contains heavy volatile oils (18-20 %) which include camphor resin, caryophylin, eugenol, naphthalene, vanillin etc. The main constituent is eugenol.

Uses : It is used as culinary (used in the kitchen) in sauce, pickles, curry powder, flavouring agent, pudding, chocolate, candies. It is also used in soap, detergent and perfume. Medicinally, it is used in relieving toothache, headache, and rheumatic pain. It has importance as antiseptic, analgesic and anti-inflammatory activity.

5. Fennel (*Foeniculum* spp.*)*

It contains α –pinene, camphene, limonene, anethole and foeniculin.

Uses : It is used as flavouring agent in food. The leaves work as digestive, appetizing. The seeds are sweet, laxative, arrest bleeding. It relieves flatulence.

6. Ginger (*Curcuma* spp.) *(Aadu)*

It contains 1 – 3 % essential oils. It has characteristic pleasant and aromatic smell. The essential oil comprises of mono, sesqui and oxygenated terpenes, zingiberene, d-camphene, cineol, limonene, geraniol, linalool, gingediol etc.

Uses : Flavouring agent in food, confectionary, meat, curry powder, pickles and carbonated drinks. Ginger oil is used in perfumery. It also act as hypoglycaemic agent for the diabetic patients.

7. Saffron (*Corcus* spp.) *(Kesar)*

It contains carotenoid glycoside including α and β carotene along with zeaxanthin and lycopene as pigments which give orange colour to saffron. The glycoside crocin also impart colour. The essential oil of saffron contains stearoptene.

Uses : It is used as colouring and flavouring agent in food > It is also used in dye industry. It is medicinally used in treatment of hysteria and sudden changes in moods. It provides strength. It has anti-tumor and antioxidant properties.

8. Coriander (*Coriandrum* spp.)

The major content is cinnamaldehyde, eugenol, benzaldehyde, rutin, linalool, pinene, thymol, di-pentene etc.

Uses : It is used as culinary agent in cookery, flavouring agent. Its medical uses are many including the treatment of bronchial asthma, bronchitis, small pox, conjunctivitis. The leaves are stimulant and tonic.

9. Asafoetida (*Ferula spp.) (Hing)*

It contains 10-17 % essential oils and 6-10% sulphur containing compounds. These include umbelliferone, ferulic acid, pinene etc.

Uses : It is used as condiment in cooking. It is antispasmodic, expectorant. Useful in respiratory problems. Also used in the treatment of hysteria, syphilis, excessive flatulence and bronchitis.

10. Fenugreek (*Trigonella* spp.)

Alkaloid named trignelline is present in fenugreek. The saponin of trigonella contains sapogenin, diosgenin, gitogenin, tigogenin etc. A glycoside called fenugrin is also present.

Uses : It is known to increase flow of milk in cattle. It is used to cure fatigue, gastric troubles, gout, and flatulence. It reduces blood sugar, enlargement of spleen. Diosgenin is a starting material for the synthesis of hormone for contraception.

11. Garlic (*Allium* spp.)

The chief constituent is diallyl sulphide. It contains compound having sulphur which are responsible for the smell e.g. allicin, allisatin I and II etc.

Uses : It's a flavouring agent in curry, *chutnies* and many more Indian dishes. It is stimulant, carminative, anti-rheumatic, and antioxidant. It lowers the cholesterol having antibacterial and anti-fungal activities. It has sedative effects too.

12. Mustard (*Brassica* spp.)

The major alkaloid present in mustard is sinigrin, sinapine, and a glycoside called myrosin.

Uses : It is used as culinary in the kitchen as cooking oil and spice in the food preparations.

It has medical uses too. If externally used, it act as counter-irritant but if used internally, it causes the vomiting. It is digestive, laxative and helpful in sciatica, urticaria and inflammatory swelling.

13. Dill (*Anethum spp.*) *(suva dana)*

It contains 20-30% of carvone apart from eugenol, pinene, limonene, thymol etc.

Uses : It is a carminative medicine, stomachic, stimulatory having an insecticidal properties. It is flavouring agent in pickles, salads and tomato juice. It is being given to the babies up to 2 years of age for digestive purpose (gripe water).

14. Pepper (*Piperene* spp.)

It consists of volatile oils, resins and alkaloid piperine. The essential oils contain α and β pinene, limonene, piperonal. The oleoresin contain Piperine, chavocine etc.

Uses : It is indispensable in sauce, soups, condiments and pickles. It is stimulant, pungent, aromatic, and digestive. It acts as appetizer which increase the flow of saliva and gastric juice. It is useful in digestive disorder, anti-inflammatory. It works well in toothache, muscular pain.

15. Chilli (*Capsicum* spp.)

The volatile oil content is 0.16 to 39.0 %. The pungent principle is capsaicinoids. Which is a mixture of capsaicin, dihydro capsaicin, homo and non-hydro capsaicins. Some pigments such as capsanthin, capsorubin, lutein and zeaxanthin is also present.

Uses : It has culinary purpose. Dry chilli is used as curry powder and condiment for the flavour and taste. Capsaicin has anti-inflammatory property, analgesic, treatment of headache, toothache, muscular pain. It has cholesterol lowering effect, its anti-obesity agent, digestive which increases salivary flow. It has anti-microbial property too.

16.Ajwain (Bishop's Weed) (*Carum* spp.)

Thymol is a main constituent in the seeds of ajwain.

Uses : It is stimulatory, antispasmodic, carminative. It relieves from flatulence, diarrhoea. The oil is used in sore throat and bronchitis. It is used as condiment.

17. Cumin (*Cuminum* spp.)

It contains cuminaldehyde, p-cymen, pines, cuminyl alcohol, terpeneol. The glucoside present in the seed is luteolin.

Uses : It is additive in increasing the flavour, used as condiment, culinary purpose. It is useful in dyspepsia and diarrhoea, It has industrial use in perfumery and flavouring liquor.

18. Basil *(Tulsi)* (*Ocimum* spp.)

It consists of methyl cinnamate, linalool, terpenic constituent such as ocimene. It contains eugenol too. Because of the essential oils, it has a property to repel the insects (You don't find much damage of insects on this crop).

Uses : It has culinary use. It is popular in French cooking. It has many medicinal properties. It is useful in cough, cold, fever. It is anti-pyretic, expectorant, stimulant, antihelmentic.

19. Onion (*Allium* spp.)

The chief constituent essential oil is allyl propyl disulphide. The volatile oil also contains methanol and propanealdehyde.

Uses : It has a regular place in everybody's houses except *Jains* and *Swaminarayan* religion believing people. It has culinary use finding place in variety of dishes. It has strong anti-microbial activity. It gives considerable relief in neuralgia, headache, migraine and mild indigestion. It excites appetite for food. It works in cold and inflammatory conditions, gout, constipation etc.

20. Horse Radish *(Muli)* (*Armoracia* spp.)

The roots contain pungent acid and vesicating oils The pungency is due to glycoside sinigrin and the myrosin which react when roots are crushed and mixed with water to give allyl isothiocyanate.

Uses : It is used as condiment which is digestive, stimulant with diuretic property (The drug which increase the flow of urine). It is counter-irritant in painful joints. It has anti-microbial property too.

21. Curry Leaf *(Mitho Limdo)* (*Murraya spp.)*

It contains alkaloids such as koenimbine, mehanimbine. The leaves contain cyclomehanimbin, curryangine, curryanine etc. It also has a residual glycoside called koenigin.

Uses : It is mild laxative, useful in the treatment of morning sickness, nausea, flatulence, vomiting. It is also considered as hair tonic (premature greying of hair) and hypoglycaemic.

Applications of Oleoresins

1. Oleoresins serve as convenient, hygienic and standardised substitute for spice powder in food and seasoning formulations.
2. They are extensively used in processed foods, snacks, sauces, sausages, sea foods and vegetable preparations.
3. They are used in alcoholic and non-alcoholic beverages.
4. They have medicinal properties too.

Purified oleoresins are used in health/functional foods and pharmaceuticals.

Different types of oleoresins produced from different spices & their uses.

S. No	Name of spice	Oleoresins	Amount ppm	Uses
1.	*Cuminum cyminum L,*	Cumin	<15	Powerful scent, digestive disorders, build immunity, improve blood circulation lymphatic congestion
2.	*Crocus sativus L,*	Saffron	<12	Flavoring &coloring agent, Ayurvedic medicine, remedies for everything ex,asthama, lowers cholesterol, anticancer
3.	*Capsicum annum L,*	Paprika	-	Natural Coloring agent, antioxidant
4.	*Common onion*	Onion	-	Antimicrobial, anathematic, digestive, diuretic, curative, blood supply & cleaner, skin clear, high Vit. A,B,C. promotes strong bones, antirheumatic, antiseptic, antisclerotic, antispasmodic, antiviral, antibacterial, carminative, depurative.
5.	*Trigonella foenumgraecum.*	Fenugreek	<10	Spices/curry powder, seasoning for fish dishes, candey, ice cream, soft drinks, and rich in Vit. Protein, minerals. Reduce blood pressure sugar level.
6.	*Foeniculum vulgare*	Fennel	<15	Scent & flavour, anti-toxic oil, counterbalancing alcohol poisoning, rehabilation of alcoholism, regularize M.C. period, quick relief of indigestion & nausea. decreas apetite.
7.	*Coriandom sativum L,*	Coriander	<15	In medicine, reduce flatulence, improves appetites,

Contd...

Table Contd...

				reliveving spasm within the gut & counters the effect of nerve pain, perfumes, and cosmetics, dentifrices, digestive, antispasmodic, and anti-rheumatic.
8.	*Piper nigrum*	Black pepper	<10	Condiment ,flavouring, perfumery industries
9.	*Elettaria cardamomum*	Cardamom	-	Antiseptic, antispasmodic, aphrodisiaic, carminative, cephalic, digestive, diuretic, stimulant, tonic (nerve)
10	*Pimpinella anisum*	Anise	<15	Culinary medicinal purpose, cough syrups & sore throats medicine, flavouring scented soaps & perfumes
11	*Apium graveolens*	Celery	<10	Favour of soft drinks& unpleasant medicaments, stimulants, carminative, nervine, sedative & even in tonic
12	*Capsicum annum*	Capsicum oleo	<20	Powerful irritant & carminative, treatment of stomach ache, anti-bacterial, police smoke preparation.
13	*Clove*	Clove	-	Antihelmintic, antibiotic, antieminitic, anti-ineuralgic, antioxidant, antiseptic, antiviral, carminative, counter irritant, expectorant, larvicidal, stimulant, stomachic, antirheumatic, dental component, tooth paste, cosmetics, perfumery, printing ink, digestive, skin care, varnish

Contd...

Table Contd...

14	*Alllium sativum*	Garlic	-	Powerful antibacterial, flavouring agent.
15	*Zinger officinale*	Ginger	<10	Flavouring agent in all types of food, aromatic, carminative, stomachic, stimulant
16	*Myristica/mace.*	Nutmeg	<10	Analgesic, antiseptic, antirheumatic, antiseptic, antispasmodic, carminative, digestive, gastric secretory stimulant, larvicidal, flavouring, soaps, perfumes, detergents, nervous system disorders curation, emmenagegue.
17	*Rosemarinus officinalis*	Rosemary	-	Antioxidant, flavouring, cosmetics, liniments, hair lotions & carminative
18	*Curcuma long*	Turmeric	<10	Pharmacological & anti-inflammatory actions.
19	Dhana	Coriander	-	Seasoning agent for sausages& meat products, baked goods, condiments, chewing gums, alcoholic & non-alcoholic beverages, curry mix.
20	Shaha jira	Carway seed	-	Seasoning of processed meat,non-alcoholic beverages, baked goods, sauces, chewing gums.

References

1. A rapid method for Determination of Gum in Guar (*Cyamopsis Tetoganeloba* (L.) Taub.) . Proccedure of the First of the ICAR Guar Res. Workshop Jan. 11-12,1997, pp. 117-123.
2. Anonymous 1967. Recommended methods for the evaluation of drugs. *Analyst,* 92, pp. 593-96.
3. Arimura G, R Ozawa, T Shimoda, T Nishioka, W Boland, J Takabyashi *Nature* 406:512–515.
4. Armbruster WS, JJ Howard, TP Clausen, EM Debevec, JC Loquvam, M Matsuki, B Cerendolo, F Andel. *Am Nat* 149:461–484.
5. Ashby MN, PA Edwards. *J Biol Chem* : 265:13157–13164.
6. Ayasse M, FP Schiestl, HF Paulus, C Lofstedt, B Hansson, F Ibarra, W Francke. *Evolution* 54:1995–2006.
7. Back KW, J Chappell. *Proc Natl Acad Sci.,* 93:6841–6845.
8. Baldwin IT, JC Schultz. *Science* 221:277–279.
9. Barkman TJ, JH Beaman, DA Gage. *Phytochemistry* 44:875–882.
10. Barnola, L.F., Hasega Wa, M., and A. Cedeno. *Biochem. Syst. Ecol.* 22: 437-445.
11. Becerra JX. *Science* : 276:253–256.
12. Bell, E.A and Charlwood, B.V. Secondary Plant Products.

13. Berenbaum MR. *J Chem Ecol* : 12:809–812.

14. Bergstrom G, HEM Dobson, I Groth. *Plant Syst Evol* : 195:221–242.

15. Bhatnagar, R., Shukla, Y. M. and Talati, J.G. Biochemical Methods for Agricultural Sciences.

16. Bissots, N.G.S and Nwauri, J. Quaternary Alkaloids of Tinospora species. *Planta Med.* 48 : 275-79.

17. Bloom AJ, FS Chapin, HA Mooney. *Annu Rev Ecol Syst* 16:363–392.

18. Bohlmann J, CL Steele, R Croteau. *J Biol Chem* 272: 21784–21792.

19. Bohlmann J, G Meyer-Gauen, R Croteau 1998 *Proc Natl Acad Sci* 95: 4126–4133.

20. Boland W, A Gabler, M Gilbert, ZF Feng. *Tetrahedron* 54:14725–14736.

21. BPC (1973). *British Pharmaceutical Codex*. The Pharmaceutical Press, London. P. 438.

22. Bryant JP, FS Chapin, DR Klein. *Oikos* 40:357–368.

23. Buchanan RA, Cull IM, Otey FH and Russel CR. *Econ. Bot.,* 32 : 131.

24. Buckingham J 1998 Dictionary of Natural Products on CD-ROM. Chapman & Hall, London.

25. Calvin M, Nemethy EK, Redenbaugh K and Otvos JW. LBL, Univ. of California Preprint 12413.

26. Capell, T. and Christou, P. *Current Opinion in Biotechnology* 15: 148–154.

27. Cates, R.G. and R.A. Redak. 1998. *In:* Chemical Mediation of Coevolution. K.C. Spencer (ed.). pp. 317-344. Academic Press, San Diego.

28. Chatterjee, A.S. and Ghost, S. Tinosporine, The furaroid bitter principle of *Tinospora cordifolia*. *Phiers Science and Culture,* 26(3) : 140-141.

29. Chen AJ, PA Kroon, CD Poulter. *Protein Sci* : 3:600–607.

30. Chopra. S.L. and J. S. Kanwar, *Analytical Agricultural Chemistry,* p. 341.

31. Cohen D. *J Theor Biol* 12:119–129.

32. Coley PD, JP Bryant, FS Chapin. *Science* 230:895–899.

33. Crepet WL. The role of insect pollination in the evolution of angiosperms. p. 29–50. *Pollination Biology*. Academic Press.

34. Croise, L. and F. Lieutier. *Ann. For. Sci.* 50: 91-97.

35. Croteau R, J Gershenzon. Genetic control of monoterpene biosynthesis in mints (*Mentha*: Lamiaceae). p. 193–229 *in* BEEA Ellis, ed. Genetic Engineering of Plant Secondary Metabolism. Plenum, New York.

36. Cseke L, N Dudareva, E Pichersky. Structure and Evolution of Linalool Synthase. *Mol Biol Evol* 15:1491–1498.

37. Cvejic JH, M Rohmer. *Phytochemistry* 53:21–28.

38. D. Ernest Gunther, D. Van. The Essentail Oils: History, origin and production in plants : Volume I and II (1948) by Nostrand Company Ltd, USA.

39. Daniel M. Methods in Plant Chemistry and Economic Botany. p. 150-151. Kalyani Publishers, New Delhi.

40. De Moraes CM, WJ Lewis, PW Pare, HT Alborn, JH Tumlinson. *Nature* 393:570–573.

41. Degenhardt J, J Gershenzon. *Planta* : 210:815–822.

42. Dethier V. *Evolution* : 8:33–54.

43. Dhaka R.P.S. and Nanak Singh: A Text Book of Biochemistry.

44. Dicke M. *Physiol Entomol* : 11:251–262.

45. Dicke M, J Bruin. *Biochem Syst Ecol* : 29:981–994.

46. Dicke, M. and J.J.A. van Loon. *Exp. Appl.* : 97:237-249.

47. Dieter Hess. Plant Physiology.

48. Dobson HEM. *Oecologia* : 72:618–623.

49. Dobson HEM, LG Bergstro¨m : The Ecology and Evolution of Pollen Odors. *Plant Syst Evol* 222:63–87.

50. Dressler RL Biology of the orchid bees (*Euglossini*). *Annu Rev Ecol Syst.* 13:373–394.

51. Dudareva N, L Cseke, VM Blanc, E Pichersky. *Plant Cell* : 8:1137–1148.

52. Ehrlich PR, PH Raven. *Evolution* : 18:586–608.

53. Ellis AG, SD Johnson. *Plant Syst Evol* : 219:137–150.

54. Evans PH, JX Becerra, DL Venable, WS Bowers. *J Chem Ecol.* 26:745–754.

55. Fahn A Secretory tissues in vascular plants. *New Phytol* : 108 : 229–257.

56. Fairbairn, J.W. and Simie, S. *J.Pharm.Pharmac.*, 15:325

57. Farmer EE, CA Ryan *Proc Natl Acad Sci.* 87:7713–7716.

58. Farrell B, C Mitter. *Evolution* : 44:1389–1403.

59. Fischbach RJ, M Staudt, I Zimmer, S Rambal, JP Schnitzler. *Physiol Plant.* 114:354–360.

60. Fischer U, S Vetter, J Novak, S Glasl, J Saukel, C Franz. *Plant Breeding* 120:251–254.

61. Fordyce JA, SB Malcolm. *J Chem Ecol.* 26: 2857–2874.

62. Fraenkel GS. Raison d'e^tre of secondary plant substances. *Science* 129:1466–1470.

63. Futuyma DJ. *Plant Species Biol.* 15:1–9.

64. Gangrade S. K. All India Co-ordinated Research Project on Medicinal and Aromatic Plants, p. 372-375. 10th All India Workshop Report, Trichur.

65. Gangrade S.K. Estimation of glycyrrhizin content in *Glycyrrhiza glabra.* In AICRP on M & AP, p.165-7. 11th All India workshop held at Rajasthan Agricultural University. Udaipur.

66. Gershenzon J, ME McConkey, RB Croteau. *Plant Physiol* : 122:205–213.

67. Gershenzon J, R Croteau: Terpenoids. pp. 165–219 *in* G Rosenthal, M Berenbaum, eds. Herbivores: Their interactions with secondary metabolites. Academic Press.

68. Gomez NE, L Witte, T Hartmann. *Cordia curassavica. J Chem Ecol.* 25:1007–1027.

69. Gopal Krishnan *et al. Indian J. Phar. Sciences*, pp. 145-147.

70. Gottlieb LD. *Science* : 216:373–379.

71. Grison-Pige L, JM Bessiere, M Hossaert-McKey. *J Chem Ecol.* 28:283–295.

72. Harborne JB. Introduction to Ecological Biochemistry. 4th ed. Academic Press.

73. Hedin PA. Responses of alder and willow to attack by tent caterpillars and webworms: Evidence for pheromonal sensitivity of willows. pp. 55–68 *in*, Plant resistance to insects. American Chemical Society Symposium Series. Plenum,Washington D.C.

74. Hefendehl FW, MJ Murray 1976 Lloydia 39:39–52.

75. Herbert R.B. The Biosynthesis of Secondary Metabolites. Chapman and Hall.

76. Hopkins W.G. Biochemistry and Mode of Action of Hormones. *In* Introduction to Plant Physiology; 2e. *John Wiley & Sons, Inc.*

77. Hossaert-McKey M, M Gibernau, JE Frey : *Exp Appl.* 70:185–191.

78. Indian Herbal Pharmacopoeia. Vol. I.

79. Indian Pharmacopoeia. Ministry of Health, Government of India, p. 353.

80. Jones CG, RD Firn. On the Evolution of Plant Secondary Chemical Diversity. *Philos Trans R Soc Lond B Biol Sci.* 333:273–280.

81. Jux A, G Gleixner, W Boland. *Angew Chem Int Ed Engl.* 40: 2091–2093.

82. Kalyanasundram, N.K.; Amin, D.R. and Dalal, K.C. *Annual Report* (Rabi). AICRP on M & AP., GAU, Anand.

83. Karawya, M.S., Balba, S.I. and Afifi, M.S.A. Investigation of the carbohydrate contents of certain mucilaginous plants. *Planta Medica*, 20 (1) L: 14-23.

84. Karban R, IT Baldwin, KJ Baxter, G Laue, GW Felton. *Oecologia* 125: 66–71.

85. Kite GC. The floral odor of *Arum maculatum*. *Biochem Syst Ecol.* 23: 343–354.

86. Kite GC, WLA Hetterschieid. *Phytochemistry* 46: 71–75.

87. Kleinhentz M, H Jactel, P Menassieu. *J Chem Ecol.* 25: 2741–2756.

88. Kuzma J, R Fall. *Plant Physiol.* 101:435–440.

89. Langenheim JH. J *Chem Ecol.* 20:1223–1280.

90. Lerdau M. *Science* 298:361.

91. Lerdau M, PD Coley. *Oikos* 98:534–536.

92. Lesburg CA, GZ Zhai, DE Cane, DW Christianson. *Science* 277:1820-1824.

93. Levin RA, RA Raguso, LA McDade. *Phytochemistry* : 58:429-440.

94. Lewinsohn E, M Gijzen, TJ Savage, R Croteau. *Plant Physiol.* 96:38-43.

95. Lichtenthaler HK, M Rohmer, J Schwender. *Physiol Plant.* 101:643–652.

96. Listor, R.E. and Pride, R.R.A. *Ibid*, 11:278.

97. Litvak ME, RK Monson. *Oecologia* : 114:531–540.

98. Lu¨ cker J, HJ Bouwmeester, W Schwab, J Blaas, LHW van der Plas, HA Verhoeven. *Plant J.* 27:315–324.

99. Mant JG, FP Schiestl, R Peakall, PH Weston. *Evolution* : 56:888–898.

100. Martin D, D Tholl, J Gershenzon, J Bohlmann. *Plant Physiol* 129:1003-1018.

101. Mattiacci L, BA Rocca, N Scascighini, M D'Alessandro, A Hern, S Dorn. *J Chem Ecol.* 27:2233–2252.

102. McGarvey DJ, R Croteau. *Plant Cell* 7: 1015–1026.

103. McKey D. *Am Nat* 108:305–320.

104. Misawa, M. Plant tissue culture : An alternative for production of useful metabolites. FAO Agric Service Bull., 108 : 1-87. Rome.

105. Mishra S.N. Qualitative and Quantitative Evaluation of Hydrolytic Products of Mucilage derived from Isabgol. 10th All India Workshop Report: 390-392.

106. Mishra S.N. Quick method for evaluation of steroidal sapogenine in Safed musli (Chlorophytum sp.) powder. In "12th All India Workshop Report" on Medicinal & Aromatic Plants, pp. 288-289.

107. Mishra,S.N. and Pacnori, M. *In* "10th All India Workshop Report" held at Trichur. pp. 382-85.

108. Mital, S.P., T.A. Thomas, B.S. Dabus and B.M. Lal, Gum content as related to seed yoeld and other character in Gum. *Indian J. Gen. Pl. Breed.* 31:228-232

109. Monson RK. *Ann Mo Bot Gard* : 83: 3–16.

110. Moore TSJ. Terpenoid biosynthesis: The basic pathway and formation of monoterpenes, sesquiterpenes, and diterpenes. pp. 339–388 *in*. *Lipid Metabolism in Plants.*

111. Morton TC, FV Vencl. *J Chem Ecol.* 24:765–785.

112. Muir S.R.; Collins G.J.; Robinson S.; Hughes S. and Bovy A. *Nature Biotechnology*: 19:470-474.

113. Murray MJ, DE Lincoln. *Genetics* 65:457-471.

114. Neish A. *Annu Rev Plant Physiol* : 11:55–80.

115. Nishizawa A, G Honda, M Tabata. *Phytochemistry* 31:139–142.

116. Pasquali G.; Goddijn J.M.; Waal Anthony de; Verpoorte R.; Schilperoort R. A.; Hoge H. C. and Memelink J. *Plant Molecular Biology* 18: 1121-1131.

117. Pellmyr O. *Oecologia* 68: 304–307.

118. Pellmyr O, LB Thien. *Taxon* 35:76–85.

119. Pellmyr O, W Tang, I Groth, G Bergstrom, LB Thien. *Biochem Syst Ecol.* 19:623–627.

120. Pettersson EM. *J Chem Ecol.* 27:2219–2231.

121. Pettersson EM, BT Sullivan, P Anderson, CW Berisford, G Birgersson. *J Chem Ecol.* 26:2507–2525.

122. Pichersky E, DR Gang. *Trends in Plant Sci.* 5:439–445.

123. Pichersky E, E Lewinsohn, R Croteau. *Arch Biochem Biophys* : 316:803–807.

124. Pichersky E, RA Raguso, E Lewinsohn, R Croteau. *Plant Physiology* 106:1533–1540.

125. Plomion C, A Yani, A Marpeau. *Genome* 39: 1123–1127.

126. Raguso RA, E Pichersky. *Plant Species Biol.* 14:95–120.

127. Rajput and Govindarajan. *Asso. Anal.Chem.* 64 : 311-318

128. Rakshaben Mishra, and Dr. Sukh Dev* *Phytochemist*, Medicinal and Aromatic Plants Project, Gujarat Agricultural University, Anand Campus, Anand , *Maltichem Research Centre, Nandesari (Dist. Baroda).

129. Rapparini F, R Baraldi, O Facini. *Phytochemistry* 57:681–687.

130. Report of the Joint Committee of the Pharmaceutical Society and the Society for Analytical Chemistry, *Analyst*, 90, 582.

131. Rhoades DF. Evolution of Plant Chemical Defense Against Herbivores. p.3-54 *in* GA Rosenthal, DH Janzen, eds. Herbivores: S102 International Journal of Plant Sciences their interactions with plant secondary plant metabolites. Academic Press, New York.

132. Robert, E.B. *Agro. J.*, 643 : 511.

133. Rosenthal GA and DH Janzen. The distribution of secondary plant compounds within plants. pp. 56–133, eds. *Herbivores*: Their interaction with secondary plant metabolites. Academic Press, New York.

134. Ruzicka L. *Experientia* 9:357–367.

135. Sato F.; Hashimoto T.; Hachiya A.; Tamura K.; Choi K; Morishige T.; Fujimoto H.; and Yamada Y. *PNAS;* 98(1):367–372.

136. Schanderl,S.H. Method in food analysis, p.709. Academic Press,New York.

137. Schiestl FP,Mayasse. *Behav Ecol Sociobiol* 48:303–307.

138. Schlatmann, J.E., Hoopen, H.J.G. and Heijnen, J.J. In *Plant Cell Culture : Secondary Metabolites*. F. Dicosmo and M. Misawa (eds.), CRC Press, NY.

139. Shepherd M, JX Chaparro, R Teasdale. *Theor Appl Genet* 99:1207–1215.

140. Simon HA. *Am Econ Rev* 49:253–283.

141. Smith, F and Montgomery, R. The Chemistry of Plant Gum and Mucilage.

142. Spurgeon SL, JW Porter. Introduction. pp. 1–46 *in* SL Spurgeon, JW Porter, eds. *Biosynthesis of Isoprenoid Compounds*. Vol 1. Wiley, New York.

143. Squillace AE. Inheritance of monoterpene composition in cortical oleoresin of slash pine. *For Sci*: 17:381–387.

144. Srivastava V.K. Chemical Evaluation of Aloe Barbadensis, pp. 164-65. NBPGR, New Delhi. In *"Eleventh All India Workshop Report on M & AP"*.

145. Steele CL, J Crock, J Bohlmann, R Croteau. *J Biol Chem*. 273:2078–2089.

146. Stipanovic R. D.,D. H. Brien and P.A. Fryxell. *Phytochemistry*,17 :1297 - 1305.

147. Studies on Galactomannans in guar some correlation for selecting for selecting grnotypes rich in Gum content. Procedure of the first ICAR Guar Res. Workshop. pp.124-130.

148. Thorsteinson A. Host selection in phytophagous insects. *Annu Rev Entomol* 5:193–218.

149. Trapp SC, RB Croteau. Genomic organization of plant terpene synthases and molecular evolutionary implications. *Genetics* 158: 811–832.

150. Trevor Robinson. The Organic Constituents of Higher Plants. 2nd Edition.

151. Varma; Talwar S. K. and Garg G. P. Chemical investigation of *Silybum marianum*, *Planta Medica*, 38: 377-378.

152. Varma Talwar S. K. and Garg G. P. *Planta Medica*, 38: 377-378.

153. Vernet P, PH Gouyon, G Valdeyron. Genetic control of the oil content in *Thymus vulgaris* L: A case of polymorphism in a biosynthetic chain. *Genetica* 69:227–231.

154. Verpoorte, R., Heijden, R.V., Schrispsema, J., Hoge, J.H.C. and Ten-Hoopen, H.J.G. (1993). Plant Cell Biotechnology for the Production of Alkaloids, Present Status and Prospects. *J. Nat. Products,* 56 : 186-207.

155. Vogel S. The Role of Scent Glands in Pollination.

156. Walton n.j. and Brown D.E. Chemicals from Plants: Perspective on Plant Secondary Products. pp. 1-25.

157. Weissbecker B, JJA Van Loon, MA Posthumus, HJ Bouwmeester, M Dicke. Identification of volatile potato sesquiterpenoids and their olfactory detection by the two-spotted stinkbug *Perillus bioculatus*. *J Chem Ecol* 26:1433–1445.

158. Wheeler GS, LM Massey, IA Southwell. Antipredator defense of biological control agent *Oxyops vitiosa* is mediated by plant volatiles sequestered from the host plant *Melaleuca quinquenervia*. *J Chem Ecol.* 28:297–315.

159. Whistler. R; Industrial Gums of Plants, Econ. Bot. 36(2), 195-202.

160. Yeoman, M.M. and Yeoman, Y. (1996). Manipulating secondary metabolism in cultured plant cells. *New Phytol.*, 134 : 552-569.

161. Zalucki MP, SB Malcolm. *J Chem Ecol.* 25:1827–1842.

162. Zangerl A, F Bazzaz. Theory and Pattern in Plant Defense Allocation. pp. 363–391 *in* R Fritz, E Simms, eds. Plant resistance to herbivores and pathogens. University of Chicago Press, Chicago.

163. Zhang W.; Franco C.; Curtin C.and Conn S.*Journal of Biomedicine and Biotechnology* 5 264–271.

Index

H

I

J

L

M

N

O

P

FSC
www.fsc.org
MIX
Papier | Fördert gute Waldnutzung
FSC® C083411

Zeitfracht Medien GmbH
Ferdinand-Jühlke-Straße 7
99095 Erfurt, Deutschland
produktsicherheit@kolibri360.de